Interventional Oncology

Peter R. Mueller · Andreas Adam

Editors

Interventional Oncology

A Practical Guide for the Interventional Radiologist

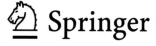
Springer

Editors
Peter R. Mueller
Department of Radiology
Massachusetts General Hospital
Boston, MA, USA
pmueller@partners.org

Andreas Adam
Department of Radiology
St. Thomas' Hospital
London, UK
andy.adam@kcl.ac.uk

ISBN 978-1-4419-1468-2   e-ISBN 978-1-4419-1469-9
DOI 10.1007/978-1-4419-1469-9
Springer New York Dordrecht Heidelberg London

Library of Congress Control Number: 2011941010

Printed on acid-free paper

Springer is part of Springer Science+Business Media (www.springer.com)

Preface

It took us a few years to get used to the words "interventional oncology." Both of us have been using interventional radiological methods to treat patients with cancer for the whole of our careers. Over the years, technological advances such as the advent of metallic stents have greatly improved the effectiveness of what we do, prolonging the survival and improving the quality of life of patients with malignant disease. Therefore, as far as we were concerned, we were practising interventional oncology before this discipline had a name.

In recent years, the term *interventional oncology* has been applied to a set of potentially curative imaging-guided interventional radiological procedures. This is helpful, as the approach to the patients treated using these methods differs in some important respects from the way that interventional radiologists have managed oncology patients requiring palliative treatments such as biliary stenting. The interventional oncologist often assumes the role of the patient's primary physician. It is necessary to explain not only the procedure being offered but also potential alternatives, such as surgery and chemotherapy, and to discuss these with the patient in some depth.

Another challenge facing the interventional oncologist is the pace of development in this field. A plethora of treatment methods has become available, and it is not easy to disentangle theoretical technical advances from substantive clinical advantages.

This book brings together some of the greatest experts in this field around the world. They are all extremely busy people, combining large clinical practices with high-flying academic careers. Most of them are personal friends of one or both of us, and we were shameless in using our friendship to recruit them as authors. Our excuse is the final outcome: this volume is an excellent account of the current state of interventional radiological methods of treating malignant tumors. We have enjoyed reading the chapters and have learned a lot from them. We are confident that our readers will find them equally useful.

Boston, MA, USA   Peter R. Mueller
London, UK   Andreas Adam

Contents

Contributors

Muneeb Ahmed, MD Assistant Professor of Radiology, Harvard Medical School, Boston, MA, USA
Section of Interventional Radiology, Beth Israel Deaconess Medical Center, Boston, MA, USA

Rony Avritscher, MD Assistant Professor of Interventional Radiology, Department of Diagnostic Radiology, The University of Texas M.D. Anderson Cancer Center, Houston, TX, USA

Michael D. Beland, MD Assistant Professor and Director of Ultrasound, Department of Diagnostic Imaging, Rhode Island Hospital, Providence, RI, USA

Xavier Buy, MD Department of Radiology, University Hospital of Strasbourg, Strasbourg, France

Laura Crocetti, MD, PhD Doctor, Division of Diagnostic Imaging and Intervention, Department of Liver Transplants, Hepatology, and Infectious Diseases, Pisa University School of Medicine, Pisa, Italy

Thomas A. DiPetrillo, MD Department of Radiation Oncology, Rhode Island Hospital, Providence, RI, USA

Ricardo Douarte, MD Department of Radiology, University Hospital of Strasbourg, Strasbourg, France

Damian E. Dupuy, MD, FACR Director of Tumor Ablation, Department of Diagnostic Imaging, Warren Alpert Medical School of Brown University, Rhode Island Hospital, Providence, RI, USA

Tomas Dvorak, MD Department of Radiation Oncology, MD Anderson Cancer Center Orlando, Orlando, FL, USA

Brian H. Eisner, MD Attending Surgeon in Urologic Surgery, Department of Urology, Massachusetts General Hospital, Boston, MA, USA

Yuman Fong, MD Vice Chair Technology Department, Department of Surgery, Memorial Sloan-Kettering Cancer Center, New York, NY, USA

Murray F. Brennan Chair in Surgery, Department of Surgery, Memorial Sloan-Kettering Cancer Center, New York, NY, USA

Afshin Gangi, MD, PhD Department of Radiology, University Hospital of Strasbourg, Strasbourg, France

Julien Garnon, MD Department of Radiology, University Hospital of Strasbourg, Strasbourg, France

Debra A. Gervais, MD Associate Radiologist, Department of Radiology, Massachusetts General Hospital, Boston, MA, USA

Shraga Nahum Goldberg, PhD Section Chief, Image-Guided Therapy and Interventional Oncology, Director, Applied Radiology Research Laboratory, Department of Radiology, Hebrew University-Hadassah Medical Center, Jerusalem, Israel

Sébastien Guihard, MD Department of Radiotherapy, Centre de lutte contre le Cancer Paul Strauss, Strasbourg, France

J. Louis Hinshaw, MD Assistant Professor, Department of Radiology, University of Wisconsin School of Medicine and Public Health, Madison, WI, USA

Theodore S. Hong, MD Director, Gastrointestinal Service, Department of Radiation Oncology, Massachusetts General Hospital, Boston, MA, USA

Shiva Jayaraman, MD, MESc, FRCSC Hepatopancreatobiliary Surgery Fellow, Department of Surgery, Memorial Sloan-Kettering Cancer Center, New York, NY, USA

Sanjeeva P. Kalva, MD Associate Director, Division of Vascular Imaging and Interventions, Department of Imaging, Massachusetts General Hospital, Harvard Medical School, Boston, MA, USA

Nicholas Kujala, MD Diagnostic Radiology Resident, Department of Diagnostic Imaging, Rhode Island Hospital, Providence, RI, USA

Riccardo Lencioni, MD Professor, Division of Diagnostic Imaging and Intervention, Department of Liver Transplants, Hepatology, and Infectious Diseases, Pisa University School of Medicine, Pisa, Italy

Meghan G. Lubner, MD Assistant Professor, Department of Radiology, University of Wisconsin School of Medicine and Public Health, Madison, WI, USA

Janet E. Murphy, MD MPH Instructor in Medicine, Harvard Medical School, Massachusetts General Hospital Cancer Center, Boston, MA, USA

Georges Noel, MD, PhD Department of Radiotherapy, Centre de lutte contre le Cancer Paul Strauss, Strasbourg, France

Rahmi Oklu, MD, PhD Division of Vascular Imaging and Interventions, Department of Imaging, Massachusetts General Hospital, Harvard Medical School, Boston, MA, USA

Sarah P. Psutka, MD Resident in Urology, PGY 4, Department of Urology, Massachusetts General Hospital, Boston, MA, USA

David P. Ryan, MD Associate Chief Clinical Director, Massachusetts General Hospital Cancer Center, Boston, MA, USA Hemotology/Oncology, Department of Medicine, Massachusetts General Hospital, Boston, MA, USA

Tarun Sabharwal, MB, BS Department of Radiology, Guy's and St. Thomas' Hospital, London, UK

Tracey G. Simon, BA Department of Diagnostic Imaging, Warren Alpert Medical School of Brown University, Rhode Island Hospital, Providence, RI, USA

Gail ter Haar, MA (Oxon), MSc, PhD, DSc (Oxon) Department of Physics, Institute of Cancer Research: Royal Marsden Hospital, Sutton, Surrey, UK

Ashraf Thabet, MD Assistant Radiologist, Department of Radiology, Massachusetts General Hospital, Boston, MA, USA

Pierre Truntzer, MD Department of Radiotherapy, Centre de lutte contre le Cancer Paul Strauss, Strasbourg, France

Georgia Tsoumakidou, MD Department of Radiology, University Hospital of Strasbourg, Strasbourg, France

Michael J. Wallace, MD Professor and Section Chief, Interventional Radiology, Department of Diagnostic Radiology, The University of Texas M.D. Anderson Cancer Center, Houston, TX, USA

Part I
Principles

Chapter 1
Principles of Medical Oncology and Chemotherapy

Janet E. Murphy and David P. Ryan

Introduction

Advances in chemotherapy, surgery, radiation therapy, and interventional oncology have made cancer treatment an increasingly complex endeavor. Multidisciplinary strategies continue to improve patient outcomes while minimizing toxicity. The role of the medical oncologist is to deliver chemotherapy and coordinate multispecialty treatment for patients diagnosed with cancer. Increasingly, medical oncologists rely on interventional oncologists to deliver targeted treatments for palliation, and at times, long-term survival. In order to optimize collaboration between disciplines, this introductory chapter will provide insight into the process that the medical oncologist undertakes when assessing a patient and planning for his/her treatment. In addition, it will provide an overview of chemotherapy, biologic/targeted therapy, and response to treatment.

Diagnosis and Staging

Human malignancy takes many forms, and the role of chemotherapy in its treatment varies. Intravenous cytotoxic chemotherapy often comprises the entire treatment, with curative intent, in leukemia, lymphoma, and germ-cell tumors such as testicular cancer. In contrast, the majority of potentially curable solid tumors require a multidisciplinary treatment approach in which chemotherapy plays a complementary role to surgery, radiation therapy, and local ablative treatments. Establishing the initial histologic diagnosis is imperative to guide the direction of therapy.

Diagnosis begins with a comprehensive patient history and physical, often followed by baseline radiologic imaging for preliminary staging and to identify the optimal site for obtaining a tissue diagnosis. Immunohistochemistry and genotype analysis play a critical role in establishing the diagnosis and therapy for a cancer, and this often impacts the decision to obtain a core biopsy rather than a fine needle aspirate. Once core biopsy of a lesion is obtained, medical oncologists rely on the expertise of our colleagues in pathology to correctly identify the cell of origin. Histologic diagnosis of malignancy starts with identification of general morphology with hematoxylin and eosin (H+E) staining. In one series, light microscopy alone categorized 60% of tumors as adenocarcinoma, 5% as squamous cell carcinoma, and the remaining 35% as the less definitive categories of poorly differentiated adenocarcinoma, poorly differentiated carcinoma, or poorly differentiated neoplasm [1].

Immunohistochemical testing using antibodies to probe cell surfaces refines the diagnosis and most often determines the origin of the malignancy. For example, staining for the cell surface protein S100 identifies malignant melanoma [2]. Cytokeratin staining identifies broad categories of adenocarcinoma, and there are over 20 commonly assayed cytokeratin markers. Figure 1.1 identifies a diagnostic algorithm based on staining for CK-7 and CK-20, two commonly used cytokeratins, in carcinoma of unknown primary.

In many malignancies, molecular features of the tumor provide prognostic and predictive information that impacts treatment. For example, breast adenocarcinoma is characterized by the presence or absence of estrogen and progesterone receptors, which are predictive of response to adjuvant selective estrogen receptor modulators (SERMs) such as tamoxifen or aromatase inhibitors (AIs) such as anastrozole [3, 4]. Overexpression of the epidermal growth factor receptor (EGFR)-family

J.E. Murphy (✉) • D.P. Ryan
Harvard Medical School, Massachusetts General Hospital Cancer Center, 55 Fruit St., Yawkey 7E, Boston, MA 02114, USA
e-mail: jemurphy@partners.org

P.R. Mueller and A. Adam (eds.), *Interventional Oncology: A Practical Guide for the Interventional Radiologist*,
DOI 10.1007/978-1-4419-1469-9_1, © Springer Science+Business Media, LLC 2012

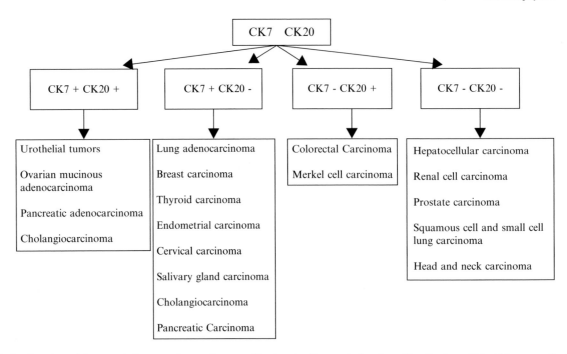

Fig. 1.1 Cytokeratin staining can help categorize malignancy (Reprinted with permission from Varadhachary GR, Abbruzzese JL, Lenzi R. Diagnostic strategies for unknown primary cancer. Cancer. 2004;100(9):1776–85.)

member protein HER2/neu predicts benefit of that anti-HER2 antibody trastuzumab (Herceptin) [5]. The benefit of trastuzumab in tumors overexpressing HER2 was recently demonstrated in locally advanced and metastatic gastric cancer as well [6]. HER2 status is assayed by two means – immunohistochemistry to assess for receptor density, and polymerase chain reaction (PCR) to assess for gene amplification, as shown in Fig. 1.2.

Oncogene mutations can predict response, or resistance, to therapy. In lung cancer, activating mutations in the EGFR predict for response to anti-EGFR tyrosine kinase inhibitors (TKIs) erlotinib (Tarceva, OSI Pharmaceuticals, Melville, New York) and gefitinib (Iressa, AstraZeneca, London, United Kingdom) in the first-line, most commonly in never-smokers [7, 8]. In contrast, activating mutations in the KRAS oncogene in colorectal cancer, present in approximately 40% of tumors, predict resistance to anti-EGFR therapy with the monoclonal antibody cetuximab [9]. Both EGFR and KRAS mutations are assessed using sequence-specific PCR-based techniques.

Once a histologic and molecular diagnosis is established, formal staging follows. Staging guidelines are disease-specific, but most solid tumors follow the American Joint Committee on Cancer (AJCC) TNM system. Notably, staging criteria differ depending on the type of cancer. T3N0M0 bladder cancer constitutes stage III disease, while T3N0M0 colon cancer is stage II, and T3N0M0 breast cancer (but also T3*N1*M0) is stage II. Exceptions to TNM staging should be noted – cancers of the brain and spinal cord are classified according to their cell type and grade; the Ann Arbor staging classification is commonly used to stage lymphomas; and staging is not relevant for most types of leukemia [10].

Patient Assessment

When a diagnosis is made and the stage is confirmed, treatment planning begins. Before selecting chemotherapy and establishing the multidisciplinary treatment approach, the oncologist must first consider the patient's larger context.

Defining Goals of Care

When malignancy is diagnosed at an earlier stage and cure is possible, most patients will opt for this approach. However, when cancer is detected at an advanced stage, the choice of therapy can be less straightforward. Consultation with the patient and his/her family is undertaken to outline options and to establish reasonable *goals of care*. Is the patient interested in

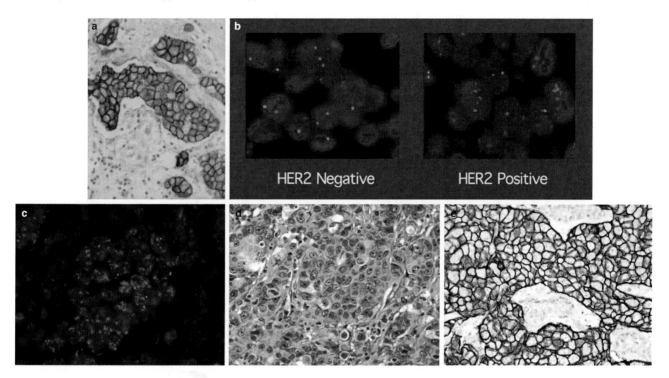

Fig. 1.2 (**a**) HE (hematoxylin and eosin) stain shows high-grade invasive ductal carcinoma of the breast with diffuse growth of pleomorphic tumor cells and frequent mitotic figures. (**b**) HER2 immunohistochemistry shows strong (3+) circular membranous staining of tumor cells. (**c**) HER2 fluorescence in-situ hybridization (FISH) shows amplification of HER2 signals (*orange*), compared with chromosome 17 signals (*green*) with amplification ratio of 9.7 [Vysis HER2 probe]. (**d**, **e**) HER2 immunohistochemistry and FISH (Images courtesy of Elena F. Brachtel, MD, Breast Pathology, Massachusetts General Hospital.)

pursuing an aggressive treatment strategy that is most likely to prolong survival, but in the interim involve potentially the greatest toxicity and the most intense need for medical follow-up? Does he/she favor a treatment that maximizes quality of life but perhaps offers less robust survival benefit? Or, does the patient wish to refrain from intensive medical intervention altogether, favoring a supportive care approach, which focuses exclusively on symptom reduction and optimizing time at home? Difficult, but important, discussions around goals are crucial at the outset of treatment, and discussions evolve with the patient's clinical course.

Identifying Medical Comorbidities

The oncologist must consider the patient's medical comorbidities in treatment planning, considering the specific toxicities of potential therapy in the context of the patient's overall health. Baseline renal or hepatic dysfunction – the latter often related to metastatic disease in the liver – often requires chemotherapy dose-reduction. Organ dysfunction may impact the choice of therapy. For example, patients with advanced colorectal cancer with liver involvement and hepatic dysfunction are often initiated on combination therapy with 5-FU/leucovorin and oxaliplatin (FOLFOX) rather than the equally efficacious 5-FU/leucovorin and irinotecan (FOLFIRI) regimen, because high bilirubin and alkaline phosphatase levels are associated with an exponential decrease in the clearance of irinotecan, and drug toxicity (neutropenia, diarrhea) correlates with serum bilirubin concentration [11]. Drugs such as doxorubicin and trastuzumab, both associated with onset of congestive heart failure, are contraindicated in patients with this preexisting condition [12, 13]. Bleomycin, which is associated with the rare but serious complication of pulmonary fibrosis, is contraindicated in patients with underlying pulmonary disease, and pulmonary function testing is compulsory prior to starting treatment [14, 15].

Medical comorbidities can impact the choice of treatment modality altogether. In patients with potentially resectable (Stage I–Stage IIIA) lung cancer, patients with significant smoking history and related comorbidities [chronic obstructive pulmonary disease (COPD) with diminished pulmonary reserve or severe cardiovascular disease] are at times deemed "medically inoperable" and their multidisciplinary treatment shifts from potentially curative surgery toward chemotherapy, radiation, and local ablation approaches, with inferior outcomes [16, 17].

Fig. 1.3 Eastern Cooperative
Oncology Group performance
status (ECOG PS) scale

0 - Asymptomatic (Fully active, able to carry on all pre-disease activities without restriction)
1 - Symptomatic but completely ambulatory (Restricted in physically strenuous activity but ambulatory and able to carry out work of a light or sedentary nature. For example, light housework, office work)
2 - Symptomatic, <50% in bed during the day (Ambulatory and capable of all self care but unable to carry out any work activities. Up and about more than 50% of waking hours)
3 - Symptomatic, >50% in bed, but not bedbound (Capable of only limited self-care, confined to bed or chair 50% or more of waking hours)
4 - Bedbound (Completely disabled. Cannot carry on any self-care. Totally confined to bed or chair)
5 - Death

Assessing Performance Status

Oncologists must continually evaluate the patient's fitness for treatment. Several validated instruments provide objective scoring of overall fitness, including the Karnofsky performance status (KPS) and the Lansky score in children. The Eastern Cooperative Oncology Group performance score (ECOG PS) is most commonly used by medical oncologists and has been demonstrated to most directly correlate with outcome [18]. ECOG PS is used to assess overall wellness, ability to conduct activities of daily living, strength, and mobility, as outlined in Fig. 1.3.

Patients with ECOG PS 0 or 1 are generally cleared for treatment without concern. Patients with ECOG PS 2 may struggle with treatment, and it becomes an individualized decision with the oncologist, patient, and family. Single-agent chemotherapy or single-agent biologic therapy with demonstrated activity (such as cetuximab therapy in head and neck cancers) may be given in the setting of a borderline patient who might be harmed by aggressive multiagent cytotoxic therapy [19]. Patients with an ECOG PS 3 or above are generally considered unfit for most therapies, and treatment may hasten morbidity and even mortality without offering potential benefit. During the course of treatment and especially in the setting of progressive metastatic disease, a patient's ECOG PS may decline, and chemotherapeutic options that were once appropriate are no longer safe. This is a very common juncture for discussion of transition to best supportive care and hospice care, in which the focus is shifted from life-prolonging treatment toward intensification of symptom control and comfort.

Patients with a small minority of disseminated but highly chemoresponsive tumors constitute an exception to the rule. For example, patients with extensive stage small cell lung cancer may be offered chemotherapy even when very ill, with potential reduction of tumor burden that results in a tremendous improvement in overall health. Hematologic malignancies (most notably lymphoma) and germ cell tumors follow this same logic.

Treatment Planning

The multidisciplinary treatment approach incorporates chemotherapy, surgery, radiation, and local treatments in a stepwise or concomitant fashion that is specific to the malignancy, stage, and patient.

Adjuvant therapy refers to treatment administered after resection of the primary tumor, but for whom odds of cure are increased with additional therapy. Selecting patients who would derive benefit from adjuvant chemotherapy means assessing recurrence risk – the goal being to screen out patients with such a low recurrence risk that the toxicity of therapy outweighs its benefit. Lymph node-negative, hormone-receptor positive breast cancer patients are assessed for adjuvant therapy based on primary tumor size and tumor grade. Equivocal cases may benefit from the use of the Recurrence Score assay (Oncotype Dx), in which the primary tumor is subjected to a 21-gene expression assay which assigns a recurrence score [20]. Figure 1.4 demonstrates a schematic of the genes that comprise the 21-gene recurrence score. A similar instrument was approved in Stage II colon cancer in 2010, and similar diagnostics are being explored in lung and other malignancies. For higher-risk patients, however, the benefit to adjuvant chemotherapy has been clearly demonstrated in multiple malignancies such as breast, lung, and colon.

QZ 269

This book is due for return on or before the last date shown below.

QZ 269

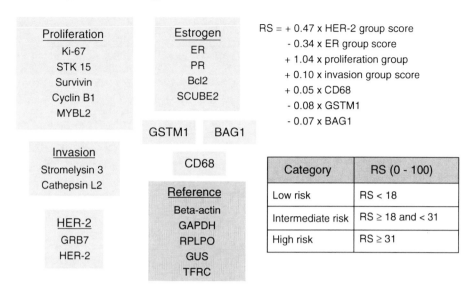

Fig. 1.4 Oncotype Dx recurrence score: schematic of a 21-gene assay

Neoadjuvant (preoperative) therapy is delivered prior to surgical resection of the primary tumor in order to reduce tumor bulk and allow for a more definitive resection. In rectal cancer, neoadjuvant chemoradiation has provided superior postoperative outcomes in terms of both local recurrence and likelihood of sphincter preservation for patients with T3/4 rectal tumors [21]. The accuracy of magnetic resonance imaging (MRI) or endoscopic ultrasound (EUS) staging for rectal cancer is critical to the multidisciplinary management of these patients [22]. For bulky stage III tumors of the breast, neoadjuvant chemotherapy improves likelihood of successful resection [23].

Palliative therapy is comprised of chemotherapy and radiation administered to the patient in whom surgical intervention with curative intent is not possible, either due to extent of metastatic disease or to medical nonoperability. Targeted treatments such as irradiating bony metastases reduce pain. Systemic chemotherapy can also reduce symptoms and prolong survival. Patients are informed that the goal of therapy is to help them live "as well as possible for as long as possible". Gemcitabine, the current mainstay of treatment for pancreatic adenocarcinoma, was demonstrated in a landmark trial that resulted in its approval to prolong life expectancy in a small subset, but more broadly offer "clinical benefit," defined as improvement in pain, performance status, or weight [24].

Introduction to Therapeutics

The treatment options in oncology have expanded tremendously over the past few decades. Cytotoxic chemotherapy remains the mainstay of treatment for some malignancies such as lung and colon cancer. In contrast, it plays little role in the treatment of renal cell carcinoma (RCC) and hepatocellular carcinoma (HCC), where treatment targeting the biochemical pathway driving the cancer (targeted therapy) has become the primary treatment modality. Regardless of method, cancer therapies share the goal of inducing cancer cell death. The mechanisms of action of each therapy will be outlined in this section.

The *fractional cell kill hypothesis*, studied most extensively in leukemia and lymphoma, is an important guiding principle for therapy. The hypothesis holds that for any given concentration of chemotherapy, a set fraction of cells will be killed, independent of the total number of cells. The same set fraction of cells will be killed with the next cycle of therapy, and so on. Of course, malignant tumors exhibit continued cell division in the midst of therapy. The number of treatments, and the interval between treatments, are determined by the theoretical time required to reduce the cell population to zero – but accounting for the tolerance of the host for *toxicity* incurred by the therapy itself [25].

The "therapeutic index" of cytotoxic chemotherapy is defined as the differential between the toxic dose and the therapeutic dose. The fundamental problem in cancer treatment – and the root of most toxicity – is the inability to differentiate malignant cells from those of the normal healthy host, resulting in a narrow therapeutic index. As most chemotherapy targets cells with rapid turnover, toxicities stem from injury to normal tissues with high turnover that are caught in the crossfire – bone marrow, hair follicles, gastrointestinal (GI) mucosa, and the reproductive organs. Managing chemotherapy-associated toxicity means both controlling symptoms and minimizing treatment delays and dose reductions.

Table 1.1 Antimetabolites commonly used in solid tumors

Group	Agent	Common cancers	Common toxicities
Pyrimidine analogs	5-Fluorouracil	Breast GI Head and neck	Diarrhea Mucositis Myelosuppression
	Capecitabine	Breast GI	Diarrhea Mucositis Myelosuppression Hand-foot syndrome
	Gemcitabine	GI Breast Lung Ovary Bladder	Flu-like syndrome Myelosuppression
Purine analogs	6-MP fludarabine	Leukemia	
Antifolates	Methotrexate	Bladder Breast	Myelosuppression Mucositis
	Pemetrexed	NSCLC Bladder Mesothelioma	Myelosuppression Fatigue Rash

GI gastrointestinal; *NSCLC* non-small cell lung cancer

The stakes of treatment interruption in the setting of toxicity are dependent on the goals of therapy. Adjuvant treatment such as dose-dense adriamycin/cyclophosphamide in breast cancer or definitive treatment with curative intent – for example, rituximab, cyclophosphamide, doxorubicin, vincristine, prednisone (R-CHOP) in lymphoma or bleomycin/etoposide/cisplatin (BEP) in testicular cancer – have the best odds of cure when delivered *on schedule* at *full dose*. For this reason, patients are given growth factor support with granulocyte-colony stimulating factor (G-CSF) for low white blood cell counts and transfused red blood cells for severe anemia. In contrast, chemotherapy that is delivered in the noncurative setting (i.e., palliative chemotherapy) is at times held or dose-reduced for toxicity. When a curative endpoint is elusive, optimizing symptom control is the top priority.

The fractional cell kill hypothesis does not hold entirely true in solid malignancy, as tumors are heterogenous, necrotic, and avascular – the very properties that require multidisciplinary approaches including interventional oncology to deliver toxic doses of therapy for local eradication. What follows is a short primer on the major classes of cytotoxic chemotherapy, primarily restricted to drugs used in the treatment of solid tumors – i.e., cancers in which interventional oncologists play a direct role in treatment. Please consult more definitive texts for detailed review of chemotherapy activity and toxicity [25, 26].

Antimetabolites (including antifolates) mimic naturally occurring components of cellular replication and metabolism. Analogs of purines and pyrimidines, the building blocks of DNA and RNA, are incorporated into growing strands, terminating replication, and ultimately resulting in cell death – though the main activity of the pyrimidine analog 5-FU is likely the inhibition of thymidylate synthetase (TS) enzyme itself. Antifolates, such as methotrexate and pemetrexed, interfere with reduction of folate to the biologically active tetrahydrofolate, an essential cofactor for DNA synthesis (Table 1.1).

The major classes of *antimicrotubule agents* are the taxanes and the vinca alkaloids. Microtubules are comprised of tubulin dimers and provide the lattice for DNA replication during mitosis, and have an equally important role in the structure of the nondividing cell. Taxanes exert their effect on the microtubule by paradoxically stabilizing the microtubule spindle apparatus and preventing depolymerization, disrupting the orderly disassembly of the spindle apparatus necessary for completing mitosis [27]. In contrast, vinca alkaloids prevent microtubule assembly by binding beta tubulin and preventing subunit dimerization and microtubule polymerization – impeding mitosis and ultimately resulting in apoptosis (Table 1.2).

Topoisomerase inhibitors exert their effects during DNA synthesis. DNA topoisomerase I is a nuclear enzyme that relieves torsional strain in DNA during replication and transcription by complexing with a single strand of DNA to allow its complementary strand to uncoil around, or pass through, the complex. Camptothecins bind to and stabilize the topoisomerase–DNA complex, preventing dissociation and resulting in double-strand breaks. Similarly, anthracyclines, once thought to intercalate DNA due to their planar structure, likely exert their main effect by binding topoisomerase II and creating strand breaks by binding and stabilizing the Topo-II–DNA complex. Etoposide binds the Topo-II complex and inhibits 5′ to 3′ reannealing after the necessary strand breaks for uncoiling are made, propagating strand breaks and leading to apoptosis (Table 1.3).

Alkylating agents and platinum analogs exert their effect by covalently altering and crosslinking the strands of DNA. As a class, they are notable for their indiscriminate tissue toxicity and steep dose–response curve – high-dose alkylators are used as conditioning (myeloablative) agents in preparation for stem cell rescue in hematologic malignancy. Classic alkylators such

Table 1.2 Antimicrotubule agents commonly used in solid tumors

Group	Agent	Common cancers	Common toxicities
Taxanes	Paclitaxel	Lung Breast Ovarian Bladder Endometrial GI	Hypersensitivity Myelosuppression/neutropenia Bradyarrhythmias Neuropathy
	Docetaxel	Breast Lung GI Head and neck	Edema/third spacing Ascites, pleural effusion Myelosuppression/neutropenia Neuropathy
Vinca alkaloids	Vinblastine	Bladder (MVAC)	Myelosuppression
	Vinorelbine	Breast Lung	Myelosuppression

GI gastrointestinal; *MVAC* methotrexate, vinblastine, adriamycin, and cisplatin

Table 1.3 Topoisomerase inhibitors commonly used in solid tumors

Group	Agent	Common cancers	Common toxicities
Anthracyclines	Doxorubicin	Breast Bladder Endometrial Sarcoma	Myelosuppression Alopecia Mucositis Cardiomyopathy MDS/AML
	Epirubicin	Esophageal/gastric Breast	
Camptothecins	Irinotecan	GI SCLC	Diarrhea Myelosuppression
	Topotecan	SCLC NSCLC Platinum-resistant ovarian Endometrial	Myelosuppression – high prevalence of Grade 4 neutropenia
Derivatives	Etoposide (VP-16)	NSCLC SCLC Ovarian Testicular	Myelosuppression LFT abnormalities MDS/AML

GI gastrointestinal; *SCLC* small cell lung cancer; *NSCLC* non-small cell lung cancer; *MDS/AML* myelodysplastic syndrome/acute myeloid leukemia; *LFT* liver function test

as the nitrogen mustards (cyclophosphamide and chlorambucil) become unstable when enzymatically activated, adding a chloroethyl group to electronegative segments of DNA. The chloroethyl moieties subsequently crosslink strands of DNA, making excision repair difficult to execute, ultimately leading to apoptosis. Nonclassical alkylators, such as dacarbazine and its derivative temozolomide, are prodrugs that when enzymatically activated, methylate the DNA base pairs guanine and adenine, leading to aberrant DNA crosslinking. Platinum compounds exert this same net effect by depositing platinum complexes within DNA (Table 1.4).

Targeted Therapy

Our expanding knowledge of cancer biology has initiated development of therapies that target biologic pathways, and their use has transformed medical oncology. Molecular targeted therapies include monoclonal antibodies (MAb) such as the anti-EGFR antibodies cetuximab and panitumumab and the antivascular endothelial growth factor (anti-VEGF) antibody bevacizumab; small molecule inhibitors of tyrosine kinases (TKIs) such as the BCR-Abl/c-kit TKI imatinib, anti-EGFR TKIs gefitinib and erlotinib, and the multitarget TKIs sunitinib and sorafenib; and the proteasome inhibitor bortezomib.

Renal cell carcinoma and hepatocellular carcinoma, two cancers in which interventional oncologists play a central role in treating, have demonstrated greatest benefit from targeted therapy where cytotoxic therapy has provided minimal or no benefit.

Table 1.4 Alkylating agents and platinum analogs commonly used in solid tumors

Group	Agent	Common cancers	Common toxicities
Nitrogen mustards	Cyclophosphamide	Breast	Myelosuppression Hemorrhagic cystitis Alopecia
	Ifosamide	Sarcoma Testicular	Myelosuppression Hematuria
Nonclassical alkylators	Dacarbazine (DTIC)	Melanoma Sarcoma	Myelosuppression LFT abnormalities
	Temozolomide	Glioblastoma Melanoma	Nausea/vomiting Headache Myelosuppression
Platinum analogs	Cisplatin	Lung Bladder Head and neck Esophagus Cervix Biliary tract Endometrial Mesothelioma Testicular	Nausea/vomiting Ototoxicity Nephrotoxicity
	Carboplatin	Lung Ovary Endometrial Head and neck Testicular	Myelosuppression Nausea/vomiting

	Oxaliplatin	GI
		Head and neck
			Transient cold-induced
			  peripheral
			  neuropathy
			Irreversible neuropathy
			Myelosuppression

GI gastrointestinal; *LFT* liver function tests

In patients with advanced, unresectable hepatocellular carcinoma in whom liver-directed therapy is also inappropriate, single-agent chemotherapy including doxorubicin, 5-FU, and cisplatin, and combination regimens with gemcitabine/oxaliplatin and cisplatin, alpha-interferon, doxorubicin, and 5-FU (PIAF) all failed to demonstrate meaningful response rates and overall outcomes [28–30]. Sorafenib, a multitargeted TKI with activity against vascular endothelial growth factor receptor (VEGFR), platelet-derived growth factor (PDGF), Raf, and c-kit was Food and Drug Administration (FDA) approved after the European Sorafenib Hepatocellular Carcinoma Assessment Randomized Protocol (SHARP) trial, a study of 602 patients with inoperable HCC, demonstrated an overall survival benefit in the sorafenib-treated patients (10.7 months versus 7.9 months with best supportive care alone) [31]. Notably, radiographic response was very low in this study (and in a Phase II study that preceded it), and survival correlated more directly with serum alpha-fetoprotein levels than with Response Evaluation Criteria in Solid Tumors (RECIST) response.

Renal cell carcinoma, with the exception of sarcomatoid and collecting duct subtypes, is generally deemed chemo-resistant, and immunotherapy with IL-2 and interferon-alpha comprised the mainstay of therapy until 2006. Advances in understanding the central role of the angiogenesis pathway highlighted the potential for targeting the VEGF and mammalian target of rapamycin (mTOR) pathways in this disease, and has led to the approval of sunitinib, sorafenib, temsirolimus, and bevacizumab in the first- and second line for treatment of advanced RCC [31–35].

Measuring the Impact of Therapy

Assessing whether treatment has had its intended effect is dependent on the stage of cancer being treated. The success of the *adjuvant* treatment of resected cancers is measured by disease nonrecurrence over a lifetime. In some cancers (e.g., triple-negative breast cancer), survival beyond 5 years portends outright cure. Paradoxically, estrogen receptor/progesterone receptor (ER/PR) positive cancers, while more indolent upfront, tend to have a longer risk-period for recurrence out to 15–20 years after adjuvant treatment [36]. Malignancies such as high-risk melanoma have a lifelong risk of recurrence.

Fig. 1.5 European Organisation for Research and Treatment of Cancer (EORTC) response evaluation criteria in solid tumors (RECIST) criteria for target lesion evaluation (October 2008)

4.3.1. Evaluation of target lesions

Complete Response (CR): Disappearance of all target lesions. Any pathological lymph nodes (whether target or non-target) must have reduction in short axis to <10 mm.

Partial Response (PR): At least a 30% decrease in the sum of diameters of target lesions, taking as reference the baseline sum diameters.

Progressive Disease (PD): At least a 20% increase in the sum of diameters of target lesions, taking as reference the *smallest sum on study* (this includes the baseline sum if that is the smallest on study). In addition to the relative increase of 20%, the sum must also demonstrate an absolute increase of at least 5 mm. (*Note:* the appearance of one or more new lesions is also considered progression).

Stable Disease (SD): Neither sufficient shrinkage to qualify for PR nor sufficient increase to qualify for PD, taking as reference the smallest sum diameters while on study.

After neoadjuvant or adjuvant treatment, monitoring serum tumor markers can provide an ongoing assessment of disease burden. For example, prostate-specific antigen (PSA) should become undetectable after radical prostatectomy, and a rise in PSA over time suggests local recurrence or metastatic disease [37]. Serum carcinoembryonic antigen (CEA) is followed in Stage II/III colorectal cancer after surgery and chemotherapy, with guidelines mandating monitoring at 3-month intervals for the first 2 years after completion of therapy, and then at 6-month intervals up to 5 years [38]. In ovarian cancer, patients with Stage III disease who have been treated with cytoreductive surgery followed by adjuvant platinum-based chemotherapy are monitored traditionally for cancer antigen 125 (CA-125) level, but recent data suggest that following patients clinically (close follow-up for symptoms) rather than with tumor markers does not impact their survival when a recurrence is detected [39]. Some, but not all, malignancies benefit from serial imaging to monitor for potential disease recurrence.

In patients with metastatic cancer, success of palliative therapy is measured by several metrics; first, clinical: assessing for symptom improvement and pain control; second, radiologic: evidence of chemotherapy response (tumor shrinkage) or disease stabilization. In the setting of a clinical trial, the European Organisation for Research and Treatment of Cancer (EORTC) RECIST criteria are used to assess response to therapy – criteria well-known to radiologists and reviewed in Fig. 1.5. The criteria mandate a two-dimensional change in the sum of target lesions greater than 30% to constitute partial response and radiologic disappearance to constitute a complete response to treatment [40]. Outside of clinical trials, medical oncologists still rely on correlative imaging to document stable disease, tumor shrinkage, or progression, but precise volumetric criteria are not as relevant.

With the advent of biologic therapy, the RECIST criteria for tumor volume assessment may be less sensitive, because the biologic mechanism of therapy may not directly induce tumor shrinkage. As mentioned above, RECIST was inadequate as a sole metric for sorafenib response in HCC in the SHARP trial. In another retrospective study of 234 patients with advanced colorectal cancer with liver metastasis treated with chemotherapy plus bevacizumab, RECIST criteria were predictive of complete or major pathologic response (documented on subsequent resection of metastases) but less sensitive for detecting minor pathologic response – as most patients fell into the "stable disease" RECIST category. In contrast, newer morphologic criteria, in which optimal response to therapy is defined as a change in metastases from heterogenous and thick, with irregular borders into bland, homogenous lesions with sharp interface with surrounding liver parenchyma, had greater sensitivity to detect minor pathologic response [41]. Positron emission tomography (PET), dynamic contrast enhanced MRI, and molecular imaging techniques will undoubtedly continue to advance our understanding of "response" in the era of targeted therapy.

As our understanding of the molecular biology of cancer therapy progresses, we are entering an era of personalized cancer medicine. Tumor genetics are used increasingly to determine both prognosis and choice of treatment. Metrics such as standard RECIST criteria, while sufficient to assess response to cytotoxic therapy, are being reevaluated in the context of targeted agents. Most importantly, patients are living longer with malignancy, and local treatment of metastatic disease is becoming more prevalent. Medical oncologists and interventional oncologists will continue to foster collaboration and improve patient outcomes in the years to come.

References

1. Varadhachary GR, Abbruzzese JL, Lenzi R. Diagnostic strategies for unknown primary cancer. Cancer. 2004;100(9):1776–85.
2. Cochran AJ, Lu HF, Li PX, Saxton R, Wen DR. S-100 protein remains a practical marker for melanocytic and other tumours. Melanoma Res. 1993;3(5):325–30.
3. Early Breast Cancer Trialists' Collaborative Group (EBCTCG). Effects of chemotherapy and hormonal therapy for early breast cancer on recurrence and 15-year survival: an overview of the randomised trials. Lancet. 2005;365(9472):1687–717.
4. Forbes JF, Cuzick J, Buzdar A, Howell A, Tobias JS, Baum M. Effect of anastrozole and tamoxifen as adjuvant treatment for early-stage breast cancer: 100-month analysis of the ATAC trial. Lancet Oncol. 2008;9(1):45–53.
5. Romond EH, Perez EA, Bryant J, et al. Trastuzumab plus adjuvant chemotherapy for operable HER2-positive breast cancer. N Engl J Med. 2005;353(16):1673–84.
6. Van Cutsem E, Kang Y, Chung H, et al. Efficacy results from the ToGA trial: a phase III study of trastuzumab added to standard chemotherapy in first-line human epidermal growth factor receptor 2-positive advanced gastric cancer. J Clin Oncol. 2009;27(Suppl):18s. Abstract LBA4509.
7. Sequist LV, Martins RG, Spigel D, et al. First-line gefitinib in patients with advanced non-small-cell lung cancer harboring somatic EGFR mutations. J Clin Oncol. 2008;26(15):2442–9.
8. Giaccone G, Gallegos Ruiz M, Le Chevalier T, et al. Erlotinib for frontline treatment of advanced non-small cell lung cancer: a phase II study. Clin Cancer Res. 2006;12(20 Pt 1):6049–55.
9. Van Cutsem E, Kohne CH, Hitre E, et al. Cetuximab and chemotherapy as initial treatment for metastatic colorectal cancer. N Engl J Med. 2009;360(14):1408–17.
10. National Cancer Institute. Cancer staging. Available at: http://www.cancer.gov/cancertopics/factsheet/Detection/staging. Accessed 8 Apr 2010.
11. Raymond E, Boige V, Faivre SS, et al. Dosage adjustment and pharmacokinetic profile of irinotecan in cancer patients with hepatic dysfunction. J Clin Oncol. 2002;20:4303–12.
12. Keefe DL. Trastuzumab-associated cardiotoxicity. Cancer. 2002;95(7):1592–600.
13. Singal PK, Iliskovic N. Doxorubicin-induced cardiomyopathy. N Engl J Med. 1998;339:900–5.
14. Sleijfer S. Bleomycin-induced pneumonitis. Chest. 2001;120(2):617–24.
15. National Comprehensive Cancer Network. NCCN guidelines for pulmonary function testing. Available at: http://www.nccn.org/professionals/physician_gls/f_guidelines.asp. Accessed 8 Apr 2010.
16. Powell JW, Dexter E, Scalzetti EM, Bogart JA. Treatment advances for medically inoperable non-small-cell lung cancer: emphasis on prospective trials. Lancet Oncol. 2009;10(9):885–94.
17. Scott WJ, Howington J, Feigenberg S, Movsas B, Pisters K. Treatment of non-small cell lung cancer stage I and stage II: ACCP evidence-based clinical practice guidelines (2nd edition). Chest. 2007;132(3 Suppl):234S–42.
18. Oken MM, Creech RH, Tormey DC, et al. Toxicity and response criteria of the Eastern Cooperative Oncology Group. Am J Clin Oncol. 1982;5(6):649–55.
19. Vermorken JB, Trigo J, Hitt R, et al. Open-label, uncontrolled, multicenter phase II study to evaluate the efficacy and toxicity of cetuximab as a single agent in patients with recurrent and/or metastatic squamous cell carcinoma of the head and neck who failed to respond to platinum-based therapy. J Clin Oncol. 2007;25(16):2171–7.
20. Mamounas EP, Tang G, Fisher B, et al. Association between the 21-gene recurrence score assay and risk of locoregional recurrence in node-negative, estrogen receptor-positive breast cancer: results from NSABP B-14 and NSABP B-20. J Clin Oncol. 2010;28(10):1677–83.
21. Sauer R, Becker H, Hohenberger W, et al. Preoperative versus postoperative chemoradiotherapy for rectal cancer. N Engl J Med. 2004;351(17):1731–40.
22. Gualdi GF, Casciani E, Guadalaxara A, d'Orta C, Polettini E, Pappalardo G. Local staging of rectal cancer with transrectal ultrasound and endorectal magnetic resonance imaging: comparison with histologic findings. Dis Colon Rectum. 2000;43(3):338–45.
23. Shenkier T, Weir L, Levine M, et al. Clinical practice guidelines for the care and treatment of breast cancer: 15. Treatment for women with stage III or locally advanced breast cancer. CMAJ. 2004;170(6):983–94.
24. Burris 3rd HA, Moore MJ, Andersen J, et al. Improvements in survival and clinical benefit with gemcitabine as first-line therapy for patients with advanced pancreas cancer: a randomized trial. J Clin Oncol. 1997;15(6):2403–13.
25. Chabner B, Longo DL, editors. Cancer chemotherapy and biotherapy: principles and practice. 3rd ed. Philadelphia: Lippincott Williams & Wilkins; 2001.
26. DeVita Jr VT, Lawrence TS, Rosenburg SA, editors. DeVita, Hellman, and Rosenberg's cancer: principles & practice of oncology. 8th ed. Philadelphia: Lippincott Williams & Wilkins; 2008.
27. Dumontet C, Sikic BI. Mechanisms of action of and resistance to antitubulin agents: microtubule dynamics, drug transport, and cell death. J Clin Oncol. 1999;17(3):1061–70.

28. Yeo W, Mok TS, Zee B, et al. A randomized phase III study of doxorubicin versus cisplatin/interferon alpha-2b/doxorubicin/fluorouracil (PIAF) combination chemotherapy for unresectable hepatocellular carcinoma. J Natl Cancer Inst. 2005;97(20):1532–8.
29. Park SH, Lee Y, Han SH, et al. Systemic chemotherapy with doxorubicin, cisplatin and capecitabine for metastatic hepatocellular carcinoma. BMC Cancer. 2006;6:3.
30. Louafi S, Boige V, Ducreux M, et al. Gemcitabine plus oxaliplatin (GEMOX) in patients with advanced hepatocellular carcinoma (HCC): results of a phase II study. Cancer. 2007;109(7):1384–90.
31. Llovet JM, Ricci S, Mazzaferro V, et al. Sorafenib in advanced hepatocellular carcinoma. N Engl J Med. 2008;359(4):378–90.
32. Motzer RJ, Hutson TE, Tomczak P, et al. Sunitinib versus interferon alfa in metastatic renal-cell carcinoma. N Engl J Med. 2007;356(2):115–24.
33. Escudier B, Eisen T, Stadler WM, et al. Sorafenib in advanced clear-cell renal-cell carcinoma. N Engl J Med. 2007;356(2):125–34.
34. Yang JC, Haworth L, Sherry RM, et al. A randomized trial of bevacizumab, an anti-vascular endothelial growth factor antibody, for metastatic renal cancer. N Engl J Med. 2003;349(5):427–34.
35. Hudes G, Carducci M, Tomczak P, et al. Temsirolimus, interferon alfa, or both for advanced renal-cell carcinoma. N Engl J Med. 2007;356(22):2271–81.
36. Berry DA, Cirrincione C, Henderson IC, et al. Estrogen-receptor status and outcomes of modern chemotherapy for patients with node-positive breast cancer. JAMA. 2006;295(14):1658–67.
37. Pound CR, Partin AW, Eisenberger MA, Chan DW, Pearson JD, Walsh PC. Natural history of progression after PSA elevation following radical prostatectomy. JAMA. 1999;281(17):1591–7.
38. National Comprehensive Cancer Network. NCCN guidelines for colorectal cancer post-treatment surveillance. Available at: http://www.nccn.org/professionals/physician_gls/f_guidelines.asp. Accessed 17 June 2011.
39. Rustin GJ, van der Burg ME, on behalf of MRC and EORTC collaborators. A randomized trial in ovarian cancer (OC) of early treatment of relapse based on CA125 level alone versus delayed treatment based on conventional clinical indicators (MRC OV05/EORTC 55955 trials). J Clin Oncol. 2009;27(Suppl):18s (suppl; Abstract 1)
40. Eisenhauer EA, Therasse P, Bogaerts J, et al. New response evaluation criteria in solid tumours: revised RECIST guideline (version 1.1). Eur J Cancer. 2009;45(2):228–47.
41. Chun YS, Vauthey JN, Boonsirikamchai P, et al. Association of computed tomography morphologic criteria with pathologic response and survival in patients treated with bevacizumab for colorectal liver metastases. JAMA. 2009;302(21):2338–44.

Chapter 2
Modern Radiation Therapy Approaches: Targeted and Ablative Strategies

Theodore S. Hong

Introduction

Modern radiation therapy is a therapeutic cancer modality that can achieve local and regional control of malignancy in addition to providing palliation. Radiation therapy exerts its anticancer effect through the accumulation of DNA damage in the tumor cells. The DNA damage leads to either acute cell death or a delayed cell death, known as mitotic catastrophe. For this reason, tumors may shrink months after the completion of radiation therapy.

Principles of Radiation Therapy

The amount of radiation, or dose, that can safely be given to a tumor, is limited by the radiation tolerance of the normal organs surrounding it. There are a number of strategies that can be used to improve the therapeutic ration of radiation therapy. The *energy* of the radiation beam determines how deeply the radiation penetrates, whereas the amount of radiation absorbed (dose) determines the biologic effects.

Most commonly, high energy megavoltage photons are used to spare skin due to its greater depth of penetration. Multiple beams can be focused from many directions to concentrate the radiation dose in the tumor and spare critical adjacent normal structures. Indeed, side effects occur when the adjacent normal tissues receive too much accumulated radiation. Both the total dose absorbed and the volume of normal tissue irradiated contribute to these side effects.

Similarly, as tumor cells can die either acutely or via a delayed mechanism, so to side effects can be either acute or late. Acute side effects are the ones that occur during the course of radiation and may persist up to a month thereafter. Tissue types prone to this type of damage are generally rapidly proliferating types, for example, mucosal surfaces that can lead to diarrhea or mucositis. In contrast, late effects may happen at any point beyond 6 weeks from the completion of therapy, rather than during treatment. Organ damage such as transverse myelitis from overtreatment of the spinal cord, radiation-induced liver disease (RILD), and radiation pneumonitis are examples of severe long-term late effects.

The field of radiation oncology primarily focuses on balancing the risks of normal tissue toxicity and the effectiveness of therapy. This chapter will focus on the newer technologies of interest to the interventional radiologist.

Intensity-Modulated Radiation Therapy

Intensity-modulated radiation therapy (IMRT) is a form of highly conformal photon-based therapy that uses modulation of the intensity across the radiation beam to create highly conformal treatment plans. In contrast to two-dimensional (2D) or three-dimensional (3D) therapy, which uses multiple static fields, IMRT provides the ability to deliver radiation to targets of unusual, concave shapes, as well as differing radiation doses within a given volume allowing dose intensification

T.S. Hong (✉)
Department of Radiation Oncology, Massachusetts General Hospital, 100 Blossom St, Boston, MA 02114, USA
e-mail: tshong1 @partners.org

P.R. Mueller and A. Adam (eds.), *Interventional Oncology: A Practical Guide for the Interventional Radiologist*,
DOI 10.1007/978-1-4419-1469-9_2, © Springer Science+Business Media, LLC 2012

Fig. 2.1 Intensity-modulated radiation therapy (IMRT) plan for a patient with pancreatic cancer. Note the conformal dose distribution

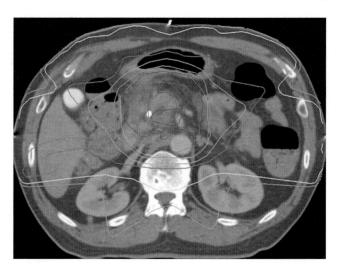

in selected areas of concern, and sparing of surrounding normal tissues. Improvements in treatment-related morbidity have been described in patients with breast, head-and-neck, and prostate cancer treated with IMRT, as compared to conventionally delivered radiation [1–3].

IMRT represents a technological advance that allows the radiation oncologist to "shape" radiation dose profiles around normal structures while fully dosing the tumor and at-risk nodal regions. Since toxicity from radiation is directly related to the volume of normal tissue irradiated, this ability for improved dose distribution provides the opportunity to reduce the overall toxicity profile associated with radiation therapy.

IMRT refers to a specific technique of linear accelerator based photon therapy whereby radiation beams are modulated in such a manner to produce highly conformal dose distributions. A primary objective of IMRT is to reduce dose to selected normal tissue structures in an effort to preserve function, while maintaining full dose delivery to tumor targets. Conventional computed tomography (CT) based radiation therapy, known as 3D-conformal radiation therapy (3D-CRT), uses static beams from two or more angles to target a tumor. These beam angles are chosen by the physician and the physicists and are modulated by a static beam modifier such as a wedge or tissue compensator. In contrast, IMRT is delivered either by multiple modulated static fields (step and shoot) or by a continuously rotating gantry (serial tomotherapy). As the radiation is delivered, specific subsections of each field, known as beamlets, are delivered at different intensities to produce highly conformal dose distribution around irregular shapes.

IMRT planning is conceptually distinct from conventional radiotherapy planning. With 3D-CRT treatment planning, the radiation oncologist will choose beam angles and shape the beam apertures using custom blocking or multileaf collimators (MLC). A generous field margin is used to account for set-up variation and physical characteristics of the beam itself. The radiation dose and profile is then calculated using broad and simple beams in a process is known as forward planning. In contrast, IMRT planning requires the up-front designation of specific targets (prostate, gross tumor, elective nodal regions) and avoidance structures (rectal wall, bladder, bowel, spinal cord, salivary glands, optic apparatus, etc.). Dose specifications are then defined for each of the targets and avoidance structures. The computer planning software then creates a series of beam angles with modulation patterns that strive to achieve the physician's dose prescription goals. This process is known as inverse planning.

IMRT is now routinely used in the treatment of disease sites where high doses are needed for cure such as prostate cancer and cancers of the head-and-neck. Increasingly, IMRT is also being used in other disease sites, such as brain tumors, lung cancer, upper gastrointestinal malignancies like pancreatic cancer (Fig. 2.1), anal cancer, and other historically difficult to treat locations. It should be noted that few head-to-head comparisons of clinical efficacy exist between 3D-CRT and IMRT.

Stereotactic Body Radiotherapy

Conventional radiation therapy is generally given in many small doses. In addition to the dose-volume predictors of radiation toxicity, how much radiation is given in a particular dose, or how the radiation is *fractionated* is also an important predictor of toxicity. Generally, radiation schedules where small doses are given over many fractions leads to fewer late effects than when large doses are given over few fractions. For this reason, most conventional curative treatments are given over daily treatments of 6–8 weeks. The typical daily dose is between 1.5 and 4 Gy/day.

Stereotactic body radiation therapy (SBRT) is a new, evolving external beam radiotherapy method used to precisely deliver a high dose of radiation to an extracranial target using one to five doses [4]. This treatment is safely deliverable due to high targeting accuracy and rapid dose falloff gradients. This technique requires intensive physics support. Specialized treatment planning is needed to achieve sharp dose falloffs. Image registration of diagnostic scans [dynamic CT imaging or magnetic resonance imaging (MRI)] is often needed to accurately identify the tumor target on the planning CT. Motion management and intensive immobilization, either invasive or noninvasive, are needed to minimize the risk of both geographical miss as well as overtreatment of normal structures. Strategies for motion management include respiratory gating, abdominal compression, or use of a "motion envelope" around the target based on a four-dimensional CT scan. Additionally, internal fiducials, such as gold seeds placed by interventional radiology under CT guidance, may also be used for targeting.

Stereotactic radiation was first developed for intracranial lesions such as brain metastases, and base of skull lesions, with a very high rate of local control and an outstanding safety profile. These sites were treated first due to the lack of internal organ motion and the ability for rigid immobilization, allowing for more accurate setup. Clinical success led investigators to develop the technology for extracranial targets. With this technology, doses of 5–25 Gy can be delivered to each treatment, in contrast to the 1.5–3 Gy mentioned above.

Multiple treatment platforms exist for delivery of SBRT. SBRT may be delivered with either photons or protons (see the next section). Commercial SBRT-specific devices, such as CyberKnife (Accuray, Sunnyvale, CA) and Novalis (Varian, Palo Alto, CA), are integrated photon SBRT delivery systems. CyberKnife uses a linear accelerator mounted on a robotic arm that allows for a delivery of a pencil beam from multiple noncoplanar angles. Unique to CyberKnife is a tumor tracking system, which uses an internally implanted fiducial that can then be tracked by the system.

Clinical Indications

SBRT is primarily used as an ablative alternative to surgery. The most commonly treated sites are the lung and the liver. However, there is increasing interest in expanding SBRT to other difficult clinical scenarios.

Lung Tumors

SBRT has been studied extensively in medically inoperable stage I non-small cell lung cancer (NSCLC). A study from Timmerman and colleagues reported the 70-patient phase II study results of SBRT in patients with medically inoperable lung cancer [5]. Patients with T2 tumors received 66 Gy divided over three fractions. Patients with T1 tumors received 60 Gy divided over three fractions. With a median follow up of 18 months, the 2-year local control was 95%, with an overall survival of 56%. Most deaths were due to intercurrent disease rather than disease progression. Of note, severe toxicity was seen in patients with tumors within 2 cm of the bronchial tree. Based on this observation, SBRT is primarily now offered to patients with peripheral tumors.

This single-institution experience was followed by a multicenter study conducted by the Radiation Therapy Oncology Group (RTOG) [6]. In this study, 59 patients with T1/2 N0 M0 NSCLC were treated to 54 Gy divided in three fractions. Patients with central tumors, as described above, were excluded. The 3-year local control was 98%. The 3-year overall survival was 56%. There were only two Grade 4 toxicities with no treatment-related deaths.

Based on these prospective results, as well as other retrospective data, SBRT is a reasonable approach for peripheral, medically inoperable non-small cell lung cancer. Ongoing studies are further characterizing the optimal treatment schedule.

Liver Tumors

SBRT represents a potential treatment modality for the management of hepatic metastases. Historically, radiotherapy for unresectable liver tumors has been limited by the risk of radiation-induced liver disease (RILD). RILD is a clinical diagnosis that occurs within 3 months of liver radiation characterized by anicteric ascites with elevated liver function tests (LFTs) with alkaline phosphatase elevated out of proportion to transaminases. However, a strong relationship between the volume of liver irradiated and the risk of RILD spurred investigators to explore the feasibility SBRT for liver tumors.

Two large prospective multi-institutional series were published in 2009. The first study by Rustohoven and colleagues [7] evaluated 47 patients with 63 lesions in a phase I/II study of SBRT. Eligibility was restricted to up to three lesions with maximal size of 6 cm. In the phase I portion, dose was escalated from 36 Gy (12 Gy/fraction) to 60 Gy (20 Gy/fraction). In the phase II portion, patients received a dose of 60 Gy. Sixty nine percent of patients had at least one prior systemic regimen. Radiation therapy was delivered with SBRT techniques in three fractions. In total, 45% of patients had extrahepatic disease at the time of study entry. The median tumor size was 2.7 cm (0.4–5.8 cm). Local control in lesions £3 cm in size was 100%, with a median survival of 20.5 months. There was only one Grade 3 toxicity noted of soft tissue breakdown in a patient whose chest wall received 48 Gy (16 Gy/fraction). There were no episodes of RILD.

Since frequently unresectable tumors are larger in size, in the second study, Lee and colleagues placed no size limit on tumor size but instead utilized an individualized approach [8]. In this multi-institutional phase I study, patients with up to four lesions (no size limit) were included. An individualized dose escalation was performed that took into account the differing volumes of normal liver irradiated given the heterogeneity in tumor size. Using the previously validated RILD risk model developed at the University of Michigan, three "isotoxic" risk groups were identified based on "effective volume" (Veff). Veff is a radiobiological model by which the heterogenous dose distribution of an organ is expressed as what fractional volume of the organ receiving the prescription dose produces the same biological effect. The three risk strata were low Veff <0.22, mid Veff 0.22–0.51, and high Veff >0.51. For the low-risk Veff stratum, the dose was escalated from 54 to 57 Gy to 60 Gy in six fractions over 2 weeks as the RILD risk was estimated to below 5%. For the mid- and high-risk Veff stratum, the dose was escalated based on an increasing normal tissue complication probability (NTCP) for RILD of 5, 10, and 20%. Patients were planned for six fractions. At the highest dose level (20% risk), the median dose/fraction was 8 Gy for the mid-risk Veff stratum and 6 Gy for the high-risk Veff stratum. In total 68 patients were treated: 13 patients in the low-risk stratum, 25 in the mid-risk, and 20 patients in the high-risk stratum. Median gross tumor volume (GTV) size was 75.2 cm^3 (range, 27.7 to 3,090 cm^3). Only one patient experienced a Grade 3 toxicity (2%). The most common side effect was fatigue (Grade 2 18%), followed by gastritis (Grade 2 4%). Subacute liver pain occurred in six patients. There were no incidents of RILD. Local control at 1 year was 71%, and median overall survival was 17.6 months.

Based on these two studies, SBRT for liver tumors may be a viable option for unresectable metastases. However, while these prospective, multi-institutional studies are compelling, the concept requires further validation. Specifically, the second study of individualized SBRT is particularly interesting as it more closely reflects the clinical reality that unresectable lesions are often larger in size with fewer competing options than the lesions described in earlier studies of liver SBRT.

Pancreatic Tumors

There has been significant interest in the use of SBRT in the management of locally advanced pancreatic cancer. Early reports suggested modest median survival with high rates of duodenal toxicity [9]. A more recent retrospective from Beth Israel Deaconess in Boston evaluated 36 patients treated with sequential gemcitabine chemotherapy and SBRT with CyberKnife [10]. With a median follow up of 24 months, the median overall survival was 14.3 months. The treatment was well-tolerated, with a 14% Grade 3 toxicity rate. Figure 2.2 shows a CyberKnife pancreas treatment plan.

One reason for the modest results with SBRT is the difficulty in visualizing the target accurately. In a study by Arvold and colleagues, 97 consecutive resected patients who underwent preoperative pancreas protocol CT were evaluated for correlation between CT size and pathologic size of the tumor [11]. Tumors were found to be larger on pathology by a median of 7 mm but up to 43 mm larger. Additionally, 79% of patients had nodal involvement not seen and 72% of patients had invasion into the duodenum, which is an avoidance structure for SBRT. Thus, the modest results may be the result of inadequate coverage of the entire tumor volume. This highlights an important consideration of SBRT – the targeting is only as reliable as the imaging.

Spinal Tumors

The spine is one of the most common sites of metastases for cancer. However, the limited tolerance of the spinal cord to radiation therapy limits the ability to give a high enough dose of radiation required for durable tumor control. Additionally, as progression happens, retreatment options are frequently limited. For this reason, SBRT is an attractive approach for tumors of the vertebral bodies.

There is limited prospective data on the use of SBRT for spinal metastases. In a phase I/II study from MD Anderson, 63 patients with 74 spinal metastases were treated with SBRT to either 30 Gy in five fractions or 27 Gy in three fractions.

Fig. 2.2 CyberKnife
(Accuray, Sunnyvale, CA)
plan for a patient with locally
advanced pancreatic cancer

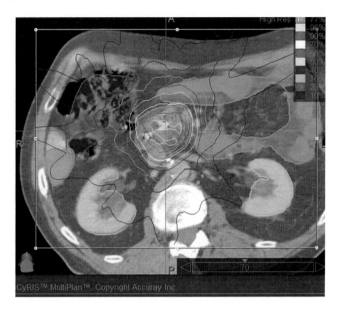

Out of 63, 35 patients had prior radiation in the sites of interest. No patient developed Grade 3 or higher toxicity. The 1-year freedom-from-radiographic progression was 84% [12]. Another phase II study from the University of Florida reported on 21 patients with 25 lesions in which 43% of patients had pain relief, and the crude local control was 96% [13].

Because of the limited data, SBRT for spine metastases is still investigational. Its greatest utility may be in the setting progression after prior radiation therapy.

Proton Beam Therapy

There has been an unprecedented interest in proton beam therapy. The basis for the advantages of proton beams lies in the physical laws that determine the absorption of energy in tissues exposed to photon or proton beams. In a specific tissue, photons are absorbed exponentially, whereas protons have a finite range dependent upon the initial proton energy. Therefore, the depth dose characteristics of the two beams are qualitatively different. Protons lose their energy in tissue mostly by coulombic interactions with electrons in the constituent atoms; however, a small fraction of energy is transferred through nuclear collisions. The energy loss per unit path length is relatively small and constant as the proton traverses the tissue until near the end of the proton range where the residual energy is lost over a short distance (approximately 0.7 cm in width at 80% of the maximum dose) and the proton comes to rest, resulting in a distinctive sharp rise in the tissue absorbed dose (energy absorbed per unit mass) – known as the Bragg peak. In physical terms, the magnitude of the transfer of energy to tissue per unit path length traversed by the protons is inversely proportional to the square of the proton velocity. The low-dose region between the entrance and the Bragg peak is called the plateau of the dose distribution, and the dose there is 30–40% of the maximum dose.

These physical characteristics lead to a lack of "exit dose." Where standard high-energy photons penetrate through the entire body, protons can stop at a depth chosen by the physician. Hence, the overall all normal tissue exposure is 30–60% less. This technology affords the opportunity for higher doses, and theoretically greater tumor control, with fewer side effects.

One flaw of proton beam therapy is the significant cost of a proton facility. A cyclotron or synchrotron, which can deliver beam to two to five rooms, is approximately 50 times the cost of a single linear accelerator. Thus, it is cost-prohibitive for most medical centers to use proton beam therapy.

Proton beam therapy has primarily been studied in intracranial/base of skull tumors and in pediatrics due to the greater importance on protecting normal tissues as well as the relatively small number of cases per year. For these patients, standard radiation schedules of 6–8 weeks are used. However, there has been growing interests in using protons for nonsurgical, potentially curative indications. Primary liver tumors (hepatocellular carcinoma and intrahepatic cholangiocarcinoma) represent one such indication, which is discussed below.

Primary Hepatoma

Many patients with primary hepatobiliary cancer are not surgical candidates due to anatomic location or size of the tumor, concurrent cirrhosis, or medical inoperability. Therefore, an important role exists for a treatment that can provide the equivalent of tumor excision, but with minimal morbidity.

The treatment of unresectable hepatocellular or locally recurrent hepatocellular cancer and cholangiocarcinoma has been palliative. Standard treatment modalities have included transarterial chemoarterial embolization (TACE), radiofrequency ablation, or systemic chemotherapy/targeted therapy with few long-term survivors. TACE is useful in patients with multiple lesions, but is not considered an ablative approach. Similarly, systemic therapy does not produce more than anecdotal complete responses.

Radiofrequency ablation (RFA) is the most commonly employed ablative technique for nonsurgical candidates at many institutions. However, the use of RFA can be limited by location. An adjacent large vessel can act as a heat sink and limit the efficacy of therapy. Treatment of dome lesions near the diaphragm carries the risk of diaphragmatic perforation, and treatment of deep lesions near bowel loops may be associated with bowel perforation. Radiofrequency ablation can be highly effective for small lesions, with local control of 75% or greater. However, this local control falls off steeply beyond 3–5 cm in maximum diameter.

Because of the limited tolerance of the liver to external beam irradiation when the whole liver is irradiated, experience with radiation has been limited. However, several studies have demonstrated that the tolerance of liver significantly increases when smaller volumes of the liver are irradiated. A study from the University of Michigan reported the results of 22 patients with unresectable hepatocellular carcinoma and cholangiocarcinoma treated by high-dose irradiation employing conformal 3D techniques using 10 MV X-rays and hepatic artery fluorodeoxyuridine. These patients were observed to have a 4-year survival of 20% and no late hepatic toxicity [14]. Total radiation doses were determined by the fraction of normal liver treated to 50% of the isocenter dose. If 33% of the normal liver received 50% of the dose, the patient was treated to 66 Gy; if 33 to 66% of the liver received 50% of the dose, the patient received 48 Gy; and if 66% of the liver received 50% of the dose, the patient received 36 Gy. Treatment was given daily at 1.8 Gy per fraction 5 days per week. The tumor response exhibits strong dose-dependence with the response rate for tumor doses above 60 Gy twice as high as for tumor doses below 50 Gy [15–17]. Similarly encouraging results of dose escalations studies using three-dimensional conformal radiotherapy have recently been reported by groups from Korea (183 patients) and Taiwan (93 patients) [18, 19]. These studies demonstrated that the overall median survival could also be significantly improved with higher doses. The chief cause of mortality was progression of underlying severe cirrhosis and not tumor or treatment-related causes.

With the lack of exit dose and greater potential for liver sparing, protons are a natural fit for primary liver tumors, especially in light of the underlying cirrhosis (Fig. 2.3). The use of protons for liver tumors has been extensively studied in Asia. Chiba and colleagues reported 162 patients with hepatocellular carcinoma (HCC) treated with proton radiotherapy. All treatments were delivered using hypo-fractionated regimens (3.5–5 Gy), and total doses ranged between 50 Gy (10 fractions) and 84 Gy (24 fractions) [20]. A total of 192 lesions were treated. Median tumor size was 3.8 cm (1.5–14.5 cm). The median dose was 72 cobalt gray equivalent (CGE) in 16 fractions. At a median follow-up interval of 31.7 months (range 3.1–133.2 months), the 5-year local control rate was 86.9% and corresponding overall survival rate was 23.5%. Survival appeared to be impacted by the level of liver dysfunction with over 50% dying without tumor progression (usually complications of liver cirrhosis). The acute side effects were limited primarily to elevation in liver enzymes (9.7%) and only five patients had Grade 2 or higher late toxicity. Among a subset of 50 patients with solitary tumors and Child Class A cirrhosis, the observed 5-year survival rate of 53.5% rivals similar to that of surgery. Similarly favorable outcomes have been observed in patients with unfavorable features and limited treatment options [21–25]. In particular, one study of 22 patients with HCC larger than 10 cm in size (median 11 cm, range 10–14 cm) treated with proton beam showed a 2-year local control of 87% with no acute or late Grade 3 toxicity [25].

Patients with portal venous thrombosis might benefit especially from proton radiotherapy, because they tend to have larger tumors and many, if not most, of these patients have few viable ablative treatment options. However, because of the size, extent, and location of the disease, conventional photon radiotherapy at higher doses may not be feasible. In a series of 35 of these patients, Sugahara and colleagues found that treatment to 50–72 CGE led to local control rates of 45% at 2 years, but with only three patients developing severe acute toxicity [26]. As noted previously, the excellent conformality of proton radiotherapy offers the possibility of retreatment if new HCCs arise within the liver further away from the originally treated HCC. The Tsukuba proton radiotherapy group has reported on the safety, feasibility, and efficacy of repeated courses of proton radiotherapy in a series of 27 patients with 68 lesions [27]. With a median interval of 24 months between the first and second courses, and a median dose of 66 CGE in 16 fractions for the retreatment, they reported a 5-year overall survival of 56% and a 5-year local control rate of 87.8%.

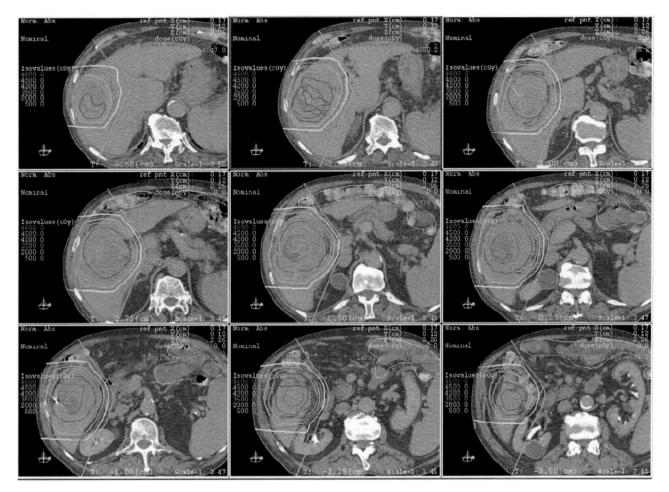

Fig. 2.3 Proton plan for a liver tumor. In contrast to the photon plans of Figs. 2.1 and 2.2, note the lack of radiation beyond the entry paths of the beam

Similarly, in a phase II trial, Kawashima and colleagues reported overall survival rates of 66% in cirrhotic patients after proton radiotherapy to 76 CGE in 3.8 CGE daily fractions [28]. In this study, 20% of patients developed hepatic insufficiency, with a rate of Grade 3 toxicity of about 40%.

Data regarding outcomes and toxicity with the use of protons in populations where hepatitis B vaccine (HBV) is nonendemic is much more limited. In a phase II trial of proton radiotherapy for HCC, Bush and colleagues treated 34 cases of unresectable HCC to 63 CGE in 15 fractions [29]. In this study, the 2-year overall survival was 55%, with local control rates of 75%. No RILD was seen in this study; however, 60% of patients were noted to have mild acute toxicity due to radiotherapy. Furthermore, less than 10% of these patients experienced a gastrointestinal bleed, which was due, in large part, to the proximity of gross disease to the colon or duodenum. Finally, of these patients, six went to liver transplant and of these two patients had a complete response after pathological review.

In summary, proton beam therapy may have a role in treating patients with underlying hepatic dysfunction, large tumors, and portal vein thrombosis not amenable to other ablative therapies. Further investigations are ongoing.

Summary

Advanced radiation techniques such as IMRT, SBRT, and proton therapy have the potential to expand the range of ablative options for the cancer patients. These modalities are complementary to the arsenal of tools available to the interventional radiologist.

References

1. Morris DE, Emami B, Mauch PM, et al. Evidence-based review of three-dimensional conformal radiotherapy for localized prostate cancer: an ASTRO outcomes initiative. Int J Radiat Oncol Biol Phys. 2005;62:3–19.

2. Donovan E, Bleakley N, Denholm E, et al. Randomised trial of standard 2D radiotherapy (RT) versus intensity modulated radiotherapy (IMRT) in patients prescribed breast radiotherapy. Radiother Oncol. 2007;82:254–64.

3. Nuttin C, A'Hern R, Rogers MS, et al. First results of a phase III multi-center randomized controlled trial of intensity modulated (IMRT) versus conventional radiotherapy (RT) in head and neck cancer (PARSPORT: ISRCTN48243537;vCRUK/03/005). J Clin Oncol. 2009;27:18s.

4. Potters L, Kavanagh B, Galvin JM, et al. American Society for Therapeutic Radiology and Oncology (ASTRO) and American College of Radiology (ACR) practice guideline for the performance of stereotactic body radiation therapy. Int J Radiat Oncol Biol Phys. 2010;76:326–32.

5. Timmerman R, McGarry R, Yiannoutsos C, et al. Excessive toxicity when treating central tumors in a phase II study of stereotactic body radiation therapy for medically inoperable early-stage lung cancer. J Clin Oncol. 2006;24:4833–9.

6. Timmerman R, Paulus R, Galvin J, et al. Stereotactic body radiation therapy for inoperable early stage lung cancer. JAMA. 2010;303:1070–6.

7. Rusthoven KE, Kavanagh BD, Cardenes H, et al. Multi-institutional phase I/II trial of stereotactic body radiation therapy for liver metastases. J Clin Oncol. 2009;27:1572–8.

8. Lee MT, Kim JJ, Diniwell R. Phase I study of individualized stereotactic body radiotherapy of liver metastases. J Clin Oncol. 2009;27:1585–91.

9. Koong AC, Le QT, Ho A, et al. Phase I study of stereotactic radiosurgery in patients with locally advanced pancreatic cancer. Int J Radiat Oncol Biol Phys. 2004;58:1017–21.

10. Mahadevan A, Jain S, Goldstein M, et al. Stereotactic body radiotherapy and gemcitabine for locally advanced pancreatic cancer. Int J Radiat Oncol Biol Phys. 2010;78(3):735–42. Epub 2010 Feb 18.

11. Arvold ND, Niemierko A, Mamon HJ, et al. Pancreatic cancer tumor size on CT scan versus pathologic specimen: implications for radiation treatment planning. Int J Radiat Oncol Biol Phys. 2011;80(5):1383–90. doi:10.1016/j.ijrobp.2010.04.058.

12. Chang EL, Shiu AS, Mendel E, et al. Phase I/II study of stereotactic body radiotherapy for spinal metastasis and its pattern of failure. J Neurosurg Spine. 2007;7:151–60.

13. Amdur RJ, Bennett J, Olivier K, et al. A prospective, phase II study demonstrating the potential value and limitation of radiosurgery for spine metastases. Am J Clin Oncol. 2009;32(5):515–20. doi:10.1097/COC.0b013e318194f70f.

14. Dawson LA, McGinn CJ, Normolle D, et al. Escalated focal liver radiation and concurrent hepatic artery flurodeoxyuridine for unresectable intrahepatic malignancies. J Clin Oncol. 2000;8:2210–8.

15. Dawson LA, Normolle D, Balter JM, et al. Analysis of radiation-induced liver disease using the Lyman NTCP model. Int J Radiat Oncol Biol Phys. 2002;53(4):810–21.

16. Dawson LA, Ten Haken RK, Lawrence TS. Partial irradiation of the liver. Semin Radiat Oncol. 2001;11:240–6.

17. McGinn CJ, Ten Haken RK, Ensminger WD, et al. Treatment of intrahepatic cancers with radiation doses based on a normal tissue complication probability model. J Clin Oncol. 1998;16:2246–52.

18. Park HC, Seong J, Han KH, et al. Dose-response relationship in local radiotherapy for hepatocellular carcinoma. Int J Radiat Oncol Biol Phys. 2002;54:150–5.

19. Cheng J. Radiation-induced liver disease after three-dimensional conformal radiotherapy for patients with hepatocellular carcinoma: dosimetric analysis and implication. Int J Radiat Oncol Biol Phys. 2002;54:156–62.

20. Chiba T, Tokuuye K, Matsuzaki Y, et al. Proton beam therapy for hepatocellular carcinoma: a retrospective review of 162 patients. Clin Cancer Res. 2005;11:3799–805.

21. Hata M, Tokuuye K, Sugahara S, et al. Proton beam therapy for hepatocellular carcinoma with limited treatment options. Cancer. 2006;107:591–8.

22. Hata M, Tokuuye K, Sugahara S, et al. Proton beam therapy for hepatocellular carcinoma with portal vein tumor thrombus. Cancer. 2005;104:794–801.

23. Hata M, Tokuuye K, Sugahara S, et al. Proton beam therapy for aged patients with hepatocellular carcinoma. Int J Radiat Oncol Biol Phys. 2007;69:805–12.

24. Mizumoto M, Tokuuye K, Sugahara S, et al. Proton beam therapy for hepatocellular carcinoma adjacent to the porta hepatis. Int J Radiat Oncol Biol Phys. 2008;71:462–7.

25. Sugahara S, Oshiro Y, Nakayama H, et al. Proton beam therapy for large hepatocellular carcinoma. Int J Radiat Oncol Biol Phys. 2010;76:460–6.

26. Sugahara D, Nakayama H, Fukuda K, et al. Proton-beam therapy for hepatocellular carcinoma associated with portal vein tumor thrombosis. Strahlenther Onkol. 2009;185:782–8.

27. Hashimoto T, Tokuuye K, Fukumitsu N, et al. Repeated proton beam therapy for hepatocellular carcinoma. Int J Radiat Oncol Biol Phys. 2006;65:196–202.

28. Kawashima M, Furuse J, Nishio T, et al. Phase II study of radiotherapy employing proton beam for hepatocellular carcinoma. J Clin Oncol. 2005;23:1839–46.

29. Bush DA, Hillebrand DJ, Slater JM, Slater JD. High-dose proton beam radiotherapy of hepatocellular carcinoma: preliminary results of a phase II trial. Gastroenterology. 2004;127:S189–93.

Chapter 3
Principles of Radiofrequency Ablation

Muneeb Ahmed and Shraga Nahum Goldberg

Introduction

As multiple subsequent chapters attest, radiofrequency (RF) ablation has become an accepted treatment option for focal primary and secondary malignancies in a wide range of organs including the liver, lung, kidney, bone, and adrenal glands [1–7]. The largest clinical experience has been for hepatic malignancies, where long-term outcomes similar to surgical resection have been reported in some matched patient populations [8]. Benefits of minimally invasive, image-guided RF ablation include reduced cost and morbidity compared to standard surgical resection, and the ability to treat patients who are not surgical candidates. However, limitations in ablative efficacy exist, including persistent growth of residual tumor at the ablation margin, the inability to effectively treat larger tumors, and variability in complete treatment based upon tumor location. Extensive investigation into potential strategies to improve ablation outcomes continues and focuses on technological development of ablative systems, improving ablative predictability and combining RF ablation with additional therapies such as chemotherapy and radiation. Given the potential complexity of treatment types and paradigms in oncology and the wider application of thermal ablation techniques, a thorough understanding of the basic principles and recent advances in thermal ablation is a necessary prerequisite for their effective clinical use.

Goals of Minimally Invasive Thermal Tumor Ablation

The overall goal of minimally invasive thermal tumor ablation for focal malignancies encompasses several specific objectives, regardless of the specific thermal ablative device that is used.

1. *Complete eradication of the primary tumor.* The primary purpose of treatment is to completely eradicate all viable malignant cells within the target tumor. Based upon tumor recurrence patterns in long-term studies in patients who have undergone surgical resection, and more recently, ablation, along with studies that have performed pathologic analysis of resection margins, there is often viable persistent microscopic tumor foci in a rim of apparently normal surrounding parenchymal tissue beyond the visible tumor margin. Therefore, tumor ablation therapies also attempt to include a 5–10 mm "ablative" margin of normal surrounding tissue in the target zone, though the required thickness of this margin is variable based upon the tumor and organ type [9, 10].
2. *Current need for multiple overlapping ablations.* Given that appropriate and complete tumor destruction only occurs when the entire target tumor is exposed to appropriate temperatures, and therefore determined by the pattern of tissue heating in the target tumor, for larger tumors (usually defined to be larger than 3–5 cm in diameter), a single ablation treatment may not be sufficient to entirely encompass the target volume [3]. Thus, an additional consideration is that multiple overlapping ablations or simultaneous use of multiple applicators may be required to successfully treat the

M. Ahmed (✉)
Section of Interventional Radiology, Beth Israel Deaconess Medical Center, Harvard Medical School, Boston, MA, USA
e-mail: mahmed@bidmc.harvard.edu

S.N. Goldberg
Department of Radiology, Hebrew University-Hadassah Medical Center, Jerusalem, Israel

Department of Radiology, Beth Israel Deaconess Medical Center, Harvard Medical School, Boston, MA, USA

P.R. Mueller and A. Adam (eds.), *Interventional Oncology: A Practical Guide for the Interventional Radiologist*,
DOI 10.1007/978-1-4419-1469-9_3, © Springer Science+Business Media, LLC 2012

entire tumor and achieve an ablative margin, though accurate targeting and probe placement can often be technically challenging [11]. Finally, growth patterns of the tumor itself can influence overall treatment outcomes, with slow growing tumors more amenable to multiple treatment sessions over longer periods of time. These principles are applicable to a wide range of ablative technologies, including both thermal and nonthermal strategies.

3. *Specificity and accuracy.* Additionally, while complete treatment of the target tumor is of primary importance, specificity and accuracy is also highly preferred, with a secondary goal of incurring as little injury as possible to surrounding nontarget normal tissue. This ability to minimize damage to normal organ parenchyma is one of the significant advantages of minimally invasive percutaneous thermal ablation and can be critical in patients who have focal tumors in the setting of limited functional organ reserve. Examples of clinical situations where this is relevant include focal hepatic tumors in patients with underlying cirrhosis and limited hepatic reserve, patients with Von Hippel Lindau syndrome who have limited renal function and required treatment of multiple renal tumors, and patients with primary lung tumors with extensive underlying emphysema and limited lung function [12–14]. Many of these patients are not surgical candidates due to limited native organ functional reserve placing them at a higher risk for postoperative complications or organ failure.

Principles of Tissue Heating in RF Ablation

1. *Mechanisms of tissue heating.* RF ablation induces irreversible cellular injury from focal high-temperature tissue heating that is generated around an RF electrode. Tissue heating occurs though two specific mechanisms.

   (a) *Energy–tissue interactions.* First, an electrode placed within the center of the target tumor delivers energy that interacts with tissue to generate focal heat immediately around it. As RF current travels from the electrode applicator to the remote grounding pad, local tissue resistance to current flow results in ion agitation and heat generation.

   (b) *Thermal conduction.* The second mechanism of tissue heating in RF ablation relies upon thermal tissue conduction [15]. Heat generated around the electrode diffuses through the tumor and results in additional high-temperature heating that is separate from the direct energy–issue interactions that occur around the electrode. The contribution of thermal conduction to overall tissue ablation is determined by several factors. Tissue heating patterns vary based upon the tumor and tissue characteristics that may affect thermal conduction. As an example, primary hepatic tumors (hepatocellular carcinoma) transmit heat better than the surrounding cirrhotic hepatic parenchyma [3, 16], and surrounding tissues such as bone can function as a thermal insulator [17].

2. *Pathophysiology of tumor and tissue heating.* The endpoint of RF ablation is adequate tissue heating so as to induce coagulation throughout the defined target area.

   (a) *Temperature thresholds.* Relatively mild increases in tissue temperature above baseline (40°C) can be tolerated by normal cellular homeostatic mechanisms. Low-temperature hyperthermia (42–45°C) results in reversible cellular injury, though this can increase cellular susceptibility to additional adjuvant therapies such as chemotherapy and radiation [18, 19]. Irreversible cellular injury occurs when cells are heated to 46°C for 60 min and occurs more rapidly as the temperature rises, so that most cell types die in a few minutes when heated at 50°C [20] (Fig. 3.1). Therefore, optimal temperatures for ablation range likely exceed 50°C. On the other end of the temperature spectrum, tissue vaporization occurs at temperatures >110°C, which in turn, limits further current deposition in RF-based systems (as compared to, for example, microwave systems that do not have this limitation).

   (b) *Pathologic changes.* Immediate cellular damage centers on protein coagulation of cytosolic and mitochondrial enzymes, and nucleic acid–histone protein complexes, which triggers cellular death over the course of several days [21]. "Heat fixation" or "coagulation necrosis" is used to describe this thermal damage, even though ultimate manifestations of cell death may not fulfill strict histopathologic criteria of coagulative necrosis [22]. This has implications with regard to clinical practice, as percutaneous biopsy and standard histopathologic interpretation may not be a reliable measure of adequate ablation [22].

   (c) *Thermal dosimetry.* The exact temperature at which cell death occurs is multifactorial and tissue-specific. Based upon prior studies demonstrating that tissue coagulation can be induced by focal tissue heating to 50°C for 4–6 min [23], this has become the standard surrogate endpoint for thermal ablation therapies in both experimental studies and in current clinical paradigms. However, studies have shown that depending on heating time, the rate of heat increase, and the tissue being heated, maximum temperatures at the edge of ablation are variable. For example, maximum temperatures at the edge of ablation zone, known as the "critical temperature," have been shown to range from 30 to 77°C for normal tissues and from 41 to 64°C for tumor models (a 23°C difference) [24, 25]. Likewise, the total amount of heat administered for a given time, known as the thermal dose, varies significantly between different

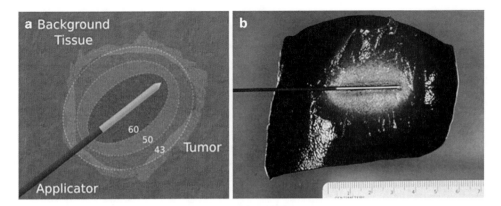

Fig. 3.1 Schematic (**a**) and pictorial (**b**) representation of focal thermal ablation therapy. Electrode applicators are positioned either with image guidance or direct visualization within the target tumor, and thermal energy is applied via the electrode. This creates a central zone of high temperatures in the tissue immediately around the electrode (they can exceed 100°C), and surrounded by more peripheral zones of sublethal tissue heating (<50°C) and background liver parenchyma (Reprinted with permission from Ahmed M, Brace CL, Lee FT, Jr, Goldberg SN. Principles of and advances in percutaneous ablation. *Radiology* 2011;258(2):351–369. Copyright the Radiological Society of North America.)

tissues [24, 25]. Thus, the threshold target temperature of 50°C should be used only as a general guideline, and indeed, one RF manufacturer uses 70°C as a more conservative endpoint for its heating algorithm (see below).

3. *Applying the principles of the Bioheat equation to achieve meaningful volumes of tumor ablation.* The ability to heat large volumes of tissue in different environments is dependent on several factors encompassing both energy delivery and local physiological tissue characteristics. The relationship between this set of parameters, as described by the Bioheat equation [26], can be simplified to describe the basic relationship guiding thermal ablation induced coagulation necrosis as: "coagulation necrosis = (energy deposited × local tissue interactions) – heat loss" [27]. Local tissues interactions include tissue perfusion, and tissue electrical and thermal conductivity, which will be discussed in greater detail in later sections.

4. *Strategies to improve RF ablation outcomes.* Based on the above relationship, several strategies to increase the ability to ablate larger tumors have been concurrently pursued. These encompass (1) technological developments, including modification of energy input algorithms and electrode design to deposit more energy into the tissue, (2) improved understanding and subsequent modification of the biophysiologic environment to increase tissue heating, and (3) incorporation of adjuvant therapies to increase uniformity of tumor cellular injury in the ablation zone, along with increasing cellular destruction in the nonlethal hyperthermic zone around the ablation.

Technologic Advancements

Technologic efforts to increase ablation size (above 1.8 cm in coagulation achievable with a single monopolar electrode [28]) have focused on modifying energy deposition algorithms and electrode designs to increase both the amount of tissue exposed to the active electrode and the overall amount of energy that can be safely deposited into the target tissue.

1. *Electrode modification.* Development of RF electrodes has contributed significantly to the ability to reliably achieve larger ablation zones. Several strategies to increase the amount of energy deposition and the overall ablation size have been balanced with the need for smaller caliber electrodes to permit the continued use of these devices in a percutaneous and minimally invasive manner.

   (a) *Multiple electrodes.* Originally, simply lengthening the electrode tip increased coagulation in an asymmetric and preferentially longitudinal geometry. Use of a single electrode inserted multiple times to perform overlapping ablations requires significantly greater time and effort, making it impractical for routine use in a clinical setting. Therefore, the use of multiple electrodes simultaneously either in a preset configuration represents a significant step forward in increasing overall ablation size. Initial work with multiple electrodes demonstrated that placement of several monopolar electrodes in a clustered arrangement (no more than 1.5 cm apart) with simultaneous RF application could increase coagulation volume by over 800% compared to a single electrode [29]. Subsequently, working to overcome the technical challenges of multiprobe application, multitined expandable RF electrodes have been developed [30]. These systems involve the deployment of a varying number of multiple thin, curved tines in the shape of an umbrella or more complex geometries from a central cannula [31, 32]. This surmounts earlier difficulties by allowing easy placement of multiple probes to create large, reproducible volumes of necrosis. Leveen, using a 12-hook array, was able to produce coagulation measuring up to 3.5 cm in diameter in in vivo porcine liver by administering increasing amounts of RF energy from a 50 W RF generator for 10 min [33]. More recently, Applebaum et al. were able to achieve >5 cm of coagulation in in vivo porcine liver using currently commercially available expandable electrodes with optimized stepped-extension and power-input algorithms [34].

(b) *Bipolar electrodes.* While the majority of conventional RF systems use monopolar electrodes (where the current runs to remotely placed grounding pads placed on the patient's thighs to complete the circuit), several studies have reported results using bipolar arrays to increase the volume of coagulation created by RF application. In these systems, applied RF current runs from an active electrode to a second grounding electrode in place of a grounding pad. Heat is generated around both electrodes, creating elliptical lesions. McGahan et al. used this method in ex vivo liver to induce necrosis of up to 4.0 cm in the long axis diameter, but could only achieve 1.4 cm of necrosis in the short diameter [35]. Though this increases the overall size of coagulation volume, the shape of necrosis is unsuitable for actual tumors, making the gains in coagulation less clinically significant. Desinger et al. have described another bipolar array that contains both the active and the return electrodes on the same 2-mm diameter probe [36]. Lee et al. used two multitined electrodes as active and return to increase coagulation during bipolar RF ablation [37]. Finally, several studies have used a multipolar (more than two) array of electrodes (multitined and single internally cooled) during RF ablation to achieve even greater volumes of coagulation [38, 39].

(c) *Electrode cooling.* One of the limitations for RF-based systems has been overheating surrounding the active electrode leading to tissue charring, rising impedance, RF circuit interruption, and ultimately limiting overall RF energy deposition. One successful strategy to address this has been the use of internal electrode cooling, where electrodes contain two hollow lumens that permit continuous internal cooling of the tip with a chilled perfusate, and the removal of warmed effluent to a collection unit outside of the body [40]. This reduces heating directly around the electrode, tissue charring, and rising impedance, allows greater RF energy deposition, and shifts the peak tissue temperature farther into the tumor, contributing to a broader depth of tissue heating from thermal conduction. In initial studies using cooling of 18 gauge single or clustered electrode needles using chilled 0°C saline perfusate, significant increases in RF energy deposition and ablation zone size were observed compared to conventional monopolar uncooled electrodes in ex vivo liver, with findings subsequently confirmed in in vivo large animal models and clinical studies [40, 41]. Similar results were observed when chilled saline was infused in combination with expandable electrode systems (referred to as an "internally cooled wet electrode"), though infusion of fluid around the electrode is more difficult to control and makes the reproducibility of results more variable [42]. Most recently, several investigators have used alternative cooling agents (e.g., argon or nitrogen gas) to achieve even greater cooling, and therefore larger zones of ablation, around the RF electrode tip [43]. As for RF-based systems, cooling of antennae shaft for microwave applicators have also been developed and reduce shaft heating (and associated complications such as skin burns) while allowing increased power deposition through smaller caliber antennae.

2. *Refinement of energy application algorithms.* The algorithm by which energy is applied during thermal ablation is dependent on the energy source, device, and type of electrode that is being used. While initial power algorithms for RF-based systems were based upon a continuous and constant high-energy input, tissue overheating and vaporization ultimately interferes with continued energy input due to high impedance to current flow from gas formation. Therefore, several strategies to maximize energy deposition have been developed and, in some cases, incorporated into commercially available devices.

(a) *Energy pulsing.* Applying high levels of energy in a pulsed manner, separated by periods of lower energy, is one such strategy that has been used with RF-based systems to increase the mean intensity of energy deposition [44]. If a proper balance between high- and low-energy deposition is achieved, preferential tissue cooling occurs adjacent to the electrode during periods of minimal energy deposition without significantly decreasing heating of deeper tissues. Thus, even greater energy can be applied during periods of high-energy deposition, thereby enabling deeper heat penetration and greater tissue coagulation [41]. Synergy between a combination of both internal cooling of the electrode and pulsing has resulted in even greater coagulation necrosis and tumor destruction than either method alone [41]. Pulsed-energy techniques have also been successfully used for microwave and laser-based systems.

(b) *Gradual "ramp-up".* Another strategy is to slowly increase (or ramp-up) the RF energy application in a continuous manner, until the impedance to RF current flow increases prohibitively [45]. This approach is often paired with multitined expandable electrodes, which have a greater contact surface area with tissue, and in which the goal is to achieve smaller ablation zones around multiple small electrode tines and more recently with internally cooled electrodes [46]. This algorithm is also often combined with a staged expansion of the electrode system such that each small ablation occurs in a slightly different location within the tumor (with the overall goal of ablating the entire target region).

(c) *Stepped-deployment.* In using expandable electrodes, tine extension in short steps with intermittent ablation (stepped-deployment) can increase achievable ablation beyond what is observed with a single-step complete tine extension algorithm from the beginning of the ablation. For example, Appelbaum et al. recently demonstrated that larger zones of coagulation (5–7 cm in diameter) can be achieved with an optimized stepped-deployment algorithm [34].

(d) *Electrode switching.* "Electrode switching" is an additional technique that is incorporated into pulsing algorithms to further increase RF tissue heating [47]. In this, multiple independently placed RF electrodes are connected to a single RF generator, and RF current is applied to a single electrode until an impedance spike is detected at which point current application is applied to the next electrode and so forth. Several studies have demonstrated significant increases in ablation zone size and a reduction in application time using this technique [47, 48]. For example, Brace et al. also show larger and more circular ablation zones with the switching application with more rapid heating being 74% faster than the sequential heating (12 vs. 46 min) [47].

(e) *High-powered RF generators.* Continued device development has also led to increases in the overall maximum amount of power that can be delivered [49, 50]. For RF-based devices, the maximum amount of RF current that can be delivered is dependent on both the generator output and the electrode surface area, as higher surface areas reduce the current density and, therefore, adequate tissue heating around the electrode cannot be achieved. While initial systems had maximum power outputs of less than 200 W, subsequent investigation suggests that higher current output and larger ablation zones can be achieved if higher-powered generators are coupled with larger-surface area electrodes. For example, Solazzo et al. used a 500-kHz (1,000 W) high-powered generator in an in vivo porcine model and achieved larger coagulation zones with a 4-cm tip cluster electrode (5.2 ± 0.8 cm) compared to a 2.5-cm cluster electrode (3.9 ± 0.3 cm) [50]. Similar gains in ablation size have been seen in higher-powered versions of microwave-based systems [51].

While many of these technological advances have been developed independently of each other, they may often be used concurrently to achieve even larger ablation zones. Furthermore, while much of this work has been based upon RF technology, specific techniques can be used for other thermal ablative therapies. For example, multiple electrodes and applicator cooling have been effectively applied in microwave-based systems, as well [52, 53].

Practical Application of Technologic Developments: Commercially Available RF Devices

Several different commercially available RF devices are commonly used and vary based on their power application algorithms and electrode designs.

1. *Selecting an RF ablation system.*

   (a) *Is one system better than another?* Zones of adequate thermal ablation can be achieved with most commercially available RF ablation devices when properly used as described in the instructions for use. Though the specific size of the ablation zone and the time required to achieve adequate ablation will likely vary between different manufacturers and devices, a recent study by Lin et al. compared four separate and commonly used devices in over 100 patients with primary and secondary hepatic tumors, and found little difference in ablation time and local tumor progression [54]. Thus, it is important for operators to be completely familiar with their device of choice, including electrode shapes and deployment techniques, power-input algorithms, and common troubleshooting issues, so as to permit thorough treatment planning and maximize optimal clinical outcomes. Ultimately, good operator technique and careful patient selection contributes at least as much to treatment success as does the specific electrode choice.

   (b) *Understanding the principles and algorithm of the selected device.* Several commonly used RF devices use different power application algorithms to deliver RF energy based upon current flow, impedance, or time. Current electrode designs are paired to specific devices and companies, and RF power algorithms are also commonly tailored to specific electrode designs (such that operators cannot interchange electrodes from one device to another and the greatest efficiencies in use are likely found by following company-recommended application protocols). Several specific electrode designs are available, most commonly divided into those that are needle-like vs. multitined expandable. Specifically, practitioners should be familiar with the shape of the coagulation zone that each system generates. For example, needle-like electrodes induce a more oval ablation zone parallel to the axis of the electrode, whereas expandable electrodes generate oval-shaped ablation zones perpendicular to the shaft of the electrode.

2. *Examples of commercially available systems [limited to the most common Food and Drug Administration (FDA) approved devices] (Fig. 3.2).*

   (a) *Cool-tip RF ablation system (Valleylab Inc., Boulder, Colorado).* The Cool-tip® RF electrode system uses a pulsed application, which inputs high amounts of current alternating frequently with "off-periods" that are triggered by rises in impedance to reduce tissue overheating around the electrode applied over a 12-min time period. The Cool-tip® RF

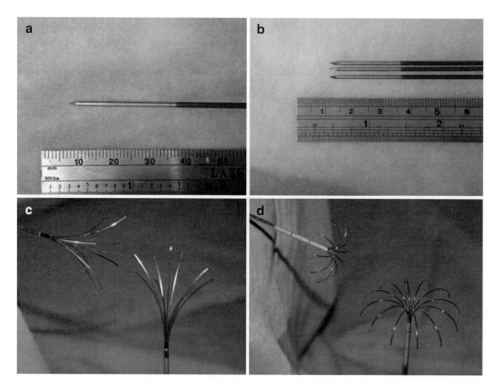

Fig. 3.2 Various radiofrequency (RF) electrode designs. Commonly used and commercially available electrode designs, including (**a**) a single internally cooled electrode with a 3-cm active tip (Cool-tip™ system, Valleylab, Boulder, Colorado), (**b**) a cluster internally cooled electrode system with three 2.5-cm active tips (Cluster™ electrode system, Valleylab, Boulder, Colorado), and two variations of an expandable electrode system (**c**: Starburst™, RITA Medical Systems, Mountain View, California; **d**: LeVeen™, Boston Scientific Corp., Natick, Massachusetts) (Reprinted with permission from Ahmed M, Brace CL, Lee FT, Jr, Goldberg SN. Principles of and advances in percutaneous ablation. *Radiology* 2011;258(2):351–369. Copyright the Radiological Society of North America.)

system uses 17 G needle-like electrodes as single, cluster, or multiple single electrodes which are internally cooled with ice water (to a temperature of <10°C). "Electrode switching" technology (described above) is currently only available with the Cool-tip® RF system.

(b) *RF 3000 ablation system (Boston Scientific, Natick, Massachusetts).* The Boston Scientific® device employs two rounds of slowly increasing power to achieve tissue heating, which occurs until tissue impedance starts to rise (thereby limiting further current input) to threshold levels, colloquially termed "roll-off." The Boston Scientific® RF system uses umbrella-shaped expandable electrodes with multiple (10–12) tines extending out from the needle shaft.

(c) *RITA system (Angiodynamics, Queensbury, New York).* Another commonly used device, the RITA system, administers RF energy to set temperature endpoints (usually 105°C as measured by sensors within the electrode tips) combined with incremental extension of an expandable electrode system. The RITA® system uses an expandable electrode system paired with slow saline drip infusion.

Understanding and Modifying the Biophysiologic Environment

An understanding of the effect of the tumor and organ biophysiologic environment on tissue heating is critical to performing successful tumor ablations, since device development is ultimately constrained by tumor and organ physiology. Most studies to date have focused on the effects of tissue characteristics, such as tissue perfusion and tissue electrical and thermal conductivity, on RF ablation.

1. *Tissue perfusion.* The foremost factor limiting thermal ablation of tumors continues to be tissue blood flow, for which the effects are twofold.

    (a) *Large vessel heat-sink effect.* Larger diameter blood vessels with higher flow act as heat sinks, drawing away either heat (or cold) from the ablative area. For example, in a study in an in vivo porcine model, Lu et al. examined the effect of hepatic vessel diameter on RF ablation outcome [55]. Using computed tomography (CT) and histopathologic

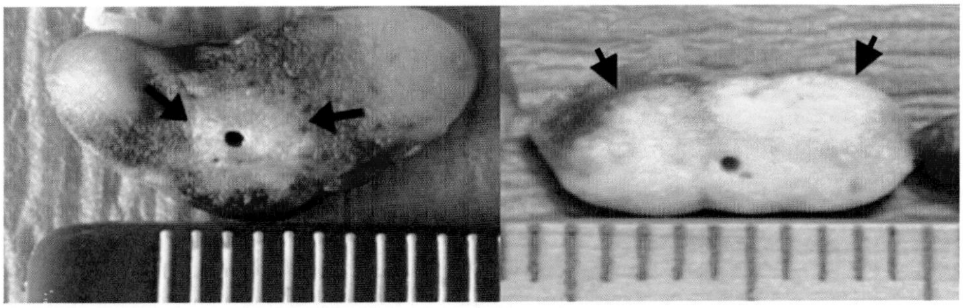

Fig. 3.3 Reducing the negative effects of tumor microvascular perfusion on tissue heating by combining antiangiogenic therapy with RF ablation. RF ablation combined with antiangiogenic therapies such as sorafenib, a vascular endothelial growth factor (VEGF) receptor inhibitor results in significantly increased tumor coagulation (right image: 9 mm, black arrows) compared to RF ablation alone (4 mm, left image, black arrows) in this small animal tumor model (Reprinted with permission from Hakime A, Hines-Peralta A, Peddi H, et al. Combination of radiofrequency ablation with antiangiogenic therapy for tumor ablation efficacy: study in mice. *Radiology* 2007; 244:464–470. Copyright the Radiological Society of North America.)

analysis, more complete thermal heating and a reduced heat-sink effect was identified when hepatic vessels within the heating zone were <3 mm in diameter. In contrast, vessels >3 mm in diameter had higher patency rates, less endothelial injury, and greater viability of surrounding hepatocytes after RF ablation. This strong predictive nature of hepatic blood flow on the extent of RF-induced coagulation has been confirmed in multiple studies where increased coagulation volumes have been obtained when hepatic blood flow is decreased, either by balloon or coil embolization or by the Pringle maneuver [56].

(b) *Microvascular perfusion.* Another effect of tissue vasculature is a result of perfusion-mediated tissue cooling (capillary vascular flow) that also functions as a heat sink. By drawing heat from the treatment zone, this effect reduces the volume of tissue that receives the required minimal thermal dose for coagulation. Along with the use of mechanical occlusion as mention above, several studies have also used pharmacologic alteration of tissue perfusion to reduce these effects. Goldberg et al. modulated hepatic blood flow using intraarterial vasopressin and high-dose halothane in conjunction with RF ablation in in vivo porcine liver [57]. Arsenic trioxide that has recently received increasing attention as a novel antineoplastic agent [58, 59] has been shown to preferentially decrease tumor blood flow and significantly increase RF-induced coagulation in a renal tumor model [58]. More recently, promising antiangiogenic therapies, such as sorafenib, are also starting to be studied as combination therapies with ablation, with similar encouraging effects in animals [60] leading to the initiation of clinical trials (Fig. 3.3). Finally, preablation intraarterial microembolization (using 100–500 micron particles, either alone or as part of performing transarterial chemoembolization) has also been used to increase the size of the ablation zone [61].

2. *Electrical conductivity.* Local electrical conductivity is a tissue characteristic that specifically influences energy deposition in RF-based systems. RF-induced tissue heating, generated by resistive heating from ionic agitation, is strongly dependent on the local electrical conductivity. To this end, the effect of local electrical conductivity on RF-induced tissue heating can occur in several ways.

(a) *Altering electrical conductivity of the target zone.* Altering the electrical environment immediately around the RF electrode with ionic agents can increase electrical conductivity prior to or during RF ablation. The increase in conductivity allows greater energy deposition and, therefore, increased coagulation volume [62, 63]. Saline may also be of benefit when attempting to ablate cavitary lesions that might not otherwise contain a sufficient current path. In general, small volumes of highly concentrated sodium ions are injected in and around the ablation site to maximize local heating effects, findings observed in both experimental and clinical studies, and subsequently incorporated into electrode development [64]. However, it should be noted that saline infusion is not always a predictable process, as fluid can migrate to unintended locations and cause complications if not used properly [65].

(b) *Effect of differing tumor and surrounding organ electrical conductivity.* Differences in electrical conductivity between the tumor and surrounding background organ can affect tissue heating at the tumor margin. Several studies have demonstrated increases in tissue heating at the tumor–organ interface when the surrounding medium is characterized by reduced lower electrical conductivity [66]. In certain clinical settings, such as treating focal tumors in either lung or bone, marked differences in electrical conductivity may result in variable heating at the tumor–organ interface, and indeed, limit heating in the surrounding organ, and may make obtaining an ablative margin difficult.

(c) *Hydrodissection.* Electrical conductivity must be taken into account when injecting additional fluid in between the target zone and adjacent nontarget organs (i.e., hydrodissection), such as diaphragm or bowel, to protect them from thermal injury. For this application, fluids with low ion content, such as 5% dextrose in water (D5W) should be used, since they have been proven to electrically force RF current away from the protected organ, decrease the size and incidence of burns on the diaphragm and bowel, and reduce pain scores in patients treated with D5W when compared to ionic solutions, such as saline [47, 48]. Ionic solutions like 0.9% saline should not be used for hydro-dissection since they actually increase RF current flow [67].

3. *Thermal conductivity*. Initial clinical studies using RF ablation for hepatocellular carcinoma in the setting of underlying cirrhosis noted an "oven" effect (i.e., increased heating efficacy for tumors surrounded by cirrhotic liver or fat, such as exophytic renal cell carcinomas), or altered thermal transmission at the junction of tumor tissue and surrounding tissue [3]. For example, very poor tumor thermal conductivity limits heat transmission centrifugally away from the electrode with marked heating in the central portion of the tumor, and limited, potentially incomplete heating in peripheral portions of the tumor. In contrast, increased thermal conductivity (such as in cystic lesions or tumors surrounded by ascites) results in fast heat transmission (i.e., heat dissipation) with potentially incomplete and heterogeneous tumor heating. Furthermore, in recent agar phantom and computer modeling studies, Liu et al. demonstrated that differences in thermal conductivity between the tumor and surrounding background tissue (specifically, decreased thermal conductivity from increased fat content of surrounding tissue) result in increased temperatures at the tumor margin. However, heating was limited in the surrounding medium, making an ablative margin difficult to achieve [68]. An understanding of the role of thermal conductivity, and tissue and tumor-specific characteristics, on tissue heating may be useful when trying to predict ablation outcome in varying clinical settings (e.g., in exophytic renal cell carcinomas surrounded by perirenal fat, lung tumors surrounded by aerated normal parenchyma, or osseous metastases surrounded by cortical bone) [16].

Combining Thermal Ablation with Adjuvant Therapies

With further long-term follow-up of patients undergoing ablation therapy, there has been an increased incidence of detection of progressive local tumor growth for all tumor types and sizes despite initial indications of adequate therapy, suggesting that there are residual foci of viable, untreated disease in a substantial, but unknown number of cases [3]. Thus, the ability to achieve complete and uniform eradication of all malignant cells remains a key barrier to clinical success, and therefore, strategies that can increase the completeness of RF tumor destruction, even for small tumors, are needed. Hence, investigators have sought to improve results by combining thermal ablation with adjuvant therapies such as radiation and chemotherapy [69, 70].

1. *Rationale for combination therapy.*

    (a) *Potential advantages of combination therapy.*

        • *Reducing residual local tumor at the treatment margin.* Improved tumor cytotoxicity is likely to reduce the local recurrence rate at the treatment site, as heterogeneity of thermal diffusion (especially in the presence of vascularity) retards uniform and complete ablation [71]. Since local control requires complete tumor destruction, ablation may be inadequate even if large zones of ablation that encompass the entire tumor are created.
        • *Improving completeness of treatment.* By killing tumor cells at lower temperatures, combined paradigms can not only increase necrosis volume, but may also create a more complete area of tumor destruction by filling in untreated gaps within the ablation zone [72].
        • *Reducing the number and duration of therapy.* Combined treatment also has the potential to achieve equivalent tumor destruction with a concomitant reduction of the duration or course of therapy (a process that currently takes hours to treat larger tumors, with many protocols requiring repeat sessions). A reduction in the time required to completely ablate a given tumor volume would permit patients with larger or greater numbers of tumors to be treated. Shorter heating time could also potentially improve their quality of life by reducing the number of patient visits and the substantial costs of prolonged procedures that require image guidance.

    (b) *Utilizing sublethal hyperthermia.* Thermal ablation when used by itself only takes advantage of temperatures that are sufficient by themselves to induce coagulation necrosis (>50°C). Yet, based upon the exponential decrease in RF tissue heating, there is a steep thermal gradient in tissues surrounding an RF electrode. Hence, there is substantial flattening of the curve below 50°C, with a much larger tissue volume encompassed by the 45°C isotherm. Modeling studies demonstrate that were the threshold for cell death to be decreased by as few as 5°C, tumor coagulation could be increased up to 1.5 cm (up to a 59% increase in spherical volume of the ablation zone) [66].

(c) *Understanding ablation geography*. Target tumors undergoing thermal ablation can be conceptually divided into three zones: (1) a central ablation area that undergoes heat-induced coagulation necrosis, (2) a peripheral rim that undergoes reversible changes from sublethal hyperthermia, and (3) surrounding tumor or normal tissue that is unaffected by focal ablation, though still exposed to adjuvant systemic therapies. The area of maximum synergy between ablation and adjuvant therapies is the peripheral rim immediately surrounding the high-temperature ablation zone.

2. *Combining thermal ablation with adjuvant chemotherapy*. Several investigators have combined thermal ablation with adjuvant chemotherapy, either with transarterial chemoembolization (TACE) or systemically administered drug-encapsulated chemotherapy [69, 73, 74].

(a) *Combined RF ablation and TACE*. While RF ablation and TACE are both independently commonly used modalities for locoregional treatment of liver tumors such as hepatocellular carcinoma (HCC), several limitations to their optimal outcomes persist. For example, RF ablation is less effective in larger tumors and difficult to use in specific locations or near larger blood vessels. In contrast, TACE can be used for larger tumors, but rates of tumor necrosis are lower (30–90% compared to >90% for RF ablation). Therefore, several experimental and clinical studies have investigated administering them in a combined manner.

- *Rationale for combination RF/TACE*. There are several potential advantages with combining RF and TACE. This includes combined two-hit cytotoxic effects of exposure to nonlethal low-level hyperthermia in periablational tumor and adjuvant chemotherapy. Alterations in tumor perfusion can potentiate the effects of either RF ablation through preablation embolization of tumor vasculature or TACE with postablation peripheral hyperemia increasing blood flow for TACE. Finally, performing TACE first can improve tumor visualization (through intratumoral iodized oil deposition) for RF ablation [47].
- *Administration paradigms*. RF ablation and TACE can be administered in varying paradigms, based upon the sequence and time between therapies.

    - *Near concurrent administration*. Mostafa et al. demonstrated, in VX2 tumors implanted in rabbit liver, that the largest treatment volumes were obtained when TACE preceded RF ablation, compared with RF before TACE or either therapy alone [61]. Ahrar et al. investigated the effects of high-temperature heating on commonly used TACE agents (doxorubicin, mitomycin-C, and cisplatin) and found minimal changes in the cytotoxic activity of the agents when exposed to clinically relevant durations of heating (>100°C for <20 min) [75]. For HCC tumors invisible on ultrasound and unenhanced CT, Lee et al. reported that 71% of tumors could be adequately visualized for subsequent RF ablation [76]. Based upon this, the optimal strategy for administration is likely performing TACE first, followed by RF ablation. This is confirmed in a recent randomized-controlled study by Morimoto et al. comparing TACE–RF (on the same day) to RF alone for intermediate-sized HCC (3.1–5.0 cm diameter), where TACE–RF resulted in lower rates of local tumor progression at 3 years [77].
    - *Sequential or alternating administration*. Another approach in combination therapy is to primarily treat the target tumor with a single modality (either TACE or RF), followed by additional adjuvant treatments using either one or both modalities for residual disease. For example, RF ablation can be performed for an initial presentation of limited disease, followed by TACE performed at a later date for residual peripheral tumor, satellite nodules, or new foci. Likewise, TACE can be performed initially to control more extensive disease with subsequent RF directed at small foci of local recurrence or new small nodules.

- *Available clinical data*. Several studies using combination therapy have reported increases in ablation size and increased treatment efficacy with combination RF/TACE, particularly as the primary treatment of large (>5 cm) unresectable tumors. For example, Yang et al. treated 103 patients with recurrent unresectable HCC after hepatectomy and reported lower intrahepatic recurrence and longer 3-year survival compared to either therapy alone [78]. The potential benefit of combining RF with TACE for small (<3 cm) remains less clear, as a recent meta-analysis of randomized-controlled studies reported no significant survival benefit for combination RF/TACE over RF alone [79]. Finally, tailoring treatment to each individual case remains important, as each modality can be adjuvantly used to "mop-up" residual disease after primary therapy.

(b) *Combined RF ablation and chemotherapy*. Several studies have investigated the use of adjuvant chemotherapy (predominantly doxorubicin-based regimens) administered around the time of RF ablation.

- *RF combined with percutaneous injection of free doxorubicin*. An initial study administered RF ablation in conjunction with percutaneous intratumoral injection of injected free doxorubicin in a rat breast adenocarcinoma model, demonstrating increases in mean tumor necrosis diameter with combination doxorubicin and RF therapy

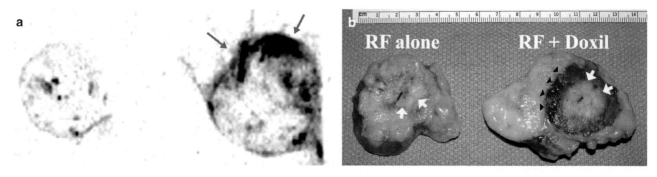

Fig. 3.4 Combination RF ablation and intravenous (IV) liposomal doxorubicin. (**a**) Autoradiography of two paired tumors from the same animal 24 h following the IV administration of tritiated liposomes, without (*left*) and with (*right*) RF ablation immediately preceding liposome injection. For the RF-ablated tumor, the central zone with little uptake corresponds to the zone of RF coagulation, with a peripheral rim of increased liposome uptake seen (small red arrows) (Reprinted with permission from He N, Wang W, Ji Z, Li C, Huang B. Microwave ablation: an experimental comparative study on internally cooled antenna versus noninternally cooled antenna in liver models. *Acad Radiol* 2010;17:894–899). (**b**) Observed effects of combined RF/IV liposomal doxorubicin therapy (*right*) compared to RF alone (*left*, 12 min RF application, 1 cm internally cooled electrode) in subcutaneous canine venereal sarcoma tumors. The central white zone (*arrows*) that corresponds to RF-induced coagulation is slightly larger (3 mm) in the combined therapy tumor, while the peripheral red zone is dramatically increased in size (0.21–0.93 cm). In the combined therapy tumor this red zone of increased tumor destruction is comprised of frank coagulative necrosis (Reprinted from Ahmed M, Liu Z, Lukyanov AN, et al. Combination radiofrequency ablation with intratumoral liposomal doxorubicin: effect on drug accumulation and coagulation in multiple tissues and tumor types in animals. *Radiology* 2005; 235:469–477. Copyright the Radiological Society of North America.)

(11.4 mm) compared to RF alone (6.7 mm) [80]. However, as initial image-guided direct intratumoral injection strategies have encountered many difficulties in clinical practice such as nonuniform drug diffusion and limited operator control on drug distribution, this method has significant limitations.

- *RF combined with intravenous (IV) liposome-encapsulated doxorubicin (Doxil®, Centocor Ortho Biotech Inc., Horsham, Pennsylvania).* Studies have combined RF ablation with doxorubicin encapsulated within a liposome [72, 81].

    - *Advantages of liposomal formulation.* Liposome particles are completely biocompatible, cause very little toxic or antigenic reaction, and are biologically inert. Incorporation of polyethylene–glycol surface modifications minimizes plasma protein absorption on liposome surfaces and subsequent recognition and uptake of liposomes by the reticuloendothelial system, which further reduces systemic phagocytosis and results in prolonged circulation time, selective agent delivery through the leaky tumor endothelium (an enhanced permeability and retention effect), as well as reduced toxicity profiles [82, 83]. Several "thermosensitive" liposomal formulations have also been developed that preferentially release their contents in hyperthermic conditions (42–45°C) [84]. As a result, this doxorubicin-containing formulation is widely accepted for clinical practice [85–87].

    - *RF/Doxil increases tumor coagulation.* Experiments in small and large animal tumor models have demonstrated significant increases in mean tumor coagulation diameter (70–100%) and volume (up to 200%) from combination RF/Doxil therapy compared to RF alone [88], with most of the gain in the larger peripheral periablative zone [81] (Fig. 3.4). In a pilot clinical study combining RF ablation (internally cooled electrode) with adjuvant liposomal doxorubicin, 10 patients with 18 intrahepatic tumors were randomized to receive either liposomal doxorubicin (20 mg Doxil) 24 h prior to RF ablation or RF ablation alone (mean tumor size undergoing ablation was 4.0 ± 1.8 cm) [72]. While no difference in the amount of tumor destruction was seen between groups immediately following RF, at 2–4 weeks, patients receiving liposomal doxorubicin had an increase in tumor destruction of 24–342% volumetric increase (median = 32%) compared to a decrease of 76–88% for treated with RF alone (a finding concordant with prior observations). Several additional and clinically beneficial findings were also observed only in the combination therapy group, including increased diameter of the treatment effect for multiple tumor types, improved completeness of tumor destruction particularly adjacent to intratumoral vessels, and increased treatment effect including the peritumoral liver parenchyma (suggesting a contribution to achieving an adequate ablative margin).

    - *RF increases intratumoral drug accumulation.* Noncoagulative hyperthermia increases intratumoral drug accumulation through increases in intratumoral blood flow and microvascular permeability likely as a result of endothelial injury and increases in vascular endothelial pore size. Animal studies have demonstrated up to a 5.6-fold increase in intratumoral doxorubicin accumulation following RF ablation, with (1) the greatest amount of intratumoral doxorubicin occurs in the zone immediately peripheral to the central RF area, and (2) smaller amounts of doxorubicin were found in the central RF-coagulated area suggesting drug deposition in areas with residual, patent vasculature [89]. These findings help explain why liposomal doxorubicin is likely to be complementary to RF ablation. The majority of the liposomes concentrated in a zone immediately peripheral to the area coagulated by RF heating and were within the region where nonlethal hyperthermia and increased destruction is observed [53]. Additionally, the patchy penetration of liposomes into the zone of coagulation implies infiltration of chemotherapy into the coagulated focus (possibly through residual patent vessels) that may improve the completeness of tumor destruction. Finally, as mentioned above, several liposomal formulations are available that have chemical structures designed to release their contents at specific hyperthermic temperatures (42–45°C), further increasing the specificity of targeting periablational tumor [90].

- *Improved cytotoxicity with combination therapy.* Several mechanisms for increased tumor destruction have also been identified, most notably increased cell stress (in part, due to upregulation of nitrative and oxidative pathways) leading to apoptosis [91]. Recently, Solazzo et al. performed immunohistochemical staining of rat breast tumors treated with RF ablation with and without adjuvant Doxil for markers of cellular stress [91]. In the periablational rim surrounding the ablation zone, combination RF/Doxil increased markers of DNA breakage and oxidative and nitrative stress early (~4 h) after RF ablation, with subsequent colocalization staining for cleaved caspase 3 (a marker for apoptosis), suggesting that these areas later underwent apoptosis. *N*-acetyl cysteine (NAC) was also administered in some animals, and reductions in both cellular stress pathways and apoptosis confirmed the causatory relationship between the two processes. Additionally, increased heat-shock protein production in a concentric ring of still-viable tumor surrounding the ablation zone, and immediately peripheral to the rim of apoptosis, had also been observed.

- *Using alternative additional agents.* This greater understanding of underlying mechanisms has led to successful investigations into adding additional adjuvant chemotherapies that specifically target cellular stress pathways.

  Paclitaxel: Recently, Yang et al. combined RF ablation with IV liposomal paclitaxel, an agent with known proapoptotic and antiheat-shock protein effects in subcutaneous rat breast adenocarcinoma tumors [92]. Combination RF–paclitaxel increased tumor coagulation and animal survival compared to RF alone, with even greater gains observed for RF–paclitaxel–Doxil. Interestingly, immunohistochemistry demonstrated reduced heat-shock protein expression and increased apoptosis for treatment combinations that included paclitaxel.

  Quercetin: Combining RF ablation with IV liposomal quercetin (a flavonoid agent with known antiheat-shock protein effects) also reduced heat-shock protein expression and increased tumor coagulation and survival [93]. Based upon these results, it is becoming clear that judicious selection of the type of chemotherapy combined with thermal therapy is necessary to potentiate and optimize the tumoricidal effects occurring in the peripheral zone of hyperthermia created by RF heating, along with tailored regimens that are tumor and organ type-specific.

- *Potential role of RF ablation in improving targeted drug delivery.* Given the effects of RF on increasing intratumoral drug delivery, the use of short courses of RF to concentrate liposomally delivered drugs could potentially expand the clinical use of this and other chemotherapeutic agents that have previously lacked efficacy due to an inability to achieve sufficient intratumoral drug concentrations. Additionally, selective intratumoral deposition of high drug concentrations could potentially allow an overall reduction of drug dosage [88], thereby reducing the potential for systemic toxicity, while maintaining delivery of high doses to the tumor target. Thus, liposomal delivery into ablated tumors has the unique potential to act as a focal targeting mechanism to guide the deposition of liposome-encapsulated agents [88, 94]. Recent improvements in imaging of liposomal delivery using gadolinium- or iohexol-labeling will likely further contribute to the utilization of targeted drug delivery [95, 96].

3. *Combining thermal ablation with adjuvant radiation.* Several studies have reported early investigation into combination RF ablation and radiation therapy with promising results [70, 97].

   (a) *Mechanisms of synergy.* There are known synergistic effects of combined external-beam radiation therapy and low-temperature hyperthermia [98]. Experimental animal studies have demonstrated increased tumor necrosis, reduced tumor growth, and improved animal survival with combined external-beam radiation and RF ablation when compared to either therapy alone [70, 99]. For example, in a rat breast adenocarcinoma model, Horkan et al. demonstrated significantly longer mean endpoint-survival for animals treated with combination RF ablation and 20-Gy external-beam radiation (94 days) compared to either radiation (40 days) or RF ablation (20 days) alone [70].

(b) *Early clinical results*. Clinical studies in primary lung malignancies confirm the synergistic effects of these therapies [97, 100]. For example, Grieco et al. reported improved survival with combination therapy in 41 patients with inoperable stage I/II nonsmall cell lung cancer treated with RF ablation and adjuvant radiation compared to either therapy alone [101]. Potential causes for the synergy include the sensitization of the tumor to subsequent radiation due to the increased oxygenation resulting from hyperthermia-induced increased blood flow to the tumor [102]. Another possible mechanism, which has been seen in animal tumor models, is an inhibition of radiation-induced repair and recovery and increased free radical formation [91]. Future work is needed to identify the optimal temperature for ablation and optimal radiation dose, as well as the most effective method of administering radiation therapy (external-beam radiation therapy, brachytherapy, or yttrium microspheres), on an organ-by-organ basis.

4. *Determining the optimal combination therapy*. Given the need to achieve complete eradication of all target tumor cells, including a 5–10 mm margin of seemingly normal liver tissue that may contain residual microscopic foci of disease, the argument for combining several modalities to achieve complete tumor cell death – similar to the multidisciplinary approach including surgery, radiation, and chemotherapy is used for the treatment of most solid cancers – cannot be overstated. Approaching each case and individual tumor with the goal of using whatever options are available within the interventional armamentarium will likely provide the highest clinical yield. Several factors should be taken into consideration when planning combination therapy such that the treatment is tailored to each case.

(a) *Tumor biology*. Certain tumors are more responsive to specific adjuvant therapies – for example, primary non-small cell lung cancer is susceptible to external-beam radiation compared to primary hepatocellular carcinoma. Marked tumor vascularity (such as is seen in HCC) limits RF tissue heating, and so optimal treatment likely includes performing adjuvant TACE first or administering adjuvant antiangiogenic therapy.

(b) *Size and number of tumors*. Smaller tumors (<3 cm) are often easily treated with a single modality (such as RF ablation), with larger tumors (>3.5 cm) requiring combination therapy. Similarly, multifocal tumors or the presence of satellite nodules around the primary tumor are also better suited to treatment with multiple modalities (e.g., RF ablation for the primary tumor and TACE for the residual peripheral satellite nodules).

(c) *Accessibility and visibility*. Tumor accessibility and visibility (i.e., can it be easily seen and reached via a percutaneous approach) should also factor into any decision on combination therapy. For example, as was noted earlier in the chapter, tumors not visible on unenhanced CT or ultrasound for RF ablation can be treated with TACE first.

Conclusion

As RF ablation is being used for an increasing number of tumor types and in varied organ settings, a thorough understanding of the basic principles and recent advances in thermal ablation is a necessary prerequisite to their effective clinical use. Several successful strategies have been used to improve thermal ablation efficacy including technological advancements in ablation devices and modifications of tissue and tumor environment. Finally, thermal ablation has been successfully combined with adjuvant chemotherapy and radiation, and future investigation will explore tailoring specific adjuvant therapies based upon a mechanistic rationale.

References

1. Gervais DA, McGovern FJ, Arellano RS, McDougal WS, Mueller PR. Renal cell carcinoma: clinical experience and technical success with radio-frequency ablation of 42 tumors. Radiology. 2003;226:417–24.
2. Kurup AN, Callstrom MR. Ablation of skeletal metastases: current status. J Vasc Interv Radiol. 2010;21:S242–50.
3. Livraghi T, Meloni F, Goldberg SN, Lazzaroni S, Solbiati L, Gazelle GS. Hepatocellular carcinoma: radiofrequency ablation of medium and large lesions. Radiology. 2000;214:761–8.
4. Solbiati L, Livraghi T, Goldberg SN, Ierace T, DellaNoce M, Gazelle GS. Percutaneous radiofrequency ablation of hepatic metastases from colorectal cancer: long term results in 117 patients. Radiology. 2001;221:159–66.
5. Venkatesan AM, Locklin J, Dupuy DE, Wood BJ. Percutaneous ablation of adrenal tumors. Tech Vasc Interv Radiol. 2010;13:89–99.
6. Zemlyak A, Moore WH, Bilfinger TV. Comparison of survival after sublobar resections and ablative therapies for stage I non-small cell lung cancer. J Am Coll Surg. 2010;211:68–72.
7. Ahmed M, Brace CL, Lee Jr FT, Goldberg SN. Principles of and advances in percutaneous ablation. Radiology. 2011;258(2):351–69.
8. McWilliams JP, Yamamoto S, Raman SS, et al. Percutaneous ablation of hepatocellular carcinoma: current status. J Vasc Interv Radiol. 2010;21:S204–13.

9. Dodd 3rd GD, Soulen MC, Kane RA, et al. Minimally invasive treatment of malignant hepatic tumors: at the threshold of a major break-through. Radiographics. 2000;20:9–27.

10. Shimada K, Sakamoto Y, Esaki M, Kosuge T. Role of the width of the surgical margin in a hepatectomy for small hepatocellular carcinomas eligible for percutaneous local ablative therapy. Am J Surg. 2008;195:775–81.

11. Dodd 3rd GD, Frank MS, Aribandi M, Chopra S, Chintapalli KN. Radiofrequency thermal ablation: computer analysis of the size of the thermal injury created by overlapping ablations. AJR Am J Roentgenol. 2001;177:777–82.

12. Gervais DA, McGovern FJ, Arellano RS, McDougal WS, Mueller PR. Radiofrequency ablation of renal cell carcinoma: part 1, Indications, results, and role in patient management over a 6-year period and ablation of 100 tumors. AJR Am J Roentgenol. 2005;185:64–71.

13. Lencioni R, Cioni D, Crocetti L, et al. Early-stage hepatocellular carcinoma in patients with cirrhosis: long-term results of percutaneous image-guided radiofrequency ablation. Radiology. 2005;234:961–7.

14. Lencioni R, Crocetti L, Cioni R, et al. Response to radiofrequency ablation of pulmonary tumours: a prospective, intention-to-treat, multi-centre clinical trial (the RAPTURE study). Lancet Oncol. 2008;9:621–8.

15. Schramm W, Yang D, Haemmerich D. Contribution of direct heating, thermal conduction and perfusion during radiofrequency and micro-wave ablation. Conf Proc IEEE Eng Med Biol Soc. 2006;1:5013–6.

16. Ahmed M, Liu Z, Humphries S, Goldberg SN. Computer modeling of the combined effects of perfusion, electrical conductivity, and thermal conductivity on tissue heating patterns in radiofrequency tumor ablation. Int J Hyperthermia. 2008;24:577–88.

17. Dupuy DE, Goldberg SN, Gazelle GS, Rosenthal DI. Cooled-tip radiofrequency ablation in the vertebral body: temperature distribution in the spinal canal. Radiology. 1997;207(P):330.

18. Seegenschmiedt M, Brady L, Sauer R. Interstitial thermoradiotherapy: review on technical and clinical aspects. Am J Clin Oncol. 1990;13:352–63.

19. Trembley B, Ryan T, Strohbehn J. Interstitial hyperthermia: physics, biology, and clinical aspects. In: Urano E, Douple E, editors. Hyperthermia and oncology, Vol. 3. Utrecht, The Netherlands: VSP; 1992: p. 11–98.

20. Larson T, Bostwick D, Corcia A. Temperature-correlated histopathologic changes following microwave thermoablation of obstructive tissues in patients with benign prostatic hyperplasia. Urology. 1996;47:463–9.

21. Zevas N, Kuwayama A. Pathologic analysis of experimental thermal lesions: comparison of induction heating and radiofrequency electro-coagulation. J Neurosurg. 1972;37:418–22.

22. Goldberg SN, Gazelle GS, Compton CC, Mueller PR, Tanabe KK. Treatment of intrahepatic malignancy with radiofrequency ablation: radiologic-pathologic correlation. Cancer. 2000;88:2452–63.

23. Goldberg SN, Gazelle GS, Halpern EF, Rittman WJ, Mueller PR, Rosenthal DI. Radiofrequency tissue ablation: importance of local tem-perature along the electrode tip exposure in determining lesion shape and size. Acad Radiol. 1996;3:212–8.

24. Mertyna P, Dewhirst MW, Halpern E, Goldberg W, Goldberg SN. Radiofrequency ablation: the effect of distance and baseline temperature on thermal dose required for coagulation. Int J Hyperthermia. 2008;24:550–9.

25. Mertyna P, Hines-Peralta A, Liu ZJ, Halpern E, Goldberg W, Goldberg SN. Radiofrequency ablation: variability in heat sensitivity in tumors and tissues. J Vasc Interv Radiol. 2007;18:647–54.

26. Pennes H. Analysis of tissue and arterial blood temperatures in the resting human forearm. J Appl Physiol. 1948;1:93–122.

27. Goldberg SN, Gazelle GS, Mueller PR. Thermal ablation therapy for focal malignancy: a unified approach to underlying principles, tech-niques, and diagnostic imaging guidance. Am J Radiol. 2000;174:323–31.

28. Goldberg SN, Gazelle GS, Dawson SL, Rittman WJ, Mueller PR, Rosenthal DI. Tissue ablation with radiofrequency: effect of probe size, gauge, duration, and temperature on lesion volume. Acad Radiol. 1995;2:399–404.

29. Goldberg SN, Gazelle GS, Dawson SL, Mueller PR, Rittman WJ, Rosenthal DI. Radiofrequency tissue ablation using multiprobe arrays: greater tissue destruction than multiple probes operating alone. Acad Radiol. 1995;2:670–4.

30. Bangard C, Rosgen S, Wahba R, et al. Large-volume multi-tined expandable RF ablation in pig livers: comparison of 2D and volumetric measurements of the ablation zone. Eur Radiol. 2010;20:1073–8.

31. Rossi S, Buscarini E, Garbagnati F. Percutaneous treatment of small hepatic tumors by an expandable RF needle electrode. AJR Am J Roentgenol. 1998;170:1015–22.

32. Siperstein AE, Rogers SJ, Hansen PD, Gitomirsky A. Laparoscopic thermal ablation of hepatic neuroendocrine tumor metastases. Surgery. 1997;122:1147–55.

33. Leveen RF. Laser hyperthermia and radiofrequency ablation of hepatic lesions. Semin Interv Radiol. 1997;12:313–24.

34. Appelbaum L, Sosna J, Pearson R, et al. Algorithm optimization for multitined radiofrequency ablation: comparative study in ex vivo and in vivo bovine liver. Radiology. 2010;254(2):430–40.

35. McGahan JP, Gu WZ, Brock JM, Tesluk H, Jones CD. Hepatic ablation using bipolar radiofrequency electrocautery. Acad Radiol. 1996;3:418–22.

36. Desinger K, Stein T, Muller G, Mack M, Vogl T. Interstitial bipolar RF-thermotherapy (REITT) therapy by planning by computer simulation and MRI-monitoring – a new concept for minimally invasive procedures. Proc SPIE. 1999;3249:147–60.

37. Lee JM, Han JK, Kim SH, et al. Bipolar radiofrequency ablation using wet-cooled electrodes: an in vitro experimental study in bovine liver. AJR Am J Roentgenol. 2005;184:391–7.

38. Seror O, N'Kontchou G, Ibraheem M, et al. Large (> or =5.0-cm) HCCs: multipolar RF ablation with three internally cooled bipolar elec-trodes–initial experience in 26 patients. Radiology. 2008;248:288–96.

39. Lee JM, Han JK, Kim HC, et al. Multiple-electrode radiofrequency ablation of in vivo porcine liver: comparative studies of consecutive monopolar, switching monopolar versus multipolar modes. Invest Radiol. 2007;42:676–83.

40. Goldberg SN, Gazelle GS, Solbiati L, Rittman WJ, Mueller PR. Radiofrequency tissue ablation: increased lesion diameter with a perfusion electrode. Acad Radiol. 1996;3:636–44.

41. Goldberg SN, Solbiati L, Hahn PF, et al. Large-volume tissue ablation with radiofrequency by using a clustered, internally-cooled electrode technique: laboratory and clinical experience in liver metastases. Radiology. 1998;209:371–9.

42. Cha J, Choi D, Lee MW, et al. Radiofrequency ablation zones in ex vivo bovine and in vivo porcine livers: comparison of the use of internally cooled electrodes and internally cooled wet electrodes. Cardiovasc Intervent Radiol. 2009;32:1235–40.

43. Hines-Peralta A, Hollander CY, Solazzo S, Horkan C, Liu ZJ, Goldberg SN. Hybrid radiofrequency and cryoablation device: preliminary results in an animal model. J Vasc Interv Radiol. 2004;15:1111–20.

44. Goldberg SN, Stein M, Gazelle GS, Sheiman RG, Kruskal JB, Clouse ME. Percutaneous radiofrequency tissue ablation: optimization of pulsed-RF technique to increase coagulation necrosis. J Vasc Interv Radiol. 1999;10:907–16.

45. Gulesserian T, Mahnken AH, Schernthaner R, et al. Comparison of expandable electrodes in percutaneous radiofrequency ablation of renal cell carcinoma. Eur J Radiol. 2006;59:133–9.

46. McGahan JP, Loh S, Boschini FJ, et al. Maximizing parameters for tissue ablation by using an internally cooled electrode. Radiology. 2010;256:397–405.

47. Brace CL, Sampson LA, Hinshaw JL, Sandhu N, Lee Jr FT. Radiofrequency ablation: simultaneous application of multiple electrodes via switching creates larger, more confluent ablations than sequential application in a large animal model. J Vasc Interv Radiol. 2009;20:118–24.

48. Laeseke PF, Sampson LA, Haemmerich D, et al. Multiple-electrode radiofrequency ablation creates confluent areas of necrosis: in vivo porcine liver results. Radiology. 2006;241:116–24.

49. Brace CL, Laeseke PF, Sampson LA, Frey TM, Mukherjee R, Lee Jr FT. Radiofrequency ablation with a high-power generator: device efficacy in an in vivo porcine liver model. Int J Hyperthermia. 2007;23:387–94.

50. Solazzo SA, Ahmed M, Liu Z, Hines-Peralta AU, Goldberg SN. High-power generator for radiofrequency ablation: larger electrodes and pulsing algorithms in bovine ex vivo and porcine in vivo settings. Radiology. 2007;242:743–50.

51. Laeseke PF, Lee Jr FT, Sampson LA, van der Weide DW, Brace CL. Microwave ablation versus radiofrequency ablation in the kidney: high-power triaxial antennas create larger ablation zones than similarly sized internally cooled electrodes. J Vasc Interv Radiol. 2009;20:1224–9.

52. Cheng Z, Xiao Q, Wang Y, Sun Y, Lu T, Liang P. 915 MHz microwave ablation with implanted internal cooled-shaft antenna: initial experimental study in in vivo porcine livers [published online ahead of print January 12, 2010]. Eur J Radiol. 2010;79(1):131–5. doi:10.1016/j.ejrad.2009.12.013.

53. He N, Wang W, Ji Z, Li C, Huang B. Microwave ablation: an experimental comparative study on internally cooled antenna versus non-internally cooled antenna in liver models. Acad Radiol. 2010;17:894–9.

54. Lin SM, Lin CC, Chen WT, Chen YC, Hsu CW. Radiofrequency ablation for hepatocellular carcinoma: a prospective comparison of four radiofrequency devices. J Vasc Interv Radiol. 2007;18:1118–25.

55. Lu DS, Raman SS, Limanond P, et al. Influence of large peritumoral vessels on outcome of radiofrequency ablation of liver tumors. J Vasc Interv Radiol. 2003;14:1267–74.

56. Patterson EJ, Scudamore CH, Owen DA, Nagy AG, Buczkowski AK. Radiofrequency ablation of porcine liver in vivo: effects of blood flow and treatment time on lesion size. Ann Surg. 1998;227:559–65.

57. Goldberg SN, Hahn PF, Halpern EF, Fogle R, Gazelle GS. Radiofrequency tissue ablation: effect of pharmacologic modulation of blood flow on coagulation diameter. Radiology. 1998;209:761–9.

58. Horkan C, Ahmed M, Liu Z, et al. Radiofrequency ablation: effect of pharmacologic modulation of hepatic and renal blood flow on coagulation diameter in a VX2 tumor model. J Vasc Interv Radiol. 2004;15:269–74.

59. Hines-Peralta A, Sukhatme V, Regan M, Signoretti S, Liu ZJ, Goldberg SN. Improved tumor destruction with arsenic trioxide and radiofrequency ablation in three animal models. Radiology. 2006;240:82–9.

60. Hakime A, Hines-Peralta A, Peddi H, et al. Combination of radiofrequency ablation with antiangiogenic therapy for tumor ablation efficacy: study in mice. Radiology. 2007;244:464–70.

61. Mostafa EM, Ganguli S, Faintuch S, Mertyna P, Goldberg SN. Optimal strategies for combining transcatheter arterial chemoembolization and radiofrequency ablation in rabbit VX2 hepatic tumors. J Vasc Interv Radiol. 2008;19:1740–8.

62. Goldberg SN, Ahmed M, Gazelle GS, et al. Radiofrequency thermal ablation with adjuvant saline injection: effect of electrical conductivity on tissue heating and coagulation. Radiology. 2001;219:157–65.

63. Aube C, Schmidt D, Brieger J, et al. Influence of NaCl concentrations on coagulation, temperature, and electrical conductivity using a perfusion radiofrequency ablation system: an ex vivo experimental study. Cardiovasc Intervent Radiol. 2007;30:92–7.

64. Miao Y, Ni Y, Yu J, Marchal G. A comparative study on validation of a novel cooled-wet electrode for radiofrequency liver ablation. Invest Radiol. 2000;35:438–44.

65. Gillams AR, Lees WR. CT mapping of the distribution of saline during radiofrequency ablation with perfusion electrodes. Cardiovasc Intervent Radiol. 2005;28:476–80.

66. Liu Z, Lobo SM, Humphries S, et al. Radiofrequency tumor ablation: insight into improved efficacy using computer modeling. AJR Am J Roentgenol. 2005;184:1347–52.

67. Laeseke PF, Sampson LA, Winter 3rd TC, Lee Jr FT. Use of dextrose 5% in water instead of saline to protect against inadvertent radiofrequency injuries. AJR Am J Roentgenol. 2005;184:1026–7.

68. Liu Z, Ahmed M, Weinstein Y, Yi M, Mahajan RL, Goldberg SN. Characterization of the RF ablation-induced 'oven effect': the importance of background tissue thermal conductivity on tissue heating. Int J Hyperthermia. 2006;22:327–42.

69. Ahmed M, Goldberg SN. Combination radiofrequency thermal ablation and adjuvant IV liposomal doxorubicin increases tissue coagulation and intratumoural drug accumulation. Int J Hyperthermia. 2004;20:781–802.

70. Horkan C, Dalal K, Coderre JA, et al. Reduced tumor growth with combined radiofrequency ablation and radiation therapy in a rat breast tumor model. Radiology. 2005;235:81–8.

71. Goldberg SN, Hahn PF, Tanabe KK, et al. Percutaneous radiofrequency tissue ablation: does perfusion-mediated tissue cooling limit coagulation necrosis? J Vasc Interv Radiol. 1998;9:101–11.

72. Goldberg SN, Kamel IR, Kruskal JB, et al. Radiofrequency ablation of hepatic tumors: increased tumor destruction with adjuvant liposomal doxorubicin therapy. AJR Am J Roentgenol. 2002;179:93–101.

73. Head HW, Dodd 3rd GD, Bao A, et al. Combination radiofrequency ablation and intravenous radiolabeled liposomal Doxorubicin: imaging and quantification of increased drug delivery to tumors. Radiology. 2010;255:405–14.

74. Kang SG, Yoon CJ, Jeong SH, et al. Single-session combined therapy with chemoembolization and radiofrequency ablation in hepatocellular carcinoma less than or equal to 5 cm: a preliminary study. J Vasc Interv Radiol. 2009;20:1570–7.

75. Ahrar K, Newman RA, Pang J, Vijjeswarapu MK, Wallace MJ, Wright KC. Dr. Gary J. Becker Young Investigator Award: relative thermo-sensitivity of cytotoxic drugs used in transcatheter arterial chemoembolization. J Vasc Interv Radiol. 2004;2004(15):901–5.

76. Lee MW, Kim YJ, Park SW, et al. Percutaneous radiofrequency ablation of small hepatocellular carcinoma invisible on both ultrasonography and unenhanced CT: a preliminary study of combined treatment with transarterial chemoembolisation. Br J Radiol. 2009;82:908–15.

77. Morimoto M, Numata K, Kondou M, Nozaki A, Morita S, Tanaka K. Midterm outcomes in patients with intermediate-sized hepatocellular carcinoma: a randomized controlled trial for determining the efficacy of radiofrequency ablation combined with transcatheter arterial chemoembolization. Cancer. 2010;166(23):5452–60.

78. Yang W, Chen MH, Wang MQ, et al. Combination therapy of radiofrequency ablation and transarterial chemoembolization in recurrent hepatocellular carcinoma after hepatectomy compared with single treatment. Hepatol Res. 2009;39:231–40.

79. Wang W, Shi J, Xie WF. Transarterial chemoembolization in combination with percutaneous ablation therapy in unresectable hepatocellular carcinoma: a meta-analysis. Liver Int. 2010;30:741–9.

80. Goldberg SN, Saldinger PF, Gazelle GS, et al. Percutaneous tumor ablation: increased coagulation necrosis with combined radiofrequency and percutaneous doxorubicin injection. Radiology. 2001;220:420–7.

81. Ahmed M, Liu Z, Lukyanov AN, et al. Combination radiofrequency ablation with intratumoral liposomal doxorubicin: effect on drug accumulation and coagulation in multiple tissues and tumor types in animals. Radiology. 2005;235:469–77.

82. Vaage J, Barbara E. Tissue uptake and therapeutic effects of stealth doxorubicin. In: Lasic D, Martin F, editors. Stealth liposomes. Boca Raton, FL: CRC Press; 1995.

83. Gabizon A, Shiota R, Papahadjopoulos D. Pharmacokinetics and tissue distribution of doxorubicin encapsulated in stable liposomes with long circulation times. J Natl Cancer Inst. 1989;81:1484–8.

84. Yarmolenko PS, Zhao Y, Landon C, et al. Comparative effects of thermosensitive doxorubicin-containing liposomes and hyperthermia in human and murine tumours. Int J Hyperthermia. 2010;26(5):485–98.

85. Ranson MR, Carmichael J, O'Byrne K, Stewart S, Smith D, Howell A. Treatment of advanced breast cancer with sterically stabilized liposomal doxorubicin: results of a multicenter phase II trial. J Clin Oncol. 1997;15:3185–91.

86. Gordon AN, Granai CO, Rose PG, et al. Phase II study of liposomal doxorubicin in platinum- and paclitaxel-refractory epithelial ovarian cancer. J Clin Oncol. 2000;18:3093–100.

87. Rivera E, Valero V, Arun B, et al. Phase II study of pegylated liposomal doxorubicin in combination with gemcitabine in patients with metastatic breast cancer. J Clin Oncol. 2003;21:3249–54.

88. Ahmed M, Monsky WE, Girnun G, et al. Radiofrequency thermal ablation sharply increases intratumoral liposomal doxorubicin accumulation and tumor coagulation. Cancer Res. 2003;63:6327–33.

89. Monsky WL, Kruskal JB, Lukyanov AN, et al. Radio-frequency ablation increases intratumoral liposomal doxorubicin accumulation in a rat breast tumor model. Radiology. 2002;224:823–9.

90. Poon RT, Borys N. Lyso-thermosensitive liposomal doxorubicin: a novel approach to enhance efficacy of thermal ablation of liver cancer. Expert Opin Pharmacother. 2009;10:333–43.

91. Solazzo S, Ahmed M, Schor-Bardach R, et al. Liposomal doxorubicin increases radiofrequency ablation-induced tumor destruction by increasing cellular oxidative and nitrative stress and accelerating apoptotic pathways. Radiology. 2010;255(1):62–74.

92. Yang W, Ahmed M, Elian M, et al. Do liposomal apoptotic enhancers increase tumor coagulation and end-point survival in percutaneous radiofrequency ablation of tumors in a rat tumor model? Radiology. 2010;257(3):685–96.

93. Yang W, Ahmed M, Tasawwar B, et al. Radiofrequency (RF) ablation combined with adjuvant liposomal quercetin-induced heat shock protein suppression increases tumor destruction and end-point survival in a rat animal model. In: Proceedings from the 27th Annual Meeting of the Society of Thermal Medicine; 2010 April 23–26; Clearwater Beach, Florida. Abstract.

94. Dromi S, Frenkel V, Luk A, et al. Pulsed-high intensity focused ultrasound and low temperature-sensitive liposomes for enhanced targeted drug delivery and antitumor effect. Clin Cancer Res. 2007;13:2722–7.

95. Danila D, Partha R, Elrod DB, Lackey M, Casscells SW, Conyers JL. Antibody-labeled liposomes for CT imaging of atherosclerotic plaques: in vitro investigation of an anti-ICAM antibody-labeled liposome containing iohexol for molecular imaging of atherosclerotic plaques via computed tomography. Tex Heart Inst J. 2009;36:393–403.

96. Erdogan S, Torchilin VP. Gadolinium-loaded polychelating polymer-containing tumor-targeted liposomes. Methods Mol Biol. 2010;605:321–34.

97. Dupuy DE, DiPetrillo T, Gandhi S, et al. Radiofrequency ablation followed by conventional radiotherapy for medically inoperable stage I non-small cell lung cancer. Chest. 2006;129:738–45.

98. Algan O, Fosmire H, Hynynen K, et al. External beam radiotherapy and hyperthermia in the treatment of patients with locally advanced prostate carcinoma. Cancer. 2000;89:399–403.

99. Solazzo S, Mertyna P, Peddi H, Ahmed M, Horkan C, Goldberg SN. RF ablation with adjuvant therapy: comparison of external beam radiation and liposomal doxorubicin on ablation efficacy in an animal tumor model. Int J Hyperthermia. 2008;24:560–7.

100. Chan MD, Dupuy DE, Mayo-Smith WW, Ng T, Dipetrillo TA. Combined radiofrequency ablation and high-dose rate brachytherapy for early-stage non-small-cell lung cancer [published online ahead of print August 24, 2010]. Brachytherapy. 2011;10(3):253–9. doi:10.1016.j.brachy.2010.07.002.

101. Grieco CA, Simon CJ, Mayo-Smith WW, DiPetrillo TA, Ready NE, Dupuy DE. Percutaneous image-guided thermal ablation and radiation therapy: outcomes of combined treatment for 41 patients with inoperable stage I/II non-small-cell lung cancer. J Vasc Interv Radiol. 2006;17:1117–24.

102. Mayer R, Hamilton-Farrell MR, van der Kleij AJ, et al. Hyperbaric oxygen and radiotherapy. Strahlenther Onkol. 2005;181:113–23.

Chapter 4
Principles of Cryoablation

Nicholas Kujala and Michael D. Beland

Introduction

In contrast to ablative therapies such as radiofrequency ablation (RFA), high intensity focused ultrasound (HIFU), or laser therapy which exploit the lethal threshold of cellular heat capacity to treat tumors, cryoablation (*cryo* – cold in Greek) is a thermal therapy option that utilizes cryogens to apply freezing temperatures to destroy target tissues. The cellular response and energy transformations of ablative therapies that initiate the spectrum of inflammation, repair, or death are distinct mechanisms depending on the ablative modality selected. This is especially true concerning cryoablation compared with the heat-based ablative modalities [1]. The concept of cooling tissues for analgesic and anti-inflammatory purposes dates back to the Egyptians [2]. Frostbite injury, which is essentially devitalized tissue, has long been known to occur secondary to prolonged or extreme low-temperature exposure. Not surprisingly, cryoablation is the oldest of the applicator-based ablative techniques [3]. Oncologic cryotherapy was first performed in England in 1845 by James Arnott. He used a self-designed apparatus to treat cancers of the skin, breast, and uterine cervix using a salt and crushed ice concoction that reached a temperature of −20°C. Although Arnott's treatments at the time were strictly palliative, he proposed that cryo-therapeutic techniques had the potential to cure [4]. In 1913, an American neurosurgeon named Irving S. Cooper developed the first liquid nitrogen surgical probe, which he used with variable success to treat movement disorders such as Parkinson disease and unresectable brain tumors. This spawned further interest in cryotherapy, which led to investigations and applications for treatments of the liver [5], prostate [6], and kidneys [7] beginning in the 1960s. The early applicators were large caliber that required open or laparoscopic access to treat visceral organs. It was not again until the 1990s that cryotherapy experienced a revival as a result of the development of safer and minimally invasive applicator systems (endoscopic and percutaneous) and enhanced imaging techniques. Improvements in ultrasonography, which allowed for real-time evaluation of cryoablation treatment, and cryoablative equipment with enhanced freezing capacity and smaller diameter cryoapplicators together have heightened cryotherapy's potential to become a more practical and well-tolerated treatment alternative to oncologic surgery in many clinical settings [8, 9].

Cryotherapy on the Molecular Level

The therapeutic goal of cryoablation is to create a localized area of cell death in targeted tissue which extends approximately 1 cm beyond the tumor margin (to approximate the goal of a complete surgical excision) while maintaining the greatest amount of vitalized tissue surrounding the lesion as is reasonably feasible. Unlike heat-induced tissue death, there is a well-defined boundary of cellular death with cryoablation. Centrally, as with RFA, coagulation necrosis defines the cryogenic lesion. A "freeze margin" circles the cryogenic lesion and consists of cells that are not destroyed during the treatment but will eventually die. Lastly, the "hypothermic zone" is a layer of tissue that experienced sublethal freezing temperatures during the treatment. Successful cryoablation treatment depends on rapidly freezing targeted tissue to lethal

N. Kujala • M.D. Beland (✉)
Department of Diagnostic Imaging, Rhode Island Hospital, Providence, RI, USA
e-mail: nkujala@lifespan.org; mbeland@lifespan.org

P.R. Mueller and A. Adam (eds.), *Interventional Oncology: A Practical Guide for the Interventional Radiologist*,
DOI 10.1007/978-1-4419-1469-9_4, © Springer Science+Business Media, LLC 2012

temperatures, slowly and completely thawing it, and repeating the "freeze–thaw" cycle. The series of events that lead to cellular death are complex and not fully understood, and the fate of cells at the periphery of the cryolesion continues to be investigated for usefulness of pretreatment synergism with cytotoxic (proapoptotic) drugs [1, 10–13].

Fast Freezing

As the treatment begins, extracellular matrix (interstitium) freezing creates a hyperosmotic environment outside of the cells, which still have intact and thermal-protective membranes. Intracellular fluid is cooled but unfrozen, and follows its osmotic gradient and diffuses out of the cell. With the loss of free water, the cells become dehydrated and undergo further hypothermic stress as the treatment continues. The process of extracellular ice accumulation exacerbates the loss of intracellular water, shrinking the cells and creating a high intracellular solute concentration. Proteins are denatured, and at approximately −10°C, the cell membrane is compromised. This allows intracellular ice formation, where mechanical shearing of organelles and membranes causes irreversible cell death. The thawing process of cryoablation permits melting of the extracellular ice, reversing the osmotic gradient and causing hypotonic extracellular water to diffuse back into cells (with intact membranes), and promoting rupture. This lethal cascade describes direct cellular injury, which is successfully achieved with rapid freezing. In addition to the toxic effects on a cellular level, cold temperatures concurrently incite vasoconstriction and local hypoperfusion, which can cause additional cell death. A "freeze phase" of approximately 5 min is generally considered adequate for these detrimental effects to take place in target tissue. However, a recent investigation by Klossner et al. [14] showed that tissue kept in the frozen state for 10 min achieved much greater cell death than a 5-min freeze. There is not a universally optimal "freeze phase" time as cryosensitivity and cooling rates are as variable as the histology of cancers [15].

Slow Thawing

The second mechanism of cell death during cryoablation is related to delayed microcirculatory failure. This process relies on vascular injury-induced ischemia of the target tissue during thawing to kill any remaining cells in the ablation zone that withstood the initial rapid freezing. Perfusion returns as the cryolesion is slowly thawed, which is believed to cause crystallization of water in a continuous fashion along the endothelium of the lumen. There is further diminished blood flow to tissue as ice accumulates within the microvasculature. Eventually, the integrity of the vessels cannot withstand the mechanical expansion and intraluminal contents leak through breaks in the endothelium into the interstitium. An inflammatory response ensues, with sequestration of platelets and microthrombotic events leading to cellular anoxia and tissue infarction [12].

This process explains why highly vascularized target tissue takes longer to ablate with cryogens. This "cold sink" phenomenon is seen when treated lesions are surrounded by abundant vascular networks, not uncommonly encountered as neovascularity is a defining characteristic of locally aggressive malignancies [3]. Local perfusion of blood at physiological temperatures counteracts the effects of cooling at the cryoapplicator site through local warming of tissue and removing the chilled blood. This can locally hinder the expansion of the cryolesion in areas of high perfusion or adjacent to larger blood vessels. This is the opposite effect of heat removal by the circulatory system, which is an obstacle in obtaining therapeutic tissue temperatures in radiofrequency ablation. While a potential obstacle to obtaining an adequate treatment margin, the cold sink effect can also be used to protect tissues that are not intended to be treated but are in close proximity to the tumor. For example, prostate cryoablation exploits this principle to prevent unwanted injury during treatments by warming the urethra through a catheter [16]. The skin can be protected when treating superficial lesions through the placement of a warming device on the skin surface (Fig. 4.1).

Freeze–Thaw Cycle Principles and Formation of a Cryolesion

Cryoablation treatments consist of at least two successive rounds of this freeze–thaw cycle. After the first cycle, the partially treated lesion of lysed cells and edema has enhanced thermal conductivity. As freezing temperatures are applied for a second time, the ice ball cools and enlarges more efficiently. The zone of coagulation necrosis is enlarged by up to 80% with the second cycle [10]. Ideally, the tissue is cooled as rapidly as reasonably possible, and is slowly and fully thawed without applying heat prior to initiating the second rapid freeze. In reality, however, the tumor size is generally much larger than the

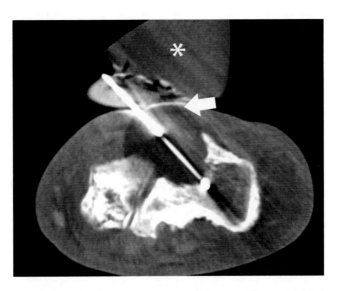

Fig. 4.1 Skin protection through warming during cryoablation of a superficial tumor. A 53-year-old female with intractable left ankle pain and inability to stand secondary to diffusely metastatic maxillary sinus cancer with painful left ankle metastasis. Computed tomography (CT) image from palliative cryoablation shows iceball surrounding cryoapplicator and extending to the skin surface (*arrow*). The skin surface was thermo-protected with a sterile glove filled with warm saline (*asterisk*) to avoid skin freezing. Following the procedure, the pain had completely resolved, and there was no skin breakdown on clinical follow-up

cryoapplicator tips (where the greatest rate of heat exchange occurs), and a full thaw without heat can require in excess of 30 min (not practical in a busy clinical setting).

The rate of tissue cooling is directly related to the probability of intracellular ice formation causing irreversible cell damage [1, 9, 10]. The latest generation of applicators can achieve cooling rates in excess of 60°C/min at the probe tip. Similar to the principles that govern the temperatures inside of the ice ball, the cooling rates of tissue are drastically affected by the distance from the applicator tips. Rates ranging from 20 to 50°C/min are sufficient to produce intracellular ice, and even slower rates are adequate in tissues with dense cellularity.

Slowly thawing target tissues that have experienced extreme cold temperatures potentiates cellular death by prolonging the time for crystallization and proliferation of ice, mechanical shearing, vasoconstriction, vascular stasis, oxidative stress, and cell dehydration. Temperatures of −15 to −40°C promote intraluminal microvascular ice formation, particularly in the narrow range of −20 to −25°C. The longer the cells experience these temperatures, the more successful the treatment can be.

Following treatment, there is a spectrum of completed cellular death and coagulation necrosis, local hemorrhage, structural damage to the tissue, inflammation, and initial sublethal damage that will progress to apoptosis or repair. Minutes to hours after complete thawing, there is tissue hyperemia and edema (inflammation). Complete cell destruction is present in the freeze margin surrounding the cryoapplicator position. Peripheral to this in the hypothermic zone is the tissue that experienced temperatures from −20 to 0°C and thus has the potential for survival. Neutrophils, lymphocytes, and macrophages are recruited to remove the infarcted and damaged tissue around the remaining collagen scaffolding. Collagen is a resilient protein that can endure a cryoablative treatment and maintain its matrix and tissue architecture. New collagen and fibroblasts are eventually all that remains in a contracted scar a few weeks to a month after treatment.

Already recognized as a mechanism of cell death with chemotherapy and radiation, apoptosis is now considered to play an integral role in cryolesion formation. Cellular-mediated programmed death occurs when sublethal thermal damage upregulates Bax protein levels. This is seen greatest in the periphery of the cryolesion and during the thawing phase. The mitochondria are integral in the upregulation of this proapoptotic protein, and creating disequilibrium of Bax and prosurvival protein Bcl-2. Of interest, Bcl-2 is overexpressed in many neoplasms, undoubtedly promoting their resistance to various treatment strategies [16, 17].

Cell death can occur with temperature ranges of −5 to −50°C. Freezing temperatures of −20°C are reported to be at the lethal threshold for noncancerous tissues, [9] and even lower for neoplasms. Experimental data on breast, prostate, lung, and liver tumors reveal potential tissue survival at temperatures greater than −40°C. Thus, ideal cryolesion temperatures range between −40 and −50°C to ensure complete freezing of intracellular and extracellular water, cell constituent damage, cessation of cellular metabolism, and ultimately cell death. There is a nonuniform temperature gradient of the lesion when the cryogen is applied. The iceball expands during the treatment, coldest at center and exponentially increasing in temperature towards its periphery, where it measures 0°C. Just 4 mm closer to the cryoapplicator, temperatures of −20°C are achieved and −40°C at 6 mm closer to the cryoapplicator [12, 18].

Cryogens, Applicators, and Delivery Systems

Cryoapplicators have evolved significantly since Cooper and Lee first developed and applied a closed loop of circulating liquid nitrogen topically in 1961. Difficulty with insulating the early probes resulted in large caliber instruments (>5 mm diameter) that limited their use beyond topical or open surgical access. Percutaneous cryoapplicator access is now performed as smaller vacuum-insulated 17-gauge needle applicators are available. As the probe size decreases so does its subsequent ice ball. Logically, more applicators are required to produce an ice ball large enough to accommodate larger tumors. Up to eight probes are available for synchronous use on standard delivery systems, with even more found on advanced platforms [19].

The two most utilized cryogens today are liquid nitrogen and argon gas. The boiling points of liquid nitrogen (−195.8°C) and argon gas (−185.7°C), which govern the achievable nadir temperature of the cryolesion, are similar and much cooler than other cryogens such as nitrous dioxide (−90°C), carbon dioxide (−79°C), and Freon-22 (−41°C). The latter cryogens have not been studied or applied as extensively in the clinical setting and, being less popular agents, will not be further considered. Although liquid nitrogen and argon gas are both used for similar purposes, their delivery systems and physical properties are quite distinct. A Cryotech LCS 3000 (Spembly, Andover, UK) apparatus weighs 172 kg is 132 cm tall, 56 cm wide, and 61 cm deep. It contains a 70-liter reservoir for storing its cryogen, liquid nitrogen. In contrast, a CRYOcare unit (Irvine, CA, USA) is an argon gas-based apparatus which weighs 79 kg and is 117 cm tall, 48 cm wide, and 64 cm deep. These systems will have multiple containers of argon gas, and also a container of helium, used for active thawing. The size and volatile cryogen storage is a clear advantage with argon systems, although their costs are typically higher.

In liquid nitrogen cryotherapy systems, pressurized gas is used to deliver liquid nitrogen to the applicator tip. At the probe tip, the liquid nitrogen phase shifts to a gas (boils), thus extracting heat from the surrounding tissues. Lower temperatures and greater freezing capacities at the probe tips are achievable with liquid nitrogen systems than with argon gas. As the rapid phase shift occurs around the applicator, a layer of gas vapor creates a natural insulation of the metal probe tip in a process known as the "Leidenfrost phenomenon." Gas begins to accumulate around the treatment zone, and the pressure gradient slows down the continuous delivery of liquid nitrogen. This "vapor blockage" [20] had been considered a limitation of liquid nitrogen delivery systems prior to the development of "gas bypass" mechanisms allowing higher ratios of delivered cryogen to impeding gas vapor.

Argon gas also undergoes a heat-extracting phase shift opposite of liquid nitrogen, converting to a liquid. It works as an effective cryogen under the "Joule–Thomson effect." The physical properties of gas as it expands are used to create freezing temperatures at the argon gas applicator tip. Argon gas, kept under high pressure (3,000 psi) in the delivery system gas cylinder, expands rapidly when it reaches a lower pressure at the probe tip. Under the laws of thermodynamics and energy conservation, the gas expansion creates increased potential energy, a corresponding decrease in kinetic energy, and thus local temperature decrease. The liquid phase that is created is considered to be a more efficient means of heat extraction [20], although the probe only cools to a temperature of −130 to −135°C. Hewitt et al. [20] demonstrated in a laboratory setting that argon-based systems have an accelerated freeze–thaw cycle relative to liquid nitrogen systems, but larger iceballs (cryolesions) are attainable with liquid nitrogen.

The development of earlier argon-based systems led to smaller probes, which made percutaneous cryoablation permissible (Fig. 4.2). Applicators, once as large as 8 mm, were reduced to 2.4 mm for argon gas delivery. Argon probes are now as small as 1.5 mm. Clinically available applicators can create a freeze zone of up to approximately 5 cm in length by 1.5–2 cm in width [3]. The smaller cryoapplicators produce relatively higher temperatures, which can be overcome by synchronous overlapping of additional probes in the treatment zone to create a comparable iceball [10]. Liquid nitrogen is restricted for use with probes greater than 3 mm in diameter. Probes of 3, 4.8, and 8 mm are used to attain freeze zones up to 5 cm.

The tumor size and contour will dictate probe size and number for cryotreatment. Smaller probes are favored for percutaneous procedures. Multiple probes, usually placed parallel to one another and 1.5 cm apart, are generally required, because smaller probes have higher nadir temperatures and their freeze radius is smaller. With multiple probes, there is the benefit of synergism and precise temperature control. A more uniform, larger, predictable iceball formation customizable to the lesion contour is also a clear advantage of using multiple probes (Fig. 4.3). Recent work has been done studying the optimal insertion depths of simultaneously applied probes. Traditionally, probes were placed at uniform depths, sometimes intentionally overshooting the target tissue and pulled back for the second freeze–thaw cycle of treatment. Probes placed at variable depths are gaining favor in treating some tumors. Complex mathematically based algorithms have been studied in an attempt for optimal localization of multiprobe applicators and thermal treatment protocol [21, 22]. Currently, most treatment planning and execution relies heavily on the experience of the operator [23].

Fig. 4.2 Iceball formation. Picture of a 2.4-mm diameter cryoapplicator with an iceball at its tip. Before applicator insertion into a patient, applicators should always be tested by briefly turning freeze cycle on, while applicator tip is submerged in sterile water. An iceball should be visible within seconds

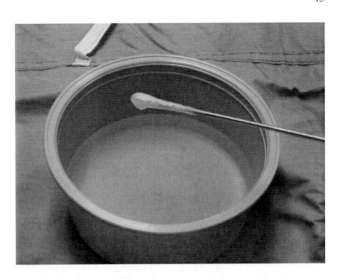

Fig. 4.3 Multiple cryoapplicators to obtain larger customized ablation zones. Picture of multiple cryoapplicators (7) being used to treat a large pelvic tumor. Note the approximate equal spacing and parallel placement to ensure uniform ablation temperatures

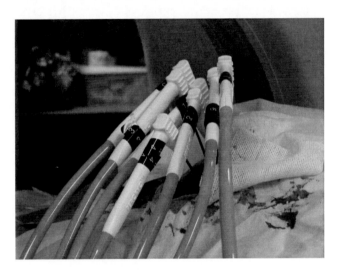

Image Monitoring

Much of the success that thermoablative techniques have had since the 1990s can be largely attributed to advancements in imaging. The real-time monitoring with ultrasound, and full-field visualization with computed tomography (CT) and magnetic resonance imaging (MRI) provided less invasive procedures, less collateral damage to adjacent organs, more accurate prediction of treatment effectiveness, and documentation of pre- and posttreatment lesion appearance for follow-up comparison. Each modality has its advantages, and combinations of each can be used during a treatment. Most importantly, the iceball size relative to the lesion should be frequently assessed to prevent damage to healthy tissue and ensure the lesion has been adequately ablated. Thermocouples (thermosensors) are used to monitor tissue temperatures in the cryolesion. They are ideally placed 1 cm from the tumor margin to increase the probability of a successful ablation zone. If lethal temperatures are achieved in the periphery beyond the tumor, it can be assumed that even lower isotherms are deeper in the iceball. In addition to monitoring the lethal freezing temperatures, they also ensure that adequate thawing has occurred [21–26].

Ultrasound

Ultrasound allows for real-time image guidance for lesion localization and cryoapplicator placement. As the iceball expands, ultrasound can determine if and when it extends beyond the lesion (a 1-cm circumferential margin is considered the standard). Since 1988, when Onik et al. [27] first experimented with animal models, the appearance of the evolving cryolesion has been well documented in cancer patients. The leading edge of the iceball (closest to the skin surface and ultrasound transducer) appears as a hyperechoic crescentic margin with posterior shadowing. The temperature of the leading edge is approximately 0°C and delineates the boundary between frozen and unfrozen tissue. Though it has excellent temporal resolution, the spacial resolution of ultrasound is inversely related to skin-to-tumor distance. In addition, the posterior extent of the iceball cannot be seen with a single static transducer and a two-dimensional image. However, the iceball generally evolves in a predictable manner. If the cryoapplicator has been positioned distal to the lesion epicenter, a successful treatment can be expected and confirmed with additional posttreatment imaging. After thawing, the treated cryolesion usually appears hyperechoic relative to normal surrounding tissue. This is not always true as many diseases manifest as increased echogenicity in organs treated with cryoablation, thus supporting the need to compare pre- and posttreatment imaging. Ultrasound is considered the most operator-dependent modality for cryolesion evaluation [26–28].

Computed Tomography

Larger field of view and circumferential visualization of the iceball are the advantages of CT over ultrasound. Growing iceballs and treated lesions appear hypodense relative to adjacent vitalized tissue on CT. There will be unavoidable artifact from the metallic applicators when intraprocedural images are taken with CT fluoroscopy units. Even with multiple probes, the size of the iceball and treated tissue are usually discernable. The plane between iceball and normal tissue has good contrast, although inferior to MRI [29]. A study by Tacke et al. [26] concluded that a greater slice thickness (5–8 mm) yielded greater contrast than thin (2 mm) slices. A disadvantage of CT is its ionizing radiation, however treatments using CT fluoroscopy units can use low-dose protocols to reduce the chance of adverse radiation effects [30–32].

Magnetic Resonance Imaging

MRI is considered the most versatile of the modalities concerning care of the patient with cryoablation. Preprocedure evaluation and planning of the disease extent is a well-known advantage of MRI. Tumor volumes are precisely measured with the multiplanar and excellent soft-tissue contrast with MRI. It can also be used for accurate positioning of cryoapplicators. Intraprocedural treatment monitoring has been shown to be an effective option, as is follow-up with contrast-enhanced MRI for residual and recurrent disease surveillance. MRI-compatible cryoapplicators and delivery systems are the first requisite for intraprocedural MRI imaging of cryoablations. MRI offers the best contrast of the three modalities used in cryoablation treatments, but at the greatest cost. The iceball is seen as a signal void on T2 weighted image (T2WI) due to T2 shortening of frozen tissue. Shortly after treatment, a T2WI hyperintense rim surrounds the treated lesion, which represents the damaged, edematous tissue. With contrast, the treatment zone is T1 hypointense and avid enhancement is seen in the periphery of the cryolesion [33]. Three-dimensional (3D) MRI techniques that allow estimates of isotherm profiles in the cryolesion have been described, which can ensure complete destruction of tumor [24, 26, 34–37].

Follow-Up

CT and MRI are the favored modalities for follow-up imaging postcryoablation. Recurrence on CT will appear as new enhancement at the margin of the nonenhancing freeze zone. Similarly, enhancement following Gadolinium administration on MRI (T1 hyperintensity) is consistent with residual or recurrent disease. If follow-up with MRI is chosen, Anderson and colleagues [28] aptly suggest the use of the same MRI scanner with the same protocol (which also implies that prior exams will be available for comparison). A 1-month follow-up period is considered adequate to allow resolution of any hemorrhage that may have occurred adjacent to the treatment zone. If no residual disease is detected with initial follow-up exams at 3 and 6 months, annual scans are then performed at some institutions [28]. There is no defined disease-free time interval in which follow-up is no longer necessary, and recurrence as far out as 3 years has been reported [38].

Uses and Applications

Liver

Patients with unresectable metastatic disease comprise the greatest volume of oncologic cryoablation in the liver (Fig. 4.4). The other major subset of patients has primary hepatocellular carcinoma in the setting of cirrhosis. As with the other visceral organs discussed below, cryoablation utilization closely paralleled the advancement in techniques for real-time monitoring with ultrasonography. Recurrence rates in patients treated with cryoablation are approximately 5%, greater than with resection. However, many of these patients were likely not surgical candidates to begin with, and a study by Seifert et al. [39] showed similar 5-year survival rates of ablation and surgical resection. Potential liver-specific complications to cryotherapy are thrombocytopenia, disseminated intravascular coagulation, biliary fistula, and multiorgan failure [9, 38, 40–43].

Renal

Cryoablation of renal tumors is one of the most common current uses of the technology [44–48]. Lesions smaller than 4 cm, and in the renal cortex, are usually given the most consideration for cryoablation. Nonsurgical candidates or patients with limited renal reserve requiring maximal nephron-sparing therapy can benefit from cryoablation. As evidence mounts for cryoablation effectiveness, it may someday be the first-line therapy for small renal cancers. Studies by Davol et al. [49] and Gill et al. [50] demonstrate 3-year cancer-free survival rates as high as 97–98%, though sometimes requiring a second ablative procedure for recurrence to achieve these rates. As with other thermal modalities, lesions close to the renal hilum are approached with caution as the risk of vascular damage is a potential complication. As expected, posterior and laterally located lesions are accessed with the greatest ease [12, 18, 28]. Treatment of central tumors places the collecting system at risk of injury and placement of a ureteral stent should be considered for warm saline instillation (Fig. 4.5).

Prostate

Technological advances have dramatically changed the scope of prostate cancer cryoablation, which is usually combined with adjunctive chemotherapy. Smaller probes, thermosensors, ultrasound improvements, and intraprocedural urethral warming catheters have significantly curtailed the dreaded complications of rectal perforation or fistula, urethral injury or stricture, and incontinence. Unfortunately, impotence is an expected outcome of complete gland cryoablation. Innovations such as ipsilateral hemi-gland ablations allow potential for preserved neurovascular integrity posttreatment. A large multicenter study of

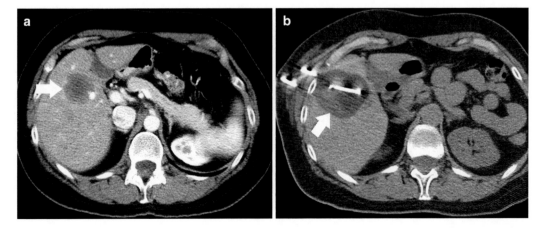

Fig. 4.4 Liver cryoablation. A 49-year-old female with primary breast cancer and metastatic disease to the liver. (**a**) Pretreatment contrast-enhanced axial CT image through the liver demonstrating a hypodense metastatic focus (*arrow*). (**b**) Intraprocedural noncontrast CT image shows portions of three cryoapplicators visible as well as the enlarging iceball (*arrow*)

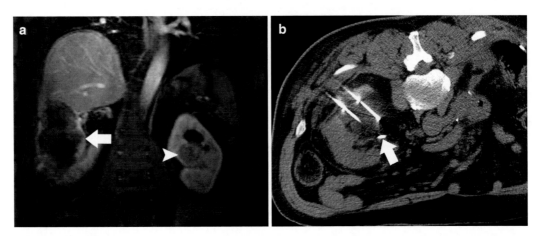

Fig. 4.5 Warm perfusion of the renal collecting system during cryoablation. A 61-year-old male who presented with bilateral renal cell carcinoma and underwent right nephrectomy prior to left renal cryoablation. (**a**) Preoperative coronal magnetic resonance imaging (MRI) shows the large surgically resected right renal mass (*arrow*) and the central left renal mass (*arrowhead*) to be treated with cryoablation. (**b**) Prone CT image obtained during cryoablation demonstrates portions of the cryoapplicators with the enlarging iceball. A left ureteral stent was placed allowing warm perfusion of the collecting system during the cryoablation to allow safe treatment of a central tumor. A portion of the ureteral stent is visible (*arrow*)

975 patients had a 63% 5-year survival rate with a median survival of 2 years. A 5-year survival rate as high as 89% (including patients with additional cryoablation treatments for recurrent disease) was reported by Donnelly et al. [51]. Cryoablation for prostate cancer treatment continues to gain favor not only for its improving safety profile but also for increasing efficacy [6, 8, 16, 52–55].

Musculoskeletal

Most experience with osseous lesions is with open surgery and adjunctive cryoablation following curettage of giant cell tumors, chondroblastomas, and chondrosarcomas. In a study by Veth et al. [56], a series of patients treated with adjunctive cryoablation of these lesions following en bloc excision had a 96–100% disease-free 2-year follow-up, including some patients requiring a repeat cryoablation. A group of patients with giant cell tumors undergoing adjunctive cryoablation had nearly an 8% recurrence, but 100 out of 102 patients were disease-free when accounting for repeat treatment. Cryoablation of aggressive primary bone lesions remains strictly for palliative purposes.

Cryotherapy as a Palliative Option

Recurrent local disease and metastatic disease is a significant cause of pain and morbidity. Many patients are not surgical candidates either by virtue of their locally invasive disease with unresectable margins or secondary to comorbidities. Promising results with palliative cryotherapy in patients with osseous or soft-tissue lesions, who also avoid long recovery times and complications of surgical resection, have been documented (Fig. 4.6). Cryoablation offers a palliative option for many of these patients with minimal recovery time [3, 57–60].

Disadvantages

Other thermal ablative therapies allow for vascular cauterization of tissue as the probes are removed, a feature that is not found with cryoapplicators. Hemostasis is a limitation of cryoablation, and highly vascularized lesions are typically reserved for other thermal ablative modalities or surgery despite the decreasing size of the cryoapplicators. In addition, despite the

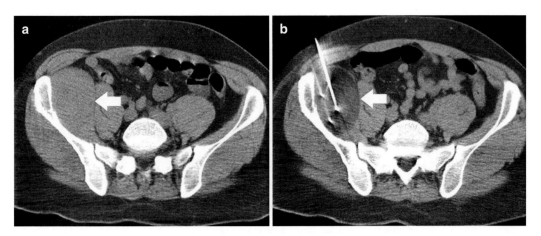

Fig. 4.6 Palliative cryoablation. A 39-year-old male with a large right iliacus metastatic lesion secondary to ocular melanoma primary with severe local pain. (**a**) Noncontrast CT image shows a large soft tissue expanding the right iliacus (*arrow*). (**b**) Supine CT image obtained during palliative cryoablation shows two of the cryoapplicators with surrounding iceball encompassing the entire tumor (*arrow*)

overlapping technique of cryoapplicators allowing larger ablation zones, very large tumors are not ideally treated with cryoablation. As 1 cm margins around the tumor are the current standard for a cryotreatment, an exponentially increasing cryolesion-to-tumor ratio can be expected with increasing tumor size [34]. Although disease recurrence rates are generally higher for lesions treated strictly with cryoablation compared to surgical resection, even a second cryoablative treatment session remains less invasive than open surgery and is preferred in some clinical settings.

Advantages

As alluded in the previous section, cryoablation is an advantageous therapeutic option for many patients with primary or metastatic disease. If clinical outcomes are shown to be comparable, cryoablation is a favored alternative to open surgery with general anesthesia, which carries many risks not associated with ablative therapies and longer recovery times. As cryoablation evolves, percutaneous access is showing promise in organs previously requiring an open or laparoscopic approach. Most cryoablative treatments are performed on an outpatient basis with local anesthesia and conscious sedation only. Postprocedural pain is believed to be reduced as a consequence of the freezing mechanism. When compared to RFA, cryoablation is advantageous in that treatment margin (iceball) monitoring is more reliable with an adequately visualized cryolesion. Cryoablation should be considered a safe and cost-effective alternative to surgery in the appropriate clinical setting.

Future Directions

Cryoablation relies heavily on image guidance for successful treatment follow-up monitoring. Although CT remains the most popular modality for guidance of cryoablation, innovation with 3D MRI estimation of isotherm distribution [34], which charts tissue temperatures in and adjacent to the treatment zone, is a promising technique for assurance of tumor ablation. At the molecular level, ionic imbalance between a necrotic and viable tissue margin can be determined using electrical impedance tomography (EIT). Although cryotherapy has been central to much of EIT research, it is not yet a routinely used method of determining ablative therapy success [61]. Investigations attempting to establish an employable mathematical model of optimize cryoapplicator placement custom-suited for individual lesions continue, which will hopefully reduce the recurrence rate of treated tumors [62]. More selective freezing of target tissues through alteration of specific thermal properties is also being investigated [63]. Many applications currently exist for oncologic cryoablation, and many more will likely surface in the coming years as minimally invasive therapy remains at the forefront of medical advancement.

References

1. Baust JG, Gage AA, Robilotto AT, Baust JM. The pathophysiology of thermoablation: optimizing cryoablation. Curr Opin Urol. 2009;19(2):127–32.
2. Cooper SM, Dawber RPR. The history of cryosurgery. JR Soc Med. 2001;94(4):196–201.
3. Beland MD, Dupuy DE, Mayo-Smith WW. Percutaneous cryoablation of symptomatic extraabdominal metastatic disease: preliminary results. AJR Am J Roentgenol. 2005;184:926–30.
4. Arnott J. On the treatment of cancer by the regulated application of an anaesthetic temperature. London: Churchill; 1851.
5. Cooper IS. Cryogenic surgery: a new method of deconstruction or extirpation of benign or malignant tissues. N Eng J Med. 1963;268:743–9.
6. Gonder M, Sloanes W, Smith V. Experimental prostate cryosurgery. Invest Urol. 1964;1:610–9.
7. Bush IM, Santoni E, Lieberman PH, Cahan WG, Whitmore WF. Some effects of freezing the rat kidney in situ. Cryobiology. 1964;2:163–70.
8. Gage AA. History of cryosurgery. Semin Surg Oncol. 1998;14:99–109.
9. Gage AA, Baust JG. Cryosurgery for tumors. J Am Coll Surg. 2007;205(2):342–56.
10. Baust JG, Gage AA. The molecular basis of cryosurgery. BJU Int. 2005;95:1187–91.
11. Baust JG, Gage AA, Clarke D, Baust JM, Van Buskirk R. Cryosurgery – a putative approach to molecular-based optimization. Cryobiology. 2004;48:190–204.
12. Carvalhal EF, Novick AC, Gill IS. Renal cryoablation application in nephron-sparing treatment. Braz J Urol. 2000;26:558–70.
13. Clarke D, Hollister WR, Baust JG, van Buskirk RG. Cryosurgical modeling: sequence of freezing and cytotoxic agent application affects cell death. Mol Urol. 1999;3:25–31.
14. Klossner DP, Clarke DM, VanBuskirk RG, et al. Cryosurgical technique: assessment of the fundamental variables using human prostate cancer model systems. Cryobiology. 2007;55:189–99.
15. Gage AA, Baust JG. Mechanisms of tissue injury in cryosurgery. Cryobiology. 1998;37:171–86.
16. Cohen J, Miller R, Shuman B. Urethral warming catheter for use during cryoablation of the prostate. Urology. 1995;45:861–4.
17. Yang WL, Addona T, Nair DG, et al. Apoptosis induced by cryo-injury in human colorectal cancer cells is associated with mitochondrial dysfunction. Int J Cancer. 2001;103:360–9.
18. Campbell SC, Krishnamurthy V, Chow G, Hale J, Myles J, Novick AC. Renal cryosurgery; experimental evaluation of treatment parameters. Urology. 1998;52:29–34.
19. Saliken JC, Cohen J, Miller R, et al. Laboratory evaluation of ice formation around a 3-mm accuprobe. Cryobiology. 1995;32:285–95.
20. Hewitt PM, Zhao J, Akhter J, Morris DL. A comparative laboratory study of liquid nitrogen and argon gas cryosurgery systems. Cryobiology. 1997;35:303–8.
21. Baissalov R, Sandison GA, Donnelly BJ, et al. A semi-empirical treatment planning model for optimization of multiprobe cryosurgery. Phys Med Biol. 2000;45:1085–98.
22. Baissalov R, Sandison GA, Reynolds D, Muldrew K. Simultaneous optimization of cryoprobe placement and thermal protocol for cryosurgery. Phys Med Biol. 2001;46:1799–814.
23. Brewer WH, Austin RS, Capps G, Neifeld JP. Intraoperative monitoring and postoperative imaging of hepatic cryosurgery. Semin Surg Oncol. 1998;14:129–55.
24. Silverman SG, Sun MR, Tuncali K, et al. Three-dimensional assessment of MRI-guided percutaneous cryotherapy of liver metastases. AJR Am J Roentgenol. 2004;183:707–12.
25. Silverman SG, Tuncali K, van Sonnenberg E, et al. Renal tumors: MR imaging-guided percutaneous cryotherapy–initial experience in 23 patients. Radiology. 2005;236:716–24.
26. Tacke J, Speetzen R, Heschel I, et al. Imaging of interstitial cryotherapy – an in vitro comparison of ultrasound, computed tomography, and magnetic resonance imaging. Cryobiology. 1999;38:250–9.
27. Onik G, Cobb C, Cohen J, et al. US characteristics of frozen prostate. Radiology. 1988;168:629–31.
28. Anderson JK, Shingleton WB, Cadedda JA. Imaging associated with percutaneous and intraoperative management of renal tumors. Urol Clin North Am. 2006;33:339–52.
29. Silverman SG, Tuncali K, Adams DF, et al. MR imaging-guided percutaneous cryotherapy of liver tumors: initial experience. Radiology. 2000;217:657–64.
30. Gupta A, Allaf ME, Kavoussi LR, et al. Computerized tomography guided percutaneous renal cryoablation with the patient under conscious sedation: initial clinical experience. J Urol. 2006;175:447–53.
31. Permpongkosol S, Sulman A, Solomon SB, et al. Percutaneous computerized tomography guided renal cryoablation using local anesthesia: pain assessment. J Urol. 2006;176:915–8.
32. Saliken JC, McKinnon JG, Gray R. CT for monitoring cryotherapy. AJR Am J Roentgenol. 1996;166:853–5.
33. McDannold NJ, Jolesz FA. Magnetic resonance image-guided thermal ablations. Top Magn Reson Imaging. 2000;11(3):191–202.
34. Mala T, Samset E, Aurdal L, et al. Magnetic resonance imaging-estimated three-dimensional temperature distribution in liver cryolesions; a study of cryolesion characteristics assumed necessary for tumor ablation. Cryobiology. 2001;43:268–75.
35. Harada J, Dohi M, Magnami T, et al. Initial experience of percutaneous renal cryosurgery under the guidance of a horizontal open MRI system. Radiat Med. 2001;19:291–6.
36. Mala T, Edwin B, Samset E, Gladhaug I, et al. Magnetic-resonance guided percutaneous cryoablation of hepatic tumours. Eur J Surg. 2001;167:610–7.
37. Samset E, Mala T, Edwin B, et al. Validation of estimated 3D temperature maps during hepatic cryo surgery. Magn Reson Imaging. 2001;19:715–21.
38. Mala T. Cryoablation of liver tumors – a review of mechanisms, techniques, and clinical outcome. Minim Invasive Ther Allied Technol. 2006;15:9–17.

39. Seifert JK, Springer A, Baier P, Junginger T. Liver resection or cryotherapy for colorectal liver metastasis: a prospective case control study. Int J Colorectal Dis. 2005;20:507–20.
40. Adam R, Hagopian EJ, Linhares M, et al. A comparison of percutaneous cryosurgery and percutaneous radiofrequency for unresectable hepatic malignancies. Arch Surg. 2002;137:1332–9. discussion 1340.
41. Crews KA, Kuhn JA, McCarty TM, et al. Cryosurgical ablation of hepatic tumors. Am J Surg. 1997;174:614–7. discussion 617–8.
42. Sarantou T, Bilchik A, Ramming K. Complications of hepatic cryosurgery. Semin Surg Oncol. 1998;14:156–62.
43. Zhou XD, Tang ZY. Cryotherapy for primary liver cancer. Semin Surg Oncol. 1998;14:171–4.
44. Permpongkosol S, Nielsen ME, Solomon SB. Percutaneous renal cryoablation. Urology. 2006;68:19–25.
45. Rodriguez R, Chan DY, Bishoff JT, et al. Renal ablative cryosurgery in selected patients with peripheral renal masses. Urology. 2000;55:25–30.
46. Hegarty NJ, Gill IS, Desai MM, et al. Probe-ablative nephron-sparing surgery: cryoablation versus radiofrequency ablation. Urology. 2006;68:7–13.
47. Kaouk JH, Aron M, Rewcastle JC, Gill IS. Cryotherapy: clinical end points and their experimental foundations. Urology. 2006;68:38–44.
48. Tuncali K, Morrison PR, Tatli S, et al. MRI-guided percutaneous cryoablation of renal tumors: use of external manual displacement of adjacent bowel loops. Eur J Radiol. 2006;59:198–202.
49. Davol PE, Fulmer BR, Rukstalis DB. Long-term results of cryoablation for renal cancer and complex renal masses. Urology. 2006;68:2–6.
50. Gill IS, Remer EM, Hasan WA, et al. Renal cryoablation: outcome at 3 years. J Urol. 2005;173:1903–7.
51. Donnelly BJ, Saliken JC, Ernst DS, et al. Prospective trial of cryosurgical ablation of the prostate: five-year results. Urology. 2002;60:645–8.
52. Bahn DK, Lee F, Badalament R, et al. Targeted cryoablation of the prostate: 7 year outcomes in the primary treatment of prostate cancer. Urology. 2002;60:3–11.
53. Chin JL, Downey DB, Mulligan M, Fenster A. Three-dimensional transrectal ultrasound guided cryoablation for localized prostate cancer in nonsurgical candidates: a feasibility study and report of early results. J Urol. 1998;159:910–6.
54. Cohen JK, Miller Jr RJ, Ahmed S, et al. Ten year biochemical disease control for prostate cancer patients treated with cryosurgery as primary therapy. Urology. 2008;71:515–8.
55. Mouraviev V, Polascik TJ. Update on cryotherapy for prostate cancer in 2006. Curr Opin Urol. 2006;16:152–6.
56. Veth R, Schreuder B, van Beem H, et al. Cryosurgery in aggressive, benign, and low-grade malignant bone tumours. Lancet Oncol. 2005;6:25–34.
57. Callstrom MR, Atwell TD, Charboneau JW, et al. Painful metastases involving bone: percutaneous image-guided cryoablation-prospective trial interim analysis. Radiology. 2006;241(2):572–80.
58. Callstrom MR, Charboneau JW. Percutaneous ablation: safe, effective treatment of bone tumors. Oncology (Williston Park). 2005;19(11 Suppl 4):22–6.
59. Wang H, Littrup PJ, Duan Y, Zhang Y, Feng H, Nie Z. Thoracic masses treated with percutaneous cryotherapy: initial experience with more than 200 procedures. Radiology. 2005;235(1):289–98.
60. Meijer S, de Rooij PD, Derksen EJ, et al. Cryosurgery for locally recurrent rectal cancer. Eur J Surg Oncol. 1992;18:255–7.
61. Davolos DM, Rubinsky B. Electrical impedance tomography of cell viability in tissue with application to cryosurgery. J Biomech Eng. 2004;126:305–9.
62. Rossi MR, Tanaka D, Shimada K, Rabin Y. Computerized planning of prostate cryosurgery using variable cryoprobe insertion depth. Cryobiology. 2010;60:71–9.
63. Yu TH, Liu J, Zhou YX. Selective freezing of target biological tissues after injection of solutions with specific thermal properties. Cryobiology. 2005;50:174–82.

Chapter 5
Principles of High-Intensity Focused Ultrasound

Gail ter Haar

Introduction

Although its use for therapeutic purposes predates diagnostic applications by several decades, ultrasound is most widely known for its imaging capabilities. The passage of ultrasound (US) through tissue can lead to biological changes that may be reversible or irreversible. The biological significance of these effects depends to a large extent on the energy in the ultrasound beam and the goal of the exposure. At diagnostic levels, any changes are largely believed to be biologically insignificant. For therapeutic ultrasound, beneficial cellular or functional effects are deliberately sought, whether these are at the cell membrane level (e.g., transient changes in permeability to facilitate drug delivery) or less subtle effects such as the localised temperatures rises that are required to achieve immediate thermal necrosis in high intensity focused ultrasound (HIFU; this technique is sometimes also referred to as FUS).

The mechanisms by which ultrasound induces such biological effects in tissue can broadly be divided into two classes – thermal and non-thermal. As the name indicates, thermal effects are those arising from the temperature rise that results from the absorption of ultrasound energy as it passes through tissue. Non-thermal (or mechanical) effects are those arising either from the formation and activity of micron-sized bubbles in the field (acoustic cavitation) or from the flow of fluids induced by the ultrasound pressure wave (acoustic streaming).

The principle behind HIFU treatments is very simple. Just as sunlight can be brought to a tight focus using a magnifying glass and used to set light to a dry leaf or piece of paper, ultrasonic beams can be focused, resulting in energy concentration in the focal region which may be sufficient to induce immediate cell death (Fig. 5.1a). The focused ultrasound beam is produced from a transducer capable of delivering high power. This may use a lens to shape the beam, a shaped crystal, a phased array, or a combination of these. The transducer parameters determine the shape and position of the focal volume [1]. Figure 5.1a shows an extracorporeal spherical bowl transducer. The HIFU treatment destroys only tissues lying within the focal region, leaving surrounding structures undamaged, forming a "trackless lesion." Figure 5.1b depicts a close up of the focal region. The acoustic field distribution at the focus is shown. The intensity exceeds that necessary to induce cyto-toxic temperature levels only in this volume. A "lesion" – region of coagulative necrosis – is seen in Fig. 5.1b. It appears as a white (cooked) ellipse lying within the undamaged (red) liver. Histology demonstrates that the margin between live and dead cells is very sharp, as shown in Fig. 5.1b (inset, bottom left). HIFU thus offers the potential for selective destruction of tissue targets at depth with no damage to overlying structures. Figure 5.1a shows a schematic of an extracorporeal treatment through the intact skin. As will be seen below, intracavitary HIFU devices are also being used.

Biological Effects

The primary intent of a HIFU treatment is the thermal ablation of the chosen target. Ablation is achieved when the temperature is maintained at 56°C for 1 s, or the thermal equivalent [2]. These thermal exposures result in instantaneous cell death from protein denaturation and damage to cytosolic and mitochondrial enzymes, and from the formation of histone complexes [3, 4]. Histologically, the damage induced is typical of coagulative necrosis. Complex cellular and sub-cellular

G. ter Haar (✉)
Department of Physics, Institute of Cancer Research: Royal Marsden Hospital, Sutton, Surrey, UK
e-mail: gail.terhaar@icr.ac.uk

P.R. Mueller and A. Adam (eds.), *Interventional Oncology: A Practical Guide for the Interventional Radiologist*,
DOI 10.1007/978-1-4419-1469-9_5, © Springer Science+Business Media, LLC 2012

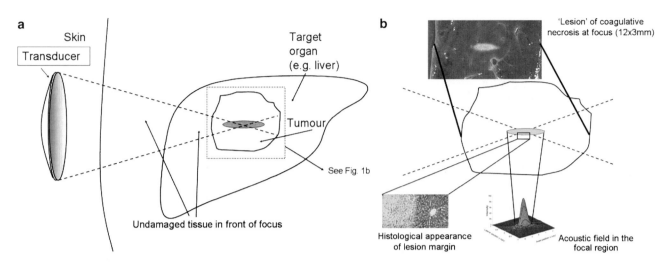

Fig. 5.1 (**a**) Schematic diagram showing the principles of high-intensity focused ultrasound (HIFU). The focus of the high-powered ultrasound beam is placed within the target volume. Exposure results in an ellipsoidal volume of thermal ablation (shown in **b**). The margin between dead and viable cells is sharp, as shown in (**b**)

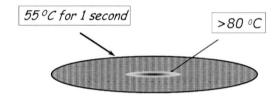

Fig. 5.2 Schematic diagram showing a HIFU lesion. At the centre of the lesion, temperatures of 80°C or higher may be achieved. The lesion margin is defined by those cells that have been subjected to 56°C for 1 s (or the thermal equivalent usually defined in terms of an equivalent time at 43°C)

changes occur. These include cell membrane, nucleic acid, cytoskeleton and mitochondrial function changes [5]. The changes in cell membrane fluidity and permeability that result from the increased temperature lead to decreased cytoplasmic streaming and impaired facilitated diffusion. Since passive diffusion is unaffected, the net result is an accumulation of intracellular metabolites, influx of extracellular fluids, cell swelling and death. Mitochondrial damage is also an important factor [5, 6]. DNA synthesis may be impaired by the denaturation of non-histone proteins resulting in the inhibition of synthesis induction by key enzymes [7]. These sub-cellular effects are likely to be of most importance at the HIFU lesion margins where the temperature reached is insufficient to cause ablation (Fig. 5.2), and the process of cell death may be more akin to that found in "low" temperature hyperthermia. Apoptosis is also seen in this tumour margin.

In addition to thermal ablation, cell killing may be the result of acoustic cavitation. It is difficult to differentiate histologically between tissue effects due to cavitation bubbles and those due to boiling, but monitoring of acoustic emissions allows their discrimination. Tissue water boiling events are accompanied by audible sounds, whereas high frequency broadband and harmonic signals (of the drive) are characteristic of acoustic cavitation. In general, intensities required to create boiling temperatures during the short HIFU pulses exceed the threshold level for inducing acoustic cavitation, and these two phenomena occur together. Histologically, the tissue is seen to contain voids where the bubble activity has created tears, mainly in extracellular spaces (Fig. 5.3c).

The classic description of the histological appearance of a HIFU lesion is as an "island" and "moat" [8]. This can be seen clearly using haematoxylin and eosin (H&E) staining (Fig. 5.3a). In the central region (the island), some regions have a "normal" appearance. These cells have undergone instantaneous "heat fixation" [9]. Swollen cells, pyknotic nuclei and reduced extracellular spaces can also be seen. There is a very sharp demarcation between damaged and normal cells at the outer edge of the "moat" region. This has been shown to be as narrow as six cells in extent (Fig. 5.3b) [10–12]. Apoptotic cells are also found in this region 6 h after exposure.

The extent of tissue destruction has been studied as a function of time after HIFU exposure. Histological studies up to 7 days after lesioning show that polymorphonuclear leucocytes and phagocytes are present at the damage boundary [12, 13]. The ultrasound-damaged cells at the lesion centre have disaggregated, with lack of distinct nuclei or cytoplasm. New granulation tissue is seen surrounding the lesion.

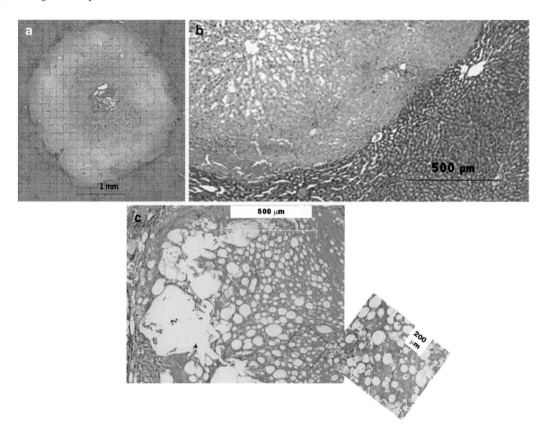

Fig. 5.3 Haematoxylin and eosin stained samples of rat liver exposed to ultrasound. Panel (**a**) shows the typical "island and moat" structure with evidence of boiling activity at the centre. Panel (**b**) shows the sharply defined margin of the lesion. Panel (**c**) shows typical holes seen when tissue has been subjected to boiling and cavitation activity (Image courtesy of Chaturika Jayadewa)

Wu et al. [9] performed histology on tissue from patients who had received HIFU therapy for their breast tumours (1.7 MHz; 5,000–15,000 W cm⁻²). Coagulative necrosis was seen in the centre of the ablated volume, and 7–14 days after treatment, a narrow band of fibrous collagen, inflammatory cells, fibroblasts and capillaries was found at the periphery. In 11 out of 23 patients, the central area retained a normal morphological appearance on H&E staining. However, electron microscopy and staining with nicotinamide adenine dinucleotide diaphorase (NADH) showed that these cells were dead. It is to be expected that in time, these cells would be broken down as a result of a combination of macrophage activity and lysosomal release.

Chen et al. [14] compared the size of HIFU lesions, as seen on magnetic resonance (MR), with that measured using H&E and triphenyl tetrazolium chloride (TTC) stains. Good agreement was found between the three techniques.

Following HIFU exposure, histology often reveals two distinct regions of damage. Tissue that has been subject to direct exposure to the HIFU focus undergoes coagulative necrosis as described above. Small blood vessels lying within this volume may be occluded, resulting in damage to tissues lying downstream that become nutrient-deprived ("indirect" damage). The size of the vessels that can be occluded depends on a number of factors, including the flow rate, but in general, total occlusion only occurs in vessels less than ~2 mm in diameter. This has been studied by a number of authors [10, 13, 15–20]. Ichihara et al. [19] were able to occlude the renal arterial branches (~0.5 mm diameter) in rabbit kidneys. Arterial wall degeneration was seen at 2 days, and a wedge shaped necrotic area that indicated lack of perfusion to this volume (2.2 MHz; 4 kW cm⁻²; 5 s; 2–10 shots).

Ishikawa et al. [21] have studied the effects of 3.2 MHz ultrasound on rat femoral vessels. They demonstrated that at an intensity of 4.3 kW cm⁻² the vessel could be occluded. These vessels are 0.1–0.2 mm in diameter. At intensities of 530 W cm⁻² and above, the vessels looked normal when studied immediately after exposure, but at 7 days vacuolar degeneration in the tunica media was seen, and elastin fibres were destroyed. Organised thrombus was seen in vessels exposed to 4.3 kW cm⁻². Increases in peak systolic velocity were seen immediately after HIFU exposure for intensities between 1.08 and 2.75 kW cm⁻². Similar damage to the adventitia has been reported by Henderson et al. [20] when using 1.54 MHz ultrasound exposures. Seket et al. [22] studied the effect of a 5.7-MHz interstitial probe operating at 40 W cm⁻² (unfocused) on porcine liver. For vessels smaller than 2 mm in diameter, they found damage (dilation, congestion and oedema), whereas larger vessels were preserved.

HIFU Sources and Equipment

A clinical HIFU system can be regarded as being comprised of two parts, one concerned with treatment delivery (principally the treatment head and its associated electronics), and the other being the treatment guidance and monitoring component.

The therapy ultrasound beam is produced from a high power piezoelectric transducer. This may, for example, be made from a piezoceramic such as lead zirconate titanate (PZT), or from a piezocomposite. Focusing can be achieved in a number of ways. A plane transducer can be used if fronted by an appropriate lens. This has the advantage that interchanging lenses will provide a range of focal lengths, but has the disadvantage that the lens may attenuate the sound energy. Most usually, the piezoelectric material is shaped into a spherical bowl, which, in turn, may be divided into a number of elements. If the bowl is driven uniformly across its surface a single, fixed focus is created, whereas careful phasing of the drive voltage applied to individual elements can allow variation in the shape and/or position of the focal volume. Division of the transducer face into many elements allows the possibility of using some of the individual elements in dual imaging and therapy mode in such a way that the head can be used for both guidance and treatment without the need to incorporate a separate imaging probe.

Another approach, used in HIFU exposure of the brain, is to mount a number of independent transducers on a former in the shape of a spherical bowl. For transrectal probes, the available geometry dictates that the therapy head is in the shape of a truncated sphere (Fig. 5.4).

The ultrasound frequency used depends largely on the target depth and on the size of the region to be ablated. For a given transducer diameter, increasing the frequency decreases the size of the focal spot, while at a fixed frequency, reducing the diameter elongates the focus. The approximately linear dependence of attenuation on frequency means that, at the lowest frequencies, the most energy reaches the target, but the absorption is the lowest. Choice of frequency is thus necessarily a compromise between the competing requirements of attenuation in overlying tissues and absorption in the target volume. The ultrasound intensity used clinically to ablate tissue varies with the application. In reading the literature, it is necessary to understand the clear distinction between the free-field focal intensity (that measured in a water bath) and the so-called in situ focal intensity (the local intensity at the focal point at the target, calculated after taking into account the attenuation of the beam by the overlying tissues). Quoted in situ intensities for HIFU treatments vary between $1–2$ kW cm^{-2} at 4 MHz and $5–20$ kW cm^{-2} at 0.8 MHz [23].

In the case of ultrasound-guided HIFU (USgHIFU), treatment monitoring and guidance is achieved using an imaging transducer that is mounted within, and integral to, the therapy ultrasound treatment head. With magnetic resonance imaging-guided HIFU (MRgHIFU or MRgFUS), this aspect is achieved using the MR scanner, with the MR compatible therapy transducer usually being mounted within a suitably converted scanner bed. Broadly speaking, there are two categories of clinical HIFU devices depending on the placing of the treatment head [1, 23]. Extracorporeal devices use sources that are sited outside the body, the sound beam being directed through the intact skin and overlying tissues to reach the target. Intracavitary devices are introduced into appropriate spaces in the body. Thus, for example, transrectal HIFU is used for treatments of the prostate, and a transoesophageal approach is being investigated for cardiac applications.

Both US and MRI (magnetic resonance imaging) have been used to provide HIFU image guidance and treatment monitoring. Each has its own advantages and disadvantages. MRI provides excellent anatomical detail, and MR thermometry based

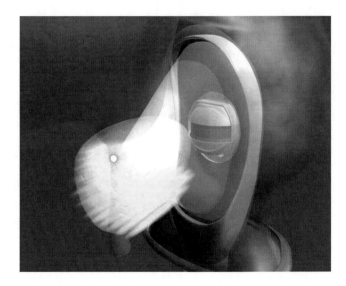

Fig. 5.4 Transrectal transducer for HIFU treatment of the prostate. In this probe, the truncated sphere can be rotated and translated as shown in order to facilitate the ablation of a clinically relevant volume (Image courtesy of E. Blanc)

Fig. 5.5 Real-time display obtained during magnetic resonance image-guided high-intensity focused ultrasound (MRgFUS) treatment of a uterine fibroid. The local thermal dose is calculated during each exposure and is displayed as *blue voxels* once the level of 240 equiv. min at 43°C is reached. This is taken as the threshold for thermal ablation. The voxels displayed in *green* have not yet reached or achieved this level

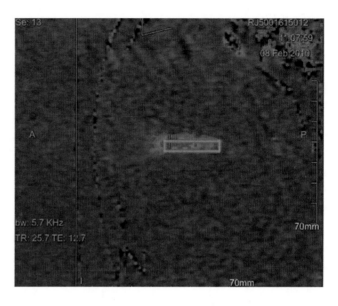

on proton resonance shift is well established [24, 25]. This allows quasi-real-time estimation of thermal dose during treatment (Fig. 5.5). However, good spatial resolution is only achieved at the expense of temporal resolution, and thus, while thermal dose provides useful feedback about treatment success locally, this is a voxel average, and as such only serves as a guide to the local thermal dose (unless appropriate corrections are made). For homogeneous tissues, this proves to be a good indicator of tissue ablation. The temporal and spatial resolution of an ultrasound image is, in general, better than that of MR images, but imaging behind gas and bone is not possible. Thus, the rib cage, for example, can make ultrasound imaging of tumours within the liver difficult. Large blood vessels are easy to visualise using Doppler ultrasound, thus facilitating their direct targeting at the start of HIFU ablation. This is sometimes a useful technique as it reduces the blood flow within a tumour, rendering it easier to achieve thermal ablation within the target volume. Ultrasound thermometry is still experimental and has not yet gained clinical acceptance. This technique relies on the fact that the speed of sound is temperature-dependent, and so there is an apparent shift in echo position when images obtained before and after heating are compared. Both ultrasound and MRI offer the possibility of elastographic imaging in which the increased stiffness of thermally ablated tissue may be visualised [26, 27]. This has not as yet been used clinically for this purpose, but appears to be a promising technique.

Treatment Delivery

A single HIFU exposure from a static transducer usually results in an ellipsoid of damage at the focus. A considerable amount of effort is being expended in designing transducers that give extended focal regions of different shapes. In order to ablate clinically relevant volumes, it is necessary to "paint out" regions by moving the focal region in such a way that confluent tissue ablation is obtained. This can be achieved by placing individual lesions side-by-side or in randomised (computer generated) patterns, or by scanning the transducer over predetermined trajectories. The most common patterns used are linear scans and spirals. Thermal models can be used to decide the combination of ultrasound focal intensity and scan speed required to produce the desired effect.

The usual treatment protocol for malignant tumours provides for ablation of the visible tumour plus a normal tissue boundary region that extends as far as the margin that would be resected by a surgeon were he to remove the tumour (Fig. 5.6).

The volume to be ablated is defined during the planning phase of treatment and is divided into slices 5–10 mm apart, depending on the focal geometry. Slices are then ablated sequentially until the whole treatment volume has been covered.

In many ways, tumours of the abdomen (such as those in the liver or kidney) provide the greatest challenge for successful HIFU treatments. The presence of the rib cage, cardiac and respiratory motion and its rich blood supply all mitigate against easy delivery of an ultrasound-based thermal therapy. Despite this, successful treatments of primary and metastatic hepatic tumours, and of renal tumours have been reported [28–31]. The ribs present a barrier to an ultrasound beam. As is well known from diagnostic ultrasound, they cast a shadow, rendering structures lying distally unimagable. With therapeutic exposures, the concern is, first, that the rib cage blocks energy that would otherwise contribute to focal heating and, second, that the high absorption at the bone surface and high local intensities created by reflection of the beam will give rise to

Fig. 5.6 Schematic showing the typical treatment plan for HIFU ablation of malignant tumours

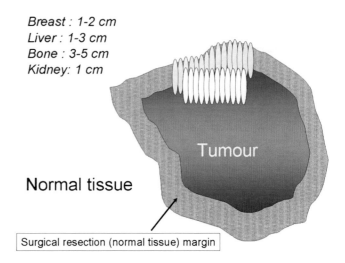

Breast : 1-2 cm
Liver : 1-3 cm
Bone : 3-5 cm
Kidney: 1 cm

Tumour

Normal tissue

Surgical resection (normal tissue) margin

damage in the adjacent soft tissue and the rib itself. A number of solutions have been proposed. Increasing the diameter of the therapy transducer spreads the ultrasound beam and reduces the incident energy density in the plane of the ribs. This is most likely to be useful for deep-seated tumours. An alternative strategy, that can be used when a multi-element transducer is used, is to switch off those elements from which the field will impinge directly on the rib – this reduces the radiating area of the transducer, but the power from the remaining elements may be increased to compensate for this. This has been proposed by a number of authors [32, 33]. In some cases, an acoustic window may be found by angling the transducer upwards below the rib cage. Zhu et al. [31] have reported the treatment of hepatocellular carcinoma following the resection of ribs to provide such an acoustic window. For 16 stage II–IV patients, the survival rate was 100% at 1 year and dropped to 55.6% 5 years after HIFU treatment.

Respiratory motion is considerable in the liver, with excursions of several centimetres being possible. In order to avoid smearing of the HIFU focus, either the exposure can be triggered to occur at the same point in the breathing cycle each time or movement can be reduced by breath holding – either with the co-operation of the conscious patient or by double intubation of the lungs by the anaesthetist, which allows selective breath hold on the lobe nearest to the liver [29].

Wu et al. [34] have shown that the use of transarterial chemoembolisation (TACE) prior to HIFU treatment of primary hepatocellular carcinoma (HCC) results in a good outcome. The embolisation reduces the blood supply to the tumour, allowing lower output powers to be used to achieve ablation. In the absence of TACE, repeated exposure of an obvious blood vessel in the region to be treated prior to volume ablation may result in a reduction of the Doppler signal (signifying a lowered blood flow) during USgHIFU and more successful ablation.

The ability of HIFU to produce highly localised trackless damage makes it an excellent candidate for treatment of conditions in the brain. The outstanding obstacle to such treatments is the poor transmission of ultrasound through the skull. Early brain HIFU treatments required the creation of an acoustic window by removing some of the skull bone [35, 36]. Sophisticated image-processing techniques are required to produce a tightly focused ultrasound beam deep within the brain without causing too much heating at the skull surface. Two MRgHIFU systems for brain treatments are currently being investigated (Fig. 5.7). The therapy ultrasound beam is generated from large area hemispherical sources on which many transducer elements are mounted. In this way, the energy density at the cranial surface can be kept to a minimum, thus reducing heating effects. Scattering of the sound beam during transit through the skull destroys the focused nature of the beam, and so time reversal or phase offsetting techniques are used to restore the energy concentration at the focus [36–38].

Clinical Systems

Extracorporeal Approach

Both US and MRI have been used to guide clinical extracorporeal HIFU treatments. The extracorporeal approach for abdominal tumours requires the focal region to be situated up to ~18 cm from the transducer, in order that deep-seated organs may be targeted. Frequencies between 0.8 and 1.7 MHz are commonly used for these treatments.

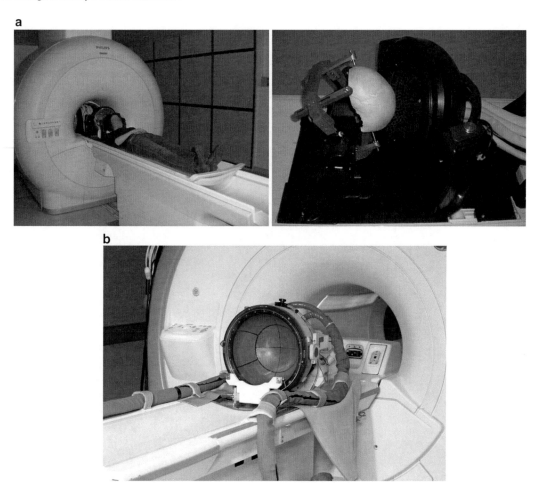

Fig. 5.7 Magnetic resonance (MR) imaging-guided systems for HIFU treatment of the brain. (**a**) System developed by SuperSonic Imagine (Aix-en-Provence, France) (Images courtesy of Claude Cohen-Bacrie and Laurent Marsac). (**b**) System developed by InSightec (ExAblate, Tirat Carmel, Israel)

Figure 5.8 shows a commercially available USgHIFU system often used for treatment of abdominal organs, and highlights the different components (JC 200, Chongqing HAIFU, Chongqing, China). The insert shows the therapy transducer with an imaging probe in its centre. The two transducers are aligned such that the imaging plane is centred on the therapy beam axis. In this device, the treatment head (a single element design) is positioned under the bed on which the patient lies. Acoustic coupling is achieved using a temperature-controlled water bath in which the treatment head sits. The treatment head can be moved under computer control to position the HIFU focus as required within the target volume. In this system, treatment is delivered either as individual exposures (shots) placed side-by-side or as linear scans such that confluent volumes are ablated. For USgHIFU, successful ablation shows up as a hyperechoic region on the US image (Fig. 5.9). This system has been widely used for the treatment of malignant tumours of the liver (both primary and secondary), kidney, breast and pancreas and for uterine fibroids.

Figure 5.10 shows the ExAblate system from InSightec (Tirat Carmel, Israel). This was the first commercially available MRgHIFU system. It differs from the US-guided system described above in that the therapy ultrasound source (also situated in the treatment couch) is designed to be MR compatible and comprises a multi-element phased array that allows electronic scanning of the focal volume. This system has been used in extensive clinical trials to investigate the role of HIFU in the treatment of uterine fibroids. In this system, individual "shots" are delivered, each in a position defined by a computerised treatment plan, until the desired volume has been "painted out."

Fig. 5.8 Extracorporeal ultrasound-guided HIFU system (Chongqing HAIFU JC 200, Chongqing, China) used for abdominal and bone treatments. The *inset* shows the therapy head (*orange*) with a central imaging probe (*green*) (Image courtesy of Professor Z. Wang)

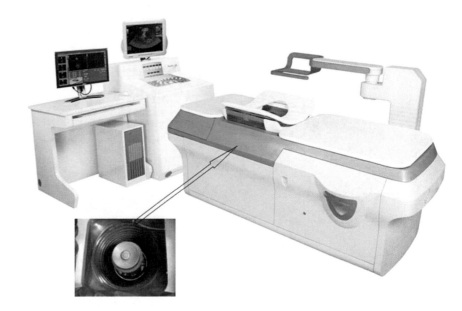

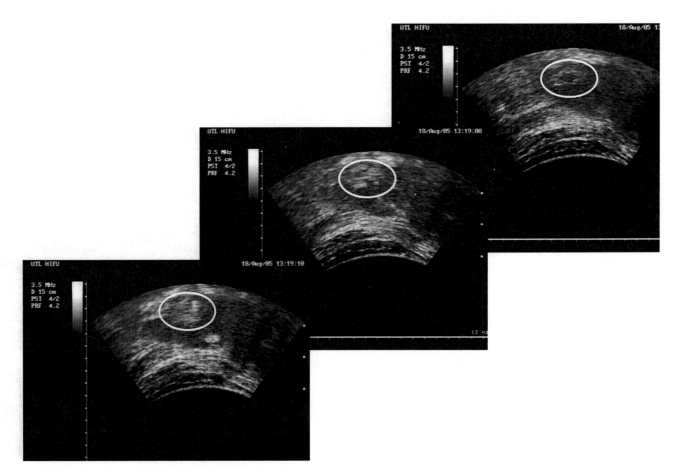

Fig. 5.9 With ultrasound-guided HIFU, the achievement of thermal ablation is currently indicated during clinical applications by the appearance of hyperechoic regions at the focus. In this figure, the ultrasound images for a sequence of exposures are shown with the build-up in area of hyperechoic regions (Image courtesy of Dr. Tom Leslie)

Fig. 5.10 The ExAblate extracorporeal system (InSightec, Tirat Carmel, Israel) (Image courtesy of Y. Medan; photo copyright InSightec Ltd.)

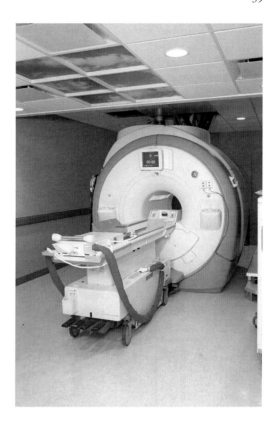

Transrectal Approach

While many patients with abdominal tumours have been treated with extracorporeal HIFU, disappointingly, with the exception of those with uterine fibroids, few have participated in properly designed prospective clinical trials. This is not the case for HIFU treatment of prostate cancer delivered transrectally. Given the prevalence and excellent record of transrectal ultrasound (TRUS) for imaging and diagnosis, interstitial USgHIFU was the natural route to follow for this application. Two clinical devices have been widely used to-date. These are the Ablatherm (EDAP TMS, Vaulx-en-Velin, France) and the Sonablate (Focus Surgery Inc., Indianapolis, Indiana) (Fig. 5.11). Conceptually, these devices are very similar, consisting of a spoon-shaped treatment head mounted on a probe that can be inserted per rectum. The HIFU and imaging transducers are mounted within the truncated spherical bowl that forms the spoon. The Sonablate transducer is double-sided, giving the potential to treat at two different focal lengths. Whole or partial gland ablations are carried out by placing ellipsoidal lesions side-by-side, taking care to achieve confluent damage while sparing the neurovascular bundles. Accurate imaging of focal prostate disease is difficult, and so whole gland treatments are most common in the absence of multiple biopsies. A number of application-specific extracorporeal devices have been developed. Theraclion (Paris, France) has produced a system specifically for treating thyroid disease, and this is currently in clinical trials (Fig. 5.12). Chongqing HAIFU (Chongqing, China) has developed a hand-held device for treating cervicitis and vulvar disease. Catheter-based devices for the treatment of oesophageal and biliary duct cancers are currently also under development, but are not as yet commercially available.

Clinical Overview

A major obstacle to more widespread clinical acceptance of HIFU at the current time is the lack of long-term clinical trials involving large numbers of patients. While many people have now been treated with HIFU around the world (>800,000), only a very small proportion of these have been under clinical trial conditions. Many of these patients have been treated in the growing number of HIFU centres in China. That said, prospective trials exist for the treatment of prostate cancer [39–42] and of uterine fibroids [43–47], with some small scale trials having been published for treatments of primary and secondary

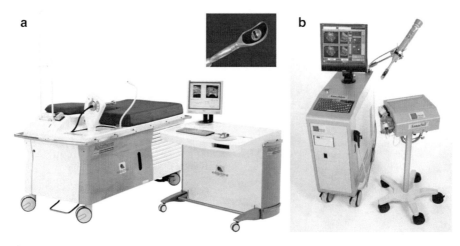

Fig. 5.11 Two transrectal devices for prostate treatments. (**a**) Ablatherm (EDAP TMS, Vaulx-en-Velin, France; image courtesy of E. Blanc). (**b**) Sonablate (Focus Surgery Inc., Indianapolis, Indiana; image courtesy of N. Sanghvi)

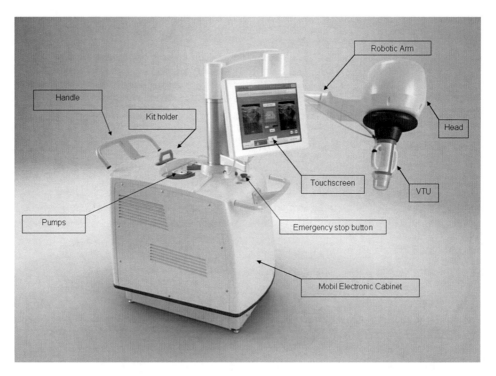

Fig. 5.12 System developed for the treatment of parathyroid disease (Theraclion, Paris, France; image courtesy of F. Lacoste)

liver cancer, and renal cancers [48]. Other clinical reports (for pain relief, breast, pancreas, brain and parathyroid treatments, for example) are largely anecdotal but provide encouraging evidence for further study [9, 34, 49–54].

MRgHIFU has been used in a number of centres for the treatment of uterine fibroids, with more than 4,000 patients having been treated, 3,000 as routine clinical practice [55]. It has been demonstrated that the greater the volume of the fibroid that does not take up MR contrast agent after ablation (non-perfused volume or NPV), the higher the probability of intervention-free follow-up [56]. Morita et al. [46] reported a mean NPV of 60% immediately after treatment, which agrees well with the $47 \pm 13\%$ at 6 months reported by Mikami et al. [45]. In a multi-centre trial, 71% of women treated on the ExAblate system under light conscious sedation, achieved the targeted symptomatic reduction (ten points on the symptom severity scale) at 6 months and 52% at 12 months [44]. Similar results have been reported by other authors.

Rabinovici et al. [57] have reported on successful pregnancies following HIFU treatments of uterine fibroids. Adverse events reported are generally transient and include mild skin burn, nausea, short-term buttock or leg pain, and transient sciatic nerve palsy, although one case of severe skin burn has been reported [58]. Ultrasound guidance of fibroid treatments is now also in clinical trial.

The vast majority of treatments of malignant tumours have been carried out under ultrasound guidance. Clinical trials of the HIFU treatment of hepatocellular carcinoma (HCC) have been published. Wu et al. [59] reported treatment of 55 patients with cirrhosis, 51 of whom had unresectable HCC, with mean tumour size 8.14 cm (range 4–14 cm). Of these patients (15 Stage II, 16 stage III$_A$, 24 stage III$_C$), the stage II patients had better outcome than the others. Overall survival rate at 6 months was 86.1%, at 12 months 61.5% and at 18 months was 35.3%. Wu et al. [50] have used transarterial chemoembolisation (TACE) 2–4 weeks prior to HIFU treatment of stage IV$_A$ HCC patients and found at 6 months that the survival increased from 13.2% for TACE alone to 85.4% for TACE+HIFU, and while there were no survivors for TACE alone at 1 year, 42.9% of TACE+HIFU patients were alive. Metastases in the liver have also been targeted with some success [28, 60].

Summary

HIFU has had a slow gestation. From its first clinical use in the 1950s for the treatment of Parkinsonism [35, 61] to the present day, there have been a number of developments. While the basics of HIFU treatments remain very much the same, technological advances have allowed the development of real-time imaging (MR and US) guidance, and of multi-element phased array sources which provide greater accuracy of treatment targeting and monitoring. This has facilitated the more widespread use of HIFU. While the evidence for clinical efficacy is accruing slowly, routine treatments using HIFU are unlikely to become more commonplace until large-scale prospective clinic trials with long-term follow-up are available.

References

1. ter Haar GR, Coussios C-C. High intensity focused ultrasound: past, present and future. Int J Hyperthermia. 2007;23:85–7.
2. Sapareto SA, Dewey WC. Thermal dose determination in cancer therapy. Int J Radiat Oncol Biol Phys. 1984;10:787–800.
3. Goldberg SN, Solbiati L, Gazelle GS, Tanabe KK, Compton CC, Muller PR. Treatment of intra hepatic malignancy with radio-frequency ablation: pathologic correlation in 16 patients. AJR Am J Roentgenol. 1998;170:1023–8.
4. Thompson S. Pathologic analysis of photothermal and photochemical effects of laser-tissue interactions. Photochem Photobiol. 1991;53:825–35.
5. Farjado LF, Egbort B, Marmor J, Hahn GM. Effects of hyperthermia on a malignant tumour. Cancer. 1980;45:613–23.
6. Yatvin MB, Cramp WA. Role of cellular membranes in hyperthermia: some observations and theories reviewed. Int J Hyperthermia. 1993;9(2):165–85.
7. Nikfarjam M, Vijayaragavan M, Christophi C. Mechanisms of focal heat destruction of liver tumours. J Surg Res. 2005;127:208–23.
8. Pond JB. The role of heat in the production of ultrasonic focal lesions. J Acoust Soc Am. 1970;47:1607–11.
9. Wu F, Wang ZB, Cao YD, et al. Heat fixation of cancer cells ablated with high intensity focused ultrasound in patients with breast cancer. Am J Surg. 2006;192:179–84.
10. Chen L, Rivens I, ter Haar G, Riddler S, Hill CR, Bensted JP. Histologic changes in rat liver tumours treated with high intensity focused ultrasound. Ultrasound Med Biol. 1993;19:67–74.
11. ter Haar GR, Robertson D. Tissue destruction with focused ultrasound in vivo. Eur Urol. 1993;23 Suppl 1:8–11.
12. Wu F, Chen WZ, Bai JB, et al. Pathological changes in human malignant carcinoma treated with high intensity focused ultrasound. Ultrasound Med Biol. 2001;27:1099–106.
13. Rowland IJ, Rivens I, Chen L, et al. MRI study of hepatic tumours following high intensity focused ultrasound surgery. Br J Radiol. 1997;70:144–53.
14. Chen L, Bouley D, Yuh E, Arceuiol D, Butts K. Study of focused ultrasound tissue damage using MRI and histology. J Magn Reson Imaging. 1999;10:146–53.
15. Delon-Martin C, Vogt C, Chignier E, Guers C, Chapelon JY, Cathignol D. Venous thrombosis generation by means of high intensity focused ultrasound. Ultrasound Med Biol. 1995;21:113–9.
16. Hynynen K, Chung AH, Colucci V, Jolesz FA. Potential adverse effects of high intensity focused ultrasound exposure on blood vessels in vivo. Ultrasound Med Biol. 1996;22:193–201.
17. Ishikawa T, Okai T, Sasaki K, et al. Functional and histological changes in rat femoral arteries by HIFU exposure. Ultrasound Med Biol. 2003;29(10):1471–7.
18. Rivens IH, Rowland IJ, Denbow M, Fisk NM, ter Haar GR, Leach MO. Vascular occlusion using focused ultrasound surgery for use in fetal medicine. Eur J Ultrasound. 1999;9:89–97.
19. Ichihara M, Sasaki K, Umemura S-I, Kushima M, Okai T. Blood flow occlusion via ultrasound image-guided high-intensity focused ultrasound and its effect on tissue perfusion. Ultrasound Med Biol. 2007;33(3):452–9.

20. Henderson PW, Lewis GK, Shaikh N, et al. A portable high-intensity focused ultrasound device for noninvasive venous ablation. J Vasc Surg. 2010;51:707–11.
21. Ishikawa T, Okai T, Sasaki K, et al. Sequential changes in rat femoral artery blood flow and tissue degeneration after exposure to high-intensity focused ultrasound. J Med Ultrasonics. 2008;35(4):177–82.
22. Seket B, Lafon C, Salomir R, et al. Morphological analysis of the interstitial ultrasonic ablation in porcine liver in vivo. Eur Surg Res. 2008;41(1):24–32.
23. ter Haar GR, Coussios C-C. High intensity focused ultrasound: physical principles and devices. Int J Hyperthermia. 2007;23:89–104.
24. Rivens IH, Shaw A, Civale J, Morris H. Treatment monitoring and thermometry for therapeutic focused ultrasound. Int J Hyperthermia. 2007;23:121–39.
25. Rieke V, Butts PK. MR thermometry. J Magn Reson Imaging. 2008;27:376–90.
26. Curiel L, Souchon R, Rouviere O, Gelet A, Chapelon J-Y. Elastography for the follow-up of high intensity focused ultrasound prostate cancer treatment: initial comparison with MRI. Ultrasound Med Biol. 2005;31:1461–8.
27. Sinkus R, Lorenzen J, Schrader D, Lorenzen M, Dargatz M, Holz D. High-resolution tensor MR elastography for breast tumour detection. Phys Med Biol. 2000;45:1649–64.
28. Illing RO, Kennedy JE, Wu F, et al. The safety and feasibility of extracorporeal high-intensity focused ultrasound (HIFU) for the treatment of liver and kidney tumours in a Western population. Br J Cancer. 2005;93:890–5.
29. Leslie TA, Kennedy JE. High intensity focused ultrasound in the treatment of abdominal and gynaecological diseases. Int J Hyperthermia. 2007;23:173–82.
30. Park MY, Jung SE, Cho SH, et al. Preliminary experience using high intensity focused ultrasound for treating liver metastasis from colon and stomach cancer. Int J Hyperthermia. 2009;25(3):180–8.
31. Zhu H, Zhou K, Zhang L, et al. High intensity focused ultrasound (HIFU) therapy for local treatment of hepatocellular carcinoma: role of partial rib resection. Eur J Radiol. 2009;72:160–6.
32. Civale J, Clarke RL, Rivens IH, ter Haar GR. The use of a segmented transducer for rib sparing in HIFU treatments. Ultrasound Med Biol. 2006;32:1753–61.
33. Hand JW, Shaw A, Sadhoo N, Rajagopal S, Dickinson RJ, Gavrilov LR. A random phased array device for delivery of high intensity focused ultrasound. Phys Med Biol. 2009;54(19):5675–93.
34. Wu F, Wang Z, Chen W-Z, et al. Extracorporeal high intensity focused ultrasound ablation in the treatment of patients with large hepatocellular carcinoma. Ann Surg Oncol. 2007;11:1061–9.
35. Fry WJ, Mosberg Jr WH, Barnard JW, Fry FJ. Production of focal destructive lesions in the central nervous system with ultrasound. J Neurosurg. 1954;11:471–8.
36. Tanter M, Pernot M, Aubry J-F, Montaldo G, Marquet F, Fink M. Compensating for bone interfaces and respiratory motion in high-intensity focused ultrasound. Int J Hyperthermia. 2007;23:141–51.
37. Hynynen K, Clement G. Clinical applications of focused ultrasound – the brain. Int J Hyperthermia. 2007;23:193–202.
38. MacDannold N, Clement G, Black P, Jolesz F, Hynynen K. Transcranial magnetic resonance imaging – guided focused ultrasound surgery of brain tumors: initial findings in 3 patients. Neurosurgery. 2010;66:323–32.
39. Illing RI, Chapman A. The clinical applications of high intensity focused ultrasound in the prostate. Int J Hyperthermia. 2007;23:183–91.
40. Uchida T, Ohkusa H, Yamashita H, et al. Five years experience of transrectal high-intensity focused ultrasound using the Sonablate device in the treatment of localized prostate cancer. Int J Urol. 2006;13:228–33.
41. Blana A, Thüroff S, Murat FJ, et al. First analysis of the long-term results with transrectal HIFU in patients with localised prostate cancer. Eur Urol. 2008;53:1194–203.
42. Rove KO, Sullivan KF, Crawford ED. High intensity focused ultrasound: ready for prime time? Urol Clin N Am. 2010;37:27–35.
43. Tempany CM, Stewart EA, McDannold N, et al. MR imaging guided focused ultrasound surgery of uterine leiomyomas: a feasibility study. Radiology. 2003;226:897–905.
44. Stewart EA, Rabinovici J, Tempany CM, et al. Clinical outcomes of focused ultrasound surgery for the treatment of uterine fibroids. Fertil Steril. 2006;85:22–9.
45. Mikami K, Murakami T, Okada A, Osuga K, Tomoda K, Nakamura H. Magnetic resonance imaging-guided focused ultrasound ablation of uterine fibroids: early clinical experience. Radiat Med. 2008;26:198–205.
46. Morita Y, Ito N, Hikida H. Non-invasive magnetic resonance imaging guided focused ultrasound treatment for uterine fibroids – early experience. Eur J Obstet Gynecol Reprod Biol. 2008;139:199–203.
47. Zaher S, Gedroyc WM, Regan L. Patient suitability for magnetic resonance guided focused ultrasound surgery of uterine fibroids. Eur J Obstet Gynecol Reprod Biol. 2009;143:98–102.
48. Wu F, Wang ZB, Chen WZ, Bai J, Zhu H, Qiao TY. Preliminary experience using high intensity focused ultrasound for the treatment of patients with advanced stage renal malignancy. J Urol. 2003;170:2237–40.
49. Klingler HC, Susani M, Seip R, Mauermann J, Sanghvi N, Marberger MJ. A novel approach to energy ablative therapy of small renal tumours: laparoscopic high-intensity focused ultrasound. Eur Urol. 2008;53:810–8.
50. Wu F, Wang Z, Zhu H, et al. Feasibility of US-guided high-intensity focused ultrasound treatment in patients with advanced pancreatic cancer: initial experience. Radiology. 2005;236:1034–40.
51. Wu F, Wang Z, Cao Y-D, et al. Expression of tumor antigens and heat shock protein 70 in breast cancer cells after high intensity focused ultrasound ablation. Ann Surg Oncol. 2007;14:1237–42.
52. Hynynen K, Pomeroy O, Smith DN, et al. MR imaging-guided focused ultrasound surgery of fibroadenomas in the breast: a feasibility study. Radiology. 2001;219:176–85.
53. Liberman B, Gianfelice D, Inbar Y, et al. Pain palliation in patients with bone metastases using MR-guided focused ultrasound surgery: a multicenter study. Ann Surg Oncol. 2008;16:140–6.
54. Gianfelice D, Gupta CH, Kucharczyk W, et al. Palliative treatment of painful bone metastases with MR imaging-guided focused ultrasound. Radiology. 2008;249:352–62.

55. Shen S-H, Fennessy F, McDannold N, Jolesz F, Tempany C. Image-guided thermal therapy of uterine fibroids. Semin Ultrasound CT MR. 2009;30:91–104.
56. Rabinovici J, Inbar Y, Revel A, Zalel Y, et al. Clinical improvement and shrinkage of uterine fibroids after thermal ablation by magnetic resonance-guided focused ultrasound surgery. Ultrasound Obstet Gynecol. 2007;30:771–7.
57. Rabinovici J, David M, Fukunishi M, et al. Pregnancy outcome following magnetic resonance guided focused ultrasound surgery (MRgFUS) for conservative treatment of uterine fibroids. Fertil Steril. 2010;93(1):199–209.
58. Leon-Villapalos J, Kaniorou-Larai M, Dziewulski P. Full thickness abdominal burn following magnetic resonance guided focused ultrasound therapy. Burns. 2005;31:1054–5.
59. Wu F, Wang ZB, Chen WZ, et al. Extracorporeal focused ultrasound surgery for treatment of human solid carcinomas: early Chinese clinical experience. Ultrasound Med Biol. 2004;30:245–60.
60. Kennedy JE, Wu F, ter Haar GR, et al. High-intensity focused ultrasound for the treatment of liver tumours. Ultrasonics. 2004;42:931–5.
61. Fry WJ, Fry FJ. Fundamental neurological research and human neurosurgery using intense ultrasound. IRE Trans Biomed Electronics. 1960;ME-7:166–81.

Chapter 6
The Role of Diagnostic Imaging in the Planning and Evaluation of Ablation Techniques

Ashraf Thabet and Debra A. Gervais

Introduction

The ability to guide minimally invasive therapy with imaging has helped foster the rise of interventional oncology in the treatment of cancer. The role of imaging, however, is not only restricted to guiding the intervention. Imaging enables tumor detection and characterization, figures prominently in cancer staging, and is ultimately used in treatment planning and targeting when percutaneous techniques are employed. Among the percutaneous techniques used in cancer treatment, thermal ablation is particularly dependent on high-quality imaging and its accurate interpretation as it is a localized therapy with success dependent on an awareness of the margins and size of the index tumor, as well as its relationship to nearby structures that may be at risk of injury. Regardless of the type of ablative therapy – whether radiofrequency electrodes, cryoprobes, or microwave antennas are used – successful thermal ablation begins with high-quality pretreatment imaging which may take the form of computed tomography (CT), magnetic resonance imaging (MRI), and/or positron emission tomography (PET).

Just as imaging is critical in the planning of thermal ablation, it is also important in assessing treatment efficacy, complications of therapy, and in guiding future treatment. Hence, radiologists who practice thermal ablation and interpret pre- and posttreatment imaging examinations will need to understand the imaging features of successfully treated tumor, of residual tumor, and of the benign ancillary findings that may be confused with treatment failure. Imaging measures of treatment success do overlap among the ablative modalities and their accurate assessment depends on comparison with high-quality pretreatment imaging.

Measures of Treatment Success

The classic hallmark of treatment success in oncologic imaging is reduction in tumor burden, as delineated by reduced tumor number and size [1]. A validated measure of tumor response to systemic therapies is the response evaluation criteria in solid tumor (RECIST), which compares the longest measured diameter of the index tumor on serial imaging examinations to determine whether there has been complete or partial response to therapy, there is stable disease, or whether there is disease progression [2]. Use of RECIST in evaluating the response to thermal ablation is challenging for several reasons. First, successful thermal ablation may produce edema and hemorrhage [1]. Hence, the zone of ablation on follow-up imaging may be larger than the index tumor and may not decrease in size over serial examinations, despite evidence of complete necrosis on biopsy [3]. Second, the zone of ablation is shaped to completely encompass and to be larger than the index tumor to obtain a treated margin that may include microscopic disease that is otherwise invisible on current imaging modalities [3]. Third, a small proportion of ablated tumors may undergo liquefactive necrosis, which may produce a paradoxical increase in size of the zone of ablation [4, 5].

Any assessment of treatment efficacy that strictly depends on tumor size may underestimate the success of thermal ablation; hence, other measures are required. Enhancement on CT or MRI requires delivery of intravenously administered contrast material to tumor. Because thermal ablation produces necrosis with loss of vascular supply, interval loss of enhancement of tumor on posttreatment imaging is a critical imaging hallmark of therapeutic success after ablation [1].

A. Thabet (✉) • D.A. Gervais
Department of Radiology, Massachusetts General Hospital, Boston, MA, USA
e-mail: athabet@partners.org

P.R. Mueller and A. Adam (eds.), *Interventional Oncology: A Practical Guide for the Interventional Radiologist*,
DOI 10.1007/978-1-4419-1469-9_6, © Springer Science+Business Media, LLC 2012

The European Association for the Study of the Liver produced a consensus statement supporting the evaluation of enhancement in the determination of liver tumor viability on imaging [6]. The persistence of enhancement, or the development of areas of enhancement in a zone of ablation where it was previously absent, raises the suspicion of viable tumor. The terms "residual disease" and "recurrent disease" have been used in the literature to describe such areas of enhancement seen on posttreatment imaging, respectively [7, 8].

Iodinated or gadolinium-based contrast agents may be contraindicated in some patients, such as those with renal dysfunction. In addition, enhancement in some cystic tumors may not be easily appreciated, as in cystic renal cell carcinoma. Other imaging measures may be needed in such patients; these may include 18-fluorine fluorodeoxyglucose (FDG) uptake on PET and diffusion-weighted imaging on MRI. In some instances, the radiologist may need to rely on changes in configuration as well as growth in size of the zone of ablation over serial imaging examinations as ways to detect viable tumor. The ultimate goal of follow-up imaging regardless of the modality used is the detection of viable tumor as early as possible, when it is at its smallest.

Liver

Pretreatment Imaging

Thermal ablation in the liver has been extensively described for hepatocellular carcinoma (HCC) as well as liver-dominant metastatic disease, such as from neuroendocrine tumor [9–11]. CT, MRI, and/or combined PET/CT may be helpful and in general, the use of the modality which best depicts the tumor is desired. Cross-sectional imaging prior to thermal ablation serves several purposes. It plays an important role in tumor detection and staging, in some instances providing information sufficient for diagnosis as in the case of HCC, when the classic MRI features are present [12]. Indeed, such imaging findings are sufficient for diagnosis of HCC in the evaluation for liver transplantation [13].

In some instances, however, biopsy may be needed. The noncirrhotic liver is home to many benign masses detectable on imaging that may become confused with malignancy, including focal nodular hyperplasia, sclerosing hemangioma, hepatic adenoma, biliary cystadenoma, and hamartoma. Because these masses may not demonstrate imaging features definite for benignity, biopsy may be indicated to establish a diagnosis in patients without cirrhosis. In addition, in some patients with a known extrahepatic primary malignancy, management may change drastically if no other metastasis has been identified; biopsy may then become critical to staging. When there is ambiguity in the characterization of a hepatic mass, biopsy is considered the reference standard diagnostic strategy, although serial follow-up imaging may be employed in cases where imaging features make suspicion for malignancy very low.

CT or MRI prior to thermal ablation is not only useful for tumor characterization and oncologic staging. As mentioned previously, thermal ablation is a local therapy, and an appreciation of tumor margin and size can be critical to treatment planning and success. A 5- to 10-mm thick margin of normal hepatic parenchyma around the index tumor is generally treated during ablation (Fig. 6.1), in a way similar to the strategy used in surgical resection in which tumor is removed with a rim of normal parenchyma [3, 8, 14]. If such a margin is not obtained, the risk of recurrence may rise as untreated microscopic disease not visible on imaging may grow [3].

In addition to tumor margin and size, the relationship of the mass to adjacent structures is evaluated, including gallbladder, diaphragm, portal and hepatic veins, kidney, and bowel. Hydrodissection may be needed to displace bowel from the ablation zone, preventing thermal injury. Similarly, evaluation of nearby structures may also be important when planning the route of the trajectory of the ablation device; for instance, a hepatic dome tumor may require transgression of the pleural space or even lung when ablation is performed using CT guidance. Knowledge of potential transgression prior to ablation will alert the radiologist to be vigilant about evaluating for pneumothorax during the procedure and to be prepared to treat it if necessary.

Posttreatment Imaging

A critical prerequisite to the evaluation of posttreatment imaging is high-quality pretreatment imaging. Ideally, such imaging is matched by both modality and technique to facilitate comparison and detection of viable tumor. Loss of interval enhancement after ablation is an imaging hallmark of treatment success on CT and MRI [1, 6, 8, 14, 15]; hence, it is useful to document enhancement prior to treatment. Similarly, some tumors may demonstrate uptake of FDG; lack of uptake after ablation on posttreatment PET may then be interpreted as nonviable tumor [1, 3, 11].

Fig. 6.1 Thermal ablation planning computed tomography (CT) in a 62-year-old man with hepatocellular carcinoma. Contrast-enhanced CT scan of the abdomen demonstrates a 1.7 cm × 1.5 cm arterially enhancing mass in segment 4. Typically, the planned margin (*black ring*) is 5–10 mm and is prescribed with respect to the three-dimensional (3D) volume of the tumor

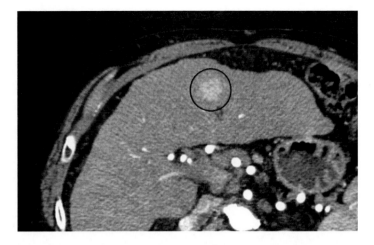

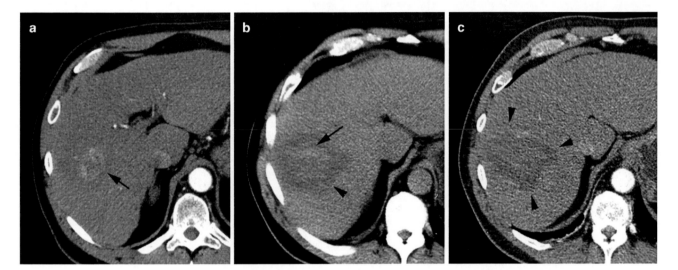

Fig. 6.2 Typical CT findings of treatment success after microwave ablation of a hepatocellular carcinoma in a 58-year-old man. (**a**) CT scan of the abdomen prior to ablation demonstrates a 3.7 cm × 3.6 cm arterially enhancing mass (*arrow*) in segment 8 of the liver. (**b**) Noncontrast CT image 1 month after microwave ablation demonstrates a hypodense zone of ablation (*arrowhead*) with areas of hyperdensity (*arrow*), corresponding to coagulated protein. (**c**) Contrast-enhanced image demonstrates no arterial enhancement in the zone of ablation (*arrowheads*)

There is little consensus among institutions in determining the frequency and length of imaging follow-up after thermal ablation in the liver. Because the goal of follow-up imaging is to detect viable tumor when it is at its smallest, the first follow-up examination may be performed at 1 month. Subsequently, serial imaging may be performed at 3- to 6-month intervals and is generally extended to at least 1 year after treatment as local recurrent disease has been reported as late as 12 months after ablation [1, 11, 14, 16].

The zone of ablation is shaped to encompass the entire index tumor and to include a surrounding margin of at least 5–10 mm of normal parenchyma [1]. The configuration of the zone of ablation will depend on several factors, including ablation method (radiofrequency or RF, cryoablation, microwave), probe design, and the potential "heat-sink" effect from nearby vessels such as portal and hepatic veins [8]. On CT, the zone of ablation is typically hypodense, although areas of hyperattenuation may be seen due to coagulated protein and blood products (Fig. 6.2). In previously enhancing masses, postcontrast CT images will optimally demonstrate no enhancement within the zone. The zone of ablation generally remains stable in size or may involute over serial examinations; an exception is the rare instance of ablation-induced liquefactive necrosis [4].

On MRI, the zone of ablation is typically variable or increased in intensity on T1-weighted images (Fig. 6.3) and will depend on the amount of denatured protein and blood products within the zone [4]. The zone of ablation is also typically T2-hypointense (Figs. 6.3 and 6.4). As in CT, lack of enhancement is an important imaging feature of nonviable tumor. Although these are the most frequent features of nonviable tumor, rarely, some tumors will undergo liquefactive necrosis and, hence, may demonstrate T2 hyperintensity [4]. This is distinguished from viable tumor by observing lack of enhancement.

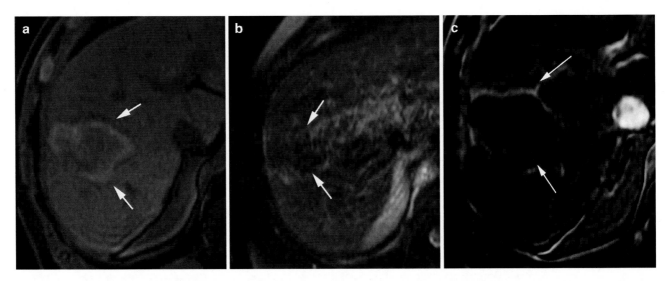

Fig. 6.3 Typical MR findings of treatment success after microwave ablation of a hepatocellular carcinoma in a 58-year-old man (same patient as in Fig. 6.3). (**a**) T1-weighted fat-saturated image from MRI performed 1 month after ablation demonstrates heterogeneity in T1 signal, consistent with coagulated protein (*arrows*). (**b**) T2-weighted fat-saturated image demonstrates hypointensity (*arrows*) in the zone of ablation. (**c**) Subtraction image after administration of gadolinium demonstrates no arterial enhancement (*arrows*) in the zone of ablation

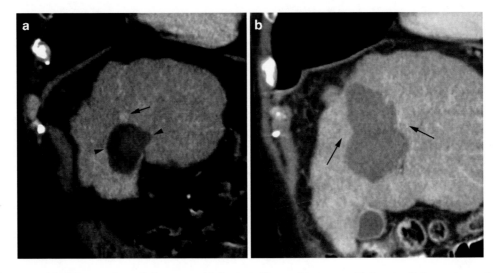

Fig. 6.4 Nodular-type residual disease after radiofrequency ablation in a 62-year-old woman with hepatocellular carcinoma (same patient as in Fig. 6.1). (**a**) Coronal image from CT of the abdomen 9 months after ablation demonstrates a new 1-cm nodular focus of enhancement (*arrow*) along the cranial aspect of the zone of ablation (*arrowheads*). (**b**) No enhancement in the zone of ablation (*arrows*) is seen 1 month after repeat RFA

The most important imaging feature of viable tumor on CT and MRI is the presence of enhancement. At least three patterns have been described after ablation: nodular-type, halo-type, and growth-type. The most common location of residual tumor after thermal ablation is at the periphery of the zone of ablation; this will often appear as nodular areas of enhancement (Fig. 6.4). Halo-type of residual disease manifests as an irregular, thick rim of enhancement around the ablation zone (Fig. 6.5). Finally, gross enlargement of the ablation zone may be documented on serial imaging and may prompt concern for viable tumor.

Other imaging features of viable tumor become particularly helpful when enhancement is not assessable. For instance, some mucinous tumors produce metastases that demonstrate little or no enhancement, as in ovarian carcinoma. Some patients will have renal dysfunction that may prevent the use of either iodinated or gadolinium-based contrast agents. As mentioned previously, CT or MRI may be performed without contrast, and close attention to changes in configuration and size of the zone of ablation may prompt suspicion for viable tumor; biopsy may be indicated in some cases. PET and PET/CT may be helpful in these circumstances; patients with preablation PET demonstrating FDG uptake may undergo follow-up imaging with PET, with interval loss of FDG uptake having been correlated with treatment success (Fig. 6.6) [1, 17, 18]. Assessment of enhancement is generally preferred over PET evaluation in most cases as the sensitivity of PET is diminished for masses less than 1 cm [1].

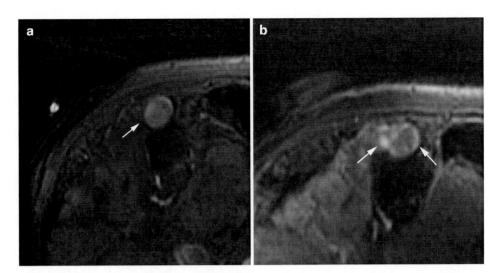

Fig. 6.5 Halo-type residual disease after radiofrequency ablation of hepatocellular carcinoma in a 53-year-old man. (**a**) Magnetic resonance imaging (MRI) demonstrates a 3.1 cm × 2.6 cm arterially enhancing mass (*arrows*) in segment 4 of the liver. (**b**) Follow-up imaging 3 months after ablation demonstrates an irregular rim of enhancement (*arrows*), suspicious for viable tumor. Follow-up imaging after repeat ablation demonstrated no further suspicious enhancement (not shown)

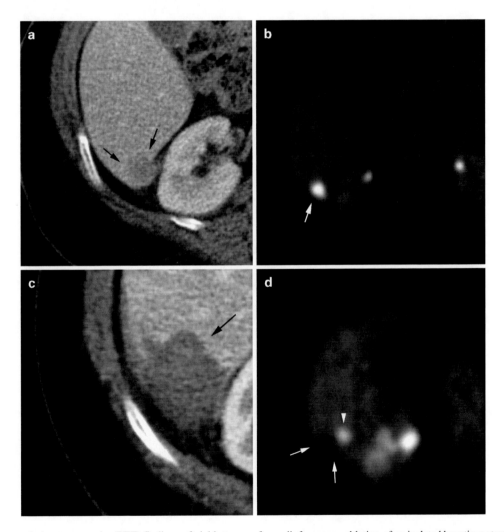

Fig. 6.6 Positron emission tomography (PET) findings of viable tumor after radiofrequency ablation of an isolated hepatic metastasis from ovarian carcinoma in a 53-year-old woman. (**a**) Contrast-enhanced CT image from a combined PET/CT examination demonstrates a 1.3 cm × 1.3 cm metastasis (*arrows*). (**b**) PET image demonstrates FDG uptake (*arrow*) in the metastasis. (**c**) CT image from PET/CT examination performed 1 month after RFA demonstrates a zone of ablation (*arrows*), which appears to encompass the index tumor. (**d**) PET image demonstrates photopenia (*arrows*) in the zone of ablation. However, a focus of FDG uptake (*arrowhead*) is seen along the medial margin, consistent with viable tumor. Follow-up imaging demonstrated interval growth and new metastases in the abdomen (not shown)

Fig. 6.7 Periablational
enhancement after repeat
thermal ablation of hepatocellular carcinoma in a
53-year-old man with hepatocellular carcinoma (same
patient as in Fig. 6.5). There
is a thin rim of enhancement
around the zone of ablation
(*arrowheads*), which is an
ancillary finding, likely due
to inflammation and
hyperemia

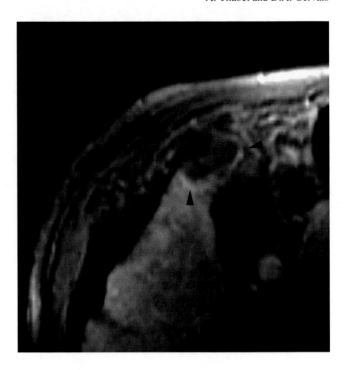

Liver transplantation may offer the best chance for cure in cirrhotic patients with hepatocellular carcinoma; in some cases, thermal ablation may be used as a bridge to transplantation [1]. The Milan criteria have been used to identify patients who may benefit most from transplantation and has been adopted by the United Network of Organ Sharing [19]. The criteria limit tumor burden to a single tumor no larger than 5 cm or to a maximum of three tumors, each no larger than 3 cm [19]. Familiarity with these criteria is important while interpreting pre- and postablation imaging, as these refer to the size of the index tumor, not the size of the zone of ablation [1].

Benign ancillary findings after thermal ablation of liver tumors may be identified on postablation imaging, and awareness of these features is important to avoid interpreting such findings as viable tumor. For example, a thin rim of enhancement on CT or MRI may be noted surrounding the zone of ablation on early follow-up examinations (Fig. 6.7). Such a thin regular rim of periablational enhancement is often due to inflammation and hyperemia; this often resolves within 6 months. It is important to distinguish benign periablational enhancement from the halo-type of residual tumor – the latter is usually thicker (>5 mm) and irregular when compared to the typically thin and regular rim of enhancement due to granulation [1, 8].

Other ancillary findings may include segmental intrahepatic biliary duct dilatation upstream from the zone of ablation [20]. Postablation arterioportal shunting may produce wedge-shaped areas of arterial enhancement peripheral to the ablation zone; this typically resolves in 6 months [16, 20]. Such areas of shunting do not demonstrate washout on portal venous phase images on CT or MR as may be seen with HCC; similarly, T2-hyperintensity in these areas is not expected on MRI, which may otherwise prompt concern for viable tumor.

Some complications of thermal ablation may be detected on follow-up imaging. Pain, fever, and leukocytosis may be secondary to abscess formation, which may occur within the liver or may result from bowel perforation; the incidence is less than 1% [21]. Patients with a bilioenteric anastamosis are at increased risk for hepatic abscess. Injury to intrahepatic bile ducts may lead to formation of biloma, which may even be incidentally detected on follow-up imaging. Other complications noted on follow-up imaging after ablation are rare, occurring in less than 1% of patients and include hepatic infarction, cholecystitis, portal vein thrombosis (of which cirrhosis is a risk factor), and diaphragmatic paresis. Transfusion-dependent intraperitoneal hemorrhage is also rare, occurring in less than 1% of patients. Tract seeding is rare with a reported rate of 0.5% [21]; poor histological differentiation of the tumor and subcapsular location may represent risk factors [22].

Kidney

Pretreatment Imaging

The increasing use of percutaneous thermal ablation in the kidney mirrors the rise in incidentally detected renal cell carcinoma (RCC). Thermal ablation has become an important alternative to surgery in RCC as a large percentage of tumors are found localized to the kidney [23]. In addition, nephron-sparing treatments have become important as tumors are found in patients who are high-risk surgical candidates, have a solitary kidney, renal dysfunction, or who have syndromes which predispose to the development of multiple tumors over a lifetime, e.g., von Hippel Lindau syndrome. Of the available ablation modalities, the greatest experience has been with radiofrequency ablation (RFA) and cryoablation [23].

In general, any solid enhancing renal mass is considered RCC until proven otherwise. However, as more cases of RCC are detected incidentally, greater proportions are detected as a small solid mass locally confined to the kidney. Although the complication rate is low, thermal ablation carries risks; hence, it may be important to document histologically that a mass is in fact RCC prior to treatment. Indeed, up to 25% of solid renal masses smaller than 3 cm may be benign [23, 24]. In addition to benign masses such as oncocytoma or lipid-poor angiomyolipoma, metastases of an extrarenal primary may also be unsuitable for thermal ablation, and biopsy may help make the distinction between a primary and secondary renal malignancy. A percutaneous image-guided biopsy may offer additional benefits as well. The biopsy procedure may offer a chance to simulate the ablation procedure, assessing the sedation requirements of the patient and how the patient handles positioning during the procedure [23].

Review of preablation imaging generally includes assessment of tumor size and margins. Thermal ablation is particularly suited to the American Joint Committee on Cancer stage T1a tumors, that is, those measuring less than 4 cm in size without nodal or distant metastases [23]. Smaller tumors are associated with a higher chance of successful treatment by ablation than the larger ones [7, 23]. Receiver operating characteristic curve analysis have shown that tumors smaller than 4 cm are associated with a 90% probability of achieving complete necrosis, but drops to 63% for tumors measuring up to 5.8 cm [7, 23]. Cryoablation differs from RFA in that the approximate zone of ablation may be monitored in real time as the ice ball is formed [23]. Hence, cryoablation is preferred by some for larger tumors as it may be associated with a lower number of required treatment sessions [23, 25]. In addition, appreciation of tumor margins is important, in an effort to treat the entire tumor [1, 23].

Evaluation of tumor location within the kidney itself is considered during review of preablation imaging. The tumor may be described as exophytic, parenchymal, central, or as mixed, having both central and exophytic components [7, 23]. Tumors with a central component approximate the collecting system, which may raise the risk of injury to these structures during ablation, including development of ureteral and infundibular strictures [23]. A renal mass which closely approximates the central collecting system and ureter may require additional protective maneuvers during ablation, as by using cool 5% dextrose in water (D5W) instilled by drip perfusion through a ureteral stent placed prior to the procedure [24, 26–28]. In addition, proximity to the central renal vasculature may expose the treatment zone to a "heat-sink" effect, raising the risk of incomplete treatment [24]. Nevertheless, there is a debate within the literature as to whether a central component reduces the likelihood of achieving complete necrosis [7, 23, 28]. Evaluation of the relationship of the tumor to other structures, particularly bowel, is also important. Most operators aim for a 1-cm distance between the target tumor and bowel [23]. As a protective maneuver, hydrodissection may be useful in some cases to displace bowel or other organs from the planned treatment zone.

Posttreatment Imaging

As with thermal ablation in the liver, evaluation of treatment efficacy begins with high-quality preablation imaging. This may consist of CT or MRI, ideally performed with contrast. PET and PET/CT currently play little role in the evaluation of RCC, since tumor cells in a large percentage of patients express little GLUT-1 transporters and, hence, may not avidly take up FDG [29, 30]. Moreover, intense urine activity could obscure adjacent small foci of residual tumor activity in those patients whose tumors are FDG-avid.

Although CT techniques vary among institutions, in general, postablation CT may include noncontrast as well as contrast-enhanced images in the nephrographic phase. In addition, excretory-phase images may be helpful to assess for complications involving the collecting system. Coronal reformations may be obtained. Similarly, MR techniques will vary among institutions, but generally may include axial T2-weighted and T2-weighted fat-saturated, axial and coronal dual echo, axial dynamic three-dimensional (3D) gradient-recalled echo before and 20, 70, and 180 s after gadolinium administration, as well as 5 min delayed spoiled gradient-recalled echo images [23]. Whether CT or MR is performed, subtraction images may be useful when assessing areas of enhancement in the ablation zone.

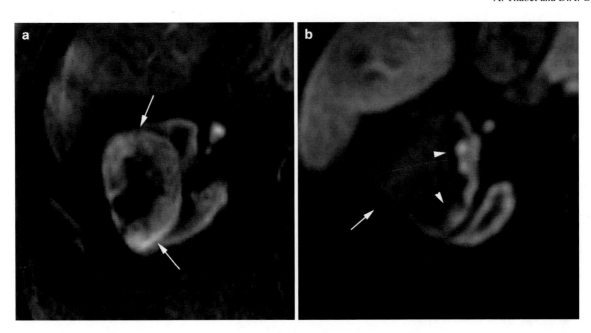

Fig. 6.8 MRI findings of viable tumor 1 month after radiofrequency ablation of biopsy-proven renal cell carcinoma in an 86-year-old woman. (**a**) A 5.6 cm×4.6 cm enhancing mass (*arrows*) is demonstrated in the right kidney. (**b**) One month after RFA, follow-up MRI demonstrates a zone of ablation (*arrow*) with a medial crescentic rim of enhancement (*arrowheads*), consistent with viable tumor

The follow-up imaging protocol will vary among institutions. Generally, the first imaging examination is performed at 1 month after ablation; earlier imaging can be performed if early onset complications are suspected, but inflammatory changes immediately after ablation may obscure evaluation for viable tumor. Subsequently, imaging may be performed at 3- to 6-month intervals for the first year, 6-month intervals for the second year, and yearly afterwards [23]. If posttreatment imaging is equivocal for viable tumor, short-interval imaging may be helpful.

Common to the assessment of both postablation CT and MR, an effort is made to evaluate whether the zone of ablation has encompassed the entire index tumor, in addition to achieving a 5- to 10-mm peripheral margin. The imaging hallmark of treatment success is interval loss of enhancement in the zone of ablation [1, 23]. Viable tumor typically manifests as peripheral nodular and/or crescentic areas of enhancement (Fig. 6.8) [1]. In cystic renal masses containing solid nodules; each nodule is separately assessed for enhancement. In patients who are unable to receive contrast material, attention to the morphology and size of the zone of ablation over serial imaging examinations becomes especially important in the detection of viable tumor [1]. The zone of ablation on CT is typically a hypodense, nonenhancing area; areas of hyperdensity on noncontrast images may be seen and are due to denatured protein and/or hemorrhage (Fig. 6.9). MR findings similarly include variable signal intensity on T1-weighted images due to denatured proteins and blood products, as well as T2-hypointensity [5].

Several benign ancillary findings after renal thermal ablation may be seen on follow-up imaging that may be confused with viable tumor. Soft-tissue stranding in fat adjacent to the zone of ablation may be identified; such stranding is typically oriented parallel to the external contour of the kidney and may coalesce over time to produce a halo appearance (Fig. 6.9) [1, 31]. Inflammatory changes in fat surrounding the kidney may represent fat necrosis, and this may occasionally lead to deviation of the axis of the kidney [1]. A change in renal axis may create a challenge when comparing the zone of ablation across serial imaging examinations; analysis of multiplanar reformations may facilitate comparison [1]. Occasionally, fatty replacement of a portion of the zone of ablation may be observed [1].

In general, the zone of ablation remains stable in size or involutes over successive examinations [1, 32, 33]. Enlargement of the zone of ablation may be considered suspicious for viable tumor. Rarely, the zone of ablation may undergo liquefactive necrosis, which may produce a paradoxical increase in size of the zone of ablation despite histological evidence of necrosis [1, 5]. On MR, liquefactive necrosis is typically T2-hyperintense, as opposed to T2-hypointensity expected in the more commonly encountered coagulation necrosis seen after RF ablation. Fat-fluid levels may also be noted [1, 5]. A feature distinguishing liquefactive necrosis from viable tumor is the lack of enhancement. However, some cases may be difficult to distinguish, and biopsy may be indicated.

Complications requiring additional intervention occur in less than 1% of patients. Hematoma in the subcapsular or perirenal space is not uncommon and rarely requires intervention [1]. Hematoma may be more common after cryoablaton compared to RFA, as the latter may provide protective coagulative effects [23]. Frank hemorrhage in the collecting system

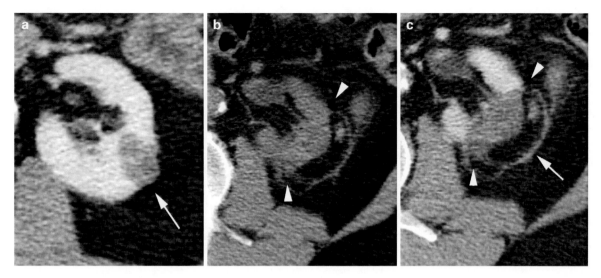

Fig. 6.9 Typical CT findings after thermal ablation of a left renal cell carcinoma (RCC) in a 65-year-old man. (**a**) A 2.4 cm×2.1 cm left renal mass is a biopsy-proven renal cell carcinoma (*arrow*). (**b**) Noncontrast CT 6 months after radiofrequency ablation (RFA) demonstrates a zone of ablation (*arrowheads*) that contains areas of hyperattenuation, corresponding to coagulated protein. (**c**) Contrast-enhanced CT demonstrates the zone of ablation (*arrowheads*) with no evidence of enhancement to suggest viable tumor. Perirenal soft tissue stranding demonstrates a typical halo appearance (*arrow*)

may be observed immediately after ablation; obscuration of the calyceal system by the index tumor has been recognized as a risk factor [1]. Follow-up CT may demonstrate a urinoma, identified as a hypodense fluid collection adjacent to or within the kidney; this may demonstrate T2-hyperintensity on MR. Excretory-phase images may be helpful in confirming excretion of contrast that enters the collection. The finding of trace contrast material within the zone of ablation but outside the collecting system alone on delayed phase images without accumulation of a urinoma may be followed [34]. Such a leak may not develop into a clinically significant urinoma in the absence of distal obstruction and, thus, may not require intervention. Ureteral strictures, however, may occur after thermal ablation and can present with hydronephrosis, which may progress over serial imaging examinations. Similarly, localized caliectasis may be identified, resulting from infundibular stricture. Urinomas and ureteral strictures may require management with percutaneous drainage and nephroureteral catheters or ureteral stents. Preablation imaging is often reviewed to identify patients at risk of such complications so that an attempt to modify that risk can be made, such as by employing ureteral thermoprotective measures as previously described.

Rarely, enhancing nodules may be seen on follow-up imaging along the path of the RF electrode or cryoprobe. Enhancing inflammatory nodules or soft tissue configured in a tram-track appearance may be seen, representing a phenomenon known as "pseudoseeding" [35]. Although these findings may enlarge on early follow-up examinations, these usually resolve [35]. Pseudoseeding has been reported after both RFA and cryoablation and occurs with an incidence of less than just under 2% [35]. Tract seeding with deposition of malignant cells, however, is exceedingly rare; one case has been reported in which a skin deposit developed at the applicator site [36]. Hence, enhancing soft tissue along the applicator tract is not diagnostic for tract seeding. If enlargement of enhancing tissue is noted on successive imaging examinations, biopsy may be helpful to exclude the possibility of viable tumor [1].

Lung

Pretreatment Imaging

Up to 80% of patients with non-small cell lung cancer (NSCLC) are not candidates for surgical resection [37, 38]. New data is emerging describing the efficacy of thermal ablation in the treatment of NSCLC, particularly in stage I patients [37, 39]. In addition, thermal ablation has been used in the treatment of unresectable pulmonary metastases, including colorectal and renal cell carcinoma [40, 41]. Among the ablation modalities available, RFA has been the most extensively studied in treatment of pulmonary malignancy [37, 39, 42].

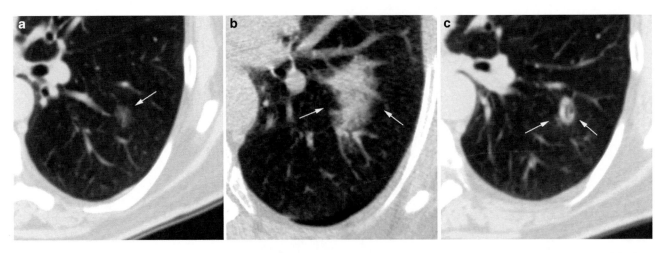

Fig. 6.10 Typical findings after radiofrequency ablation of a bronchoalveolar carcinoma in a 69-year-old woman. (**a**) CT examination of the chest reveals a 1.1 cm×1 cm left lower-lobe ground glass nodule (*arrow*) consistent with biopsy-proven bronchoalveolar carcinoma. (**b**) Immediate postablation CT image demonstrates ground glass opacities surrounding the zone of ablation (*arrows*). (**c**) Follow-up CT scan 1 month after RFA demonstrates resolution of the ground glass opacities (*arrows*)

In addition to tumor detection and staging, preablation imaging is useful in the evaluation of tumor size, margin, and location relative to other critical structures such as the hilum, heart, and bronchi. Indeed, some central masses may be better suited for radiotherapy [39]. However, contiguity with vascular structures is not a strict contraindication to ablation; in one series, RFA was performed on lung tumors directly abutting the descending aorta without complication [43]. One of the key determinants of treatment success in RFA of the lung is the ability to achieve a margin of approximately 8–10 mm [37, 39]. At least 95% of microscopic extension along tumor margin may be treated if such a margin is achieved [44]. Larger tumors are at increased risk of recurrence, and it has been suggested that this may be due to incomplete ablation [39]. In a study by Okuma et al., the most significant risk factor for local recurrence was tumor size of 2 cm or larger [45]. This data suggests that in order to minimize the risk of leaving viable tumor, the entire index tumor would need to be treated, in addition to a margin that may increase the overall ablation diameter by approximately 1.6–2 cm [39].

Hence, particular attention to proximity of critical structures is needed when contemplating lung ablation. Heat-sink effect from nearby vessels may limit RF energy deposition and lead to incomplete treatment [37, 39]. The lung provides an additional challenge to effective RFA – during impedance-controlled RFA, consideration of placement of the active tip of the RF probe within the tumor is important as exposure of active tip to aerated lung may result in incomplete treatment due to high impedances [37]. The risk of pneumothorax presents an additional challenge and, as with lung biopsy [46], may be increased in the presence of emphysema.

Posttreatment Imaging

CT and PET are the imaging workhorses in the follow-up of thermal ablation of the lung [37, 39, 47]. MRI currently plays little role given the paucity of protons in lung tissue that can be imaged, although some investigations have suggested that the use of diffusion-weighted imaging may be helpful in predicting residual disease. In a study by Okuma et al., for instance, in those patients who go on to demonstrate residual disease, the zone of ablation demonstrated a statistically significantly lower apparent diffusion coefficient on MRI performed 3 days after ablation compared to patients who did not recur [48].

Imaging follow-up is particularly important after lung RFA, as recurrence rates as high as 43% have been reported, with cases of recurrent disease detected as far out as 2 years after ablation [37]. Although imaging protocols may vary, in general, the first follow-up CT examination is performed 1 month after ablation, with and without contrast [37, 39]. Subsequently, a CT and PET/CT may be performed alternately every 3–6 months for the first year. The imaging interval may be increased to every 6–12 months afterwards.

A common finding seen immediately after RFA is a peripheral halo of ground glass opacity surrounding the zone of ablation, which typically resolves after 1 month and may represent blood products (Fig. 6.10). Absence of peripheral ground glass opacity may be a predictor of incomplete treatment (Fig. 6.11) [37, 49]. As in thermal ablation in other organs, an

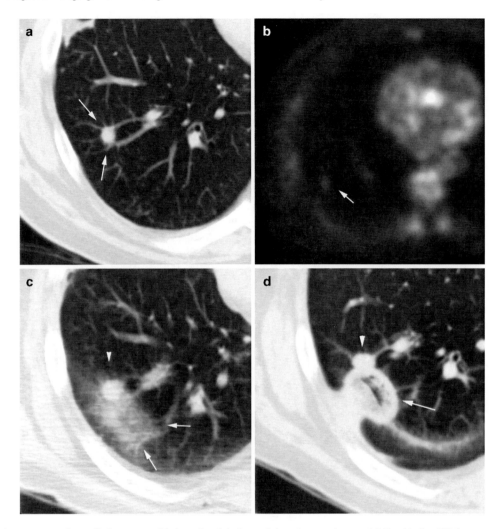

Fig. 6.11 Local recurrence after radiofrequency ablation of a right lower-lobe adenocarcinoma. (**a**) Preablation CT demonstrates a 1-cm right lower-lobe nodule (*arrows*). (**b**) PET scan demonstrates FDG uptake in the nodule (*arrow*). (**c**) CT image performed immediately after RFA demonstrates ground glass opacities (*arrows*) surrounding all but the anterior aspect (*arrowhead*) of the nodule. (**d**) CT scan performed 3 months after RFA demonstrates a nodule (*arrowhead*) anterior to the zone of ablation (*arrow*). One year after repeat RFA, PET/CT demonstrated stable zone of ablation (not shown)

important determinant of viable tumor is enhancement, with recurrence suspected if a change in attenuation greater than 15 Hounsfield units is demonstrated between noncontrast and contrast-enhanced images [37]. It is noteworthy that a thin rim of periablational enhancement may be seen up to 6 months after treatment, considered a result of inflammation and hyperemia [8, 42].

Postablation CT and PET/CT images are reviewed in an effort to detect one of several patterns of recurrence that have been described [37]. A focal area of enhancement in the zone of ablation raises the suspicion for local recurrence and is the most common recurrence pattern (Fig. 6.11). Occasionally, new nodules may develop in the same lobe as the treated tumor and has been termed "intrapulmonary recurrence" [37]. Assessment of hilar and mediastinal lymph nodes is also made to detect nodal recurrence, which may be FDG-avid [37]. Recurrence is classified as "distant," if new nodules are identified in lobes other than that containing the zone of ablation or if new nonhilar, nonmediastinal adenopathy is detected [37].

Iodinated contrast may be contraindicated in some patients due to allergy or renal dysfunction. Hence, enhancement patterns cannot be assessed and other measures of tumor progression are required. In such instances, particular attention is needed in assessing growth of the zone of ablation over serial imaging examinations. PET/CT may also play a useful adjunct in such cases, as persistent or new foci of FDG-avidity raise the suspicion of viable tumor.

Other ancillary findings after pulmonary RFA are important to recognize as benign. Not infrequently, pleural thickening (Fig. 6.12) as well as linear opacities between the pleura and zone of ablation in the path of the RF probe may be seen [42]. Pleural effusions may also be observed (Fig. 6.12) and rarely require treatment [37]. In addition to a thin periablational rim of

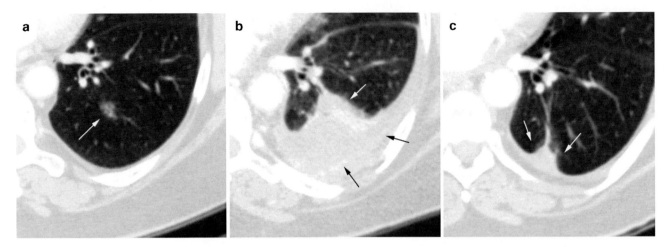

Fig. 6.12 Pleural changes after radiofrequency ablation of a left lower-lobe adenocarcinoma in a 53-year-old woman. (**a**) Preablation CT examination of the chest demonstrates a 1-cm left lower-lobe nodule, which is a biopsy-proven adenocarcinoma. (**b**) CT performed 1 month after RFA demonstrates the zone of ablation (*white arrow*) as well as pleural thickening and small pleural effusion (*black arrows*). (**c**) CT scan performed 9 months later demonstrates interval decrease in size and prominence of the zone of ablation (*arrows*), pleural effusion, and pleural thickening

Fig. 6.13 CT scan performed 1 month after repeat ablation of a right lower-lobe adenocarcinoma (same patient as in Fig. 6.12) demonstrates multiple air lucencies in the zone of ablation (*arrows*)

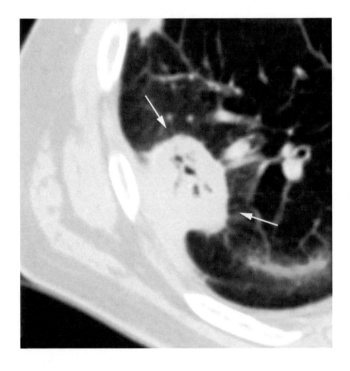

enhancement, the zone of ablation may itself enlarge up to 6 months after ablation [42]. The zone of ablation will appear larger at 1 month compared to immediate postablation images, which is not unexpected given the goal of achieving an 8- to 10-mm margin of treatment [37, 39]. In general, an increase in size after 6 months is considered suspicious for recurrence [42].

In addition, cavitation in the zone of ablation may be observed (Fig. 6.13), which may be more common when treated tumor is located within the inner two-thirds of the lung [42]. Proximity to a segmental bronchus is also associated with an increased likelihood of developing cavitation on follow-up imaging [42]. Cavitation may decrease in size over subsequent imaging examinations [42].

Several complications may occur after pulmonary RFA, some of which may be detected during follow-up imaging. During or immediately after the ablation procedure, a pneumothorax may develop, which may occur in 13–33% of patients, and 50% of patients who develop pneumothorax may require chest tube placement [39]. A chest radiograph may be routinely obtained 2–3 h after the procedure to assess for clinically silent pneumothorax [37]. Intrapulmonary hemorrhage is also a potential complication, occurring in up to 5.9% of patients [50], but is usually self-limited and requires no intervention. In less than 1% of cases, a bronchopleural fistula may also occur. Other complications that may manifest on follow-up imaging include phrenic nerve injury and pneumonia.

Other Organs

The number of reports in the literature describing thermal ablation in other organs is growing. For example, some investigators have described ablation of metastases to the adrenal gland, including from HCC, as well as of functioning adrenal adenomas [1, 15, 51]. Other targets of ablation include lymph nodes, peritoneal nodules, thyroid nodules, and breast carcinoma [52, 53]. The role of imaging before and after ablation is similar to that described above. Preablation imaging is useful in tumor detection, margin characterization, and assessment of surrounding structures, whereas postablation imaging is used to assess treatment efficacy including assessment of enhancement, growth of the ablation zone, and if applicable, FDG-avidity on PET. Further investigation is required regarding the role of thermal ablation in these organs, as well as in further defining the imaging algorithm for follow-up.

Conclusion

As thermal ablation increasingly becomes a viable alternative to surgery in the treatment of visceral malignancies such as primary and secondary hepatic malignancy, renal cell carcinoma, non-small cell lung cancer, and pulmonary metastases, radiologists increasingly need to better understand the role of imaging in ablation planning as well as in treatment follow-up. CT, MRI, and PET contribute greatly to ablation planning and follow-up, and only when there is a clear understanding of the role these modalities play will the radiologist be able to select the correct modality and interpret the imaging examination appropriately.

Preablation imaging may be used in tumor detection, characterization, and staging as well as in the evaluation of the 3D volume of the tumor and its relationship to nearby structures, which will help the interventional radiologist to formulate a treatment plan that will maximize the likelihood of achieving complete tumor necrosis while simultaneously minimizing the risk of complication. Postablation imaging is crucial to the evaluation of treatment efficacy. Familiarity with the typical imaging features of successfully ablated tumor, viable tumor, as well as benign ancillary findings that may be confused with viable tumor is essential in maximizing the radiologist's contribution to the care of the ablation patient and in assisting the oncologic team in guiding therapy and revising prognosis.

References

1. Thabet A, Kalva S, Gervais D. Percutaneous image-guided therapy of intra-abdominal malignancy: imaging evaluation of treatment response. Abdom Imaging. 2009;34:593–609.
2. Therasse P, Arbuck SG, Eisenhauer EA, et al. New guidelines to evaluate the response to treatment in solid tumors. European Organization for Research and Treatment of Cancer, National Cancer Institute of the United States, National Cancer Institute of Canada. J Natl Cancer Inst. 2000;92:205–16.
3. Goldberg SN, Gazelle GS, Compton CC, Mueller PR, Tanabe KK. Treatment of intrahepatic malignancy with radiofrequency ablation: radiologic-pathologic correlation. Cancer. 2001;88:2452–63.
4. Sironi S, Livraghi T, Meloni F, et al. Small hepatocellular carcinoma treated with percutaneous RF ablation: MR imaging follow-up. AJR Am J Roentgenol. 1999;173:1225–9.
5. Merkle EM, Nour SG, Lewin JS. MR imaging follow-up after percutaneous radiofrequency ablation of renal cell carcinoma: findings in 18 patients during first 6 months. Radiology. 2005;235:1065–71.
6. Bruix J, Sherman M, Llovet JM, et al. Clinical management of hepatocellular carcinoma. Conclusions of the Barcelona-2000 EASL conference. European Association for the Study of the Liver. J Hepatol. 2001;35:421–30.
7. Gervais DA, McGovern FJ, Arellano RS, McDougal WS, Mueller PR. Radiofrequency ablation of renal cell carcinoma: part 1, Indications, results, and role in patient management over a 6-year period and ablation of 100 tumors. AJR Am J Roentgenol. 2005;185:64–71.
8. Goldberg SN, Grassi CJ, Cardella JF, et al. Image-guided tumor ablation: standardization of terminology and reporting criteria. J Vasc Interv Radiol. 2005;16:765–78.
9. Gillams AR. Thermal ablation of liver metastases. Abdom Imaging. 2001;26:361–8.
10. Choi D, Lim HK, Rhim H, et al. Percutaneous radiofrequency ablation for early-stage hepatocellular carcinoma as a first-line treatment: long-term results and prognostic factors in a large single-institution series. Eur Radiol. 2007;17:684–92.

11. Chopra S, Dodd III GD, Chintapalli KN, et al. Tumor recurrence after radiofrequency thermal ablation of hepatic tumors: spectrum of findings on dual- phase contrast-enhanced CT. AJR Am J Roentgenol. 2001;177:381–7.
12. Hussain S, Reinhold C, Mitchell D. Cirrhosis and lesion characterization at MR Imaging. Radiographics. 2009;29:1637–52.
13. Stigliano R, Burroughs AK. Should we biopsy each liver mass suspicious for HCC before liver transplantation? No, please don't. J Hepatol. 2005;43:563–8.
14. Goldberg S, Dupuy DE. Image-guided radiofrequency tumor ablation: challenges and opportunities – Part I. J Vasc Interv Radiol. 2001;12:1021–32.
15. Goldberg S, Dupuy DE. Image-guided radiofrequency tumor ablation: challenges and opportunities – Part II. J Vasc Interv Radiol. 2001;12:1135–48.
16. Lim HK, Choi D, Lee WJ, et al. Hepatocellular carcinoma treated with percutaneous radio-frequency ablation: evaluation with follow-up multiphase helical CT. Radiology. 2001;221:447–54.
17. de Baere T, Risse O, Kuoch V, et al. Adverse events during radiofrequency treatment of 582 hepatic tumors. AJR Am J Roentgenol. 2003;181:695–700.
18. Veit P, Antoch G, Stergar H, et al. Detection of residual tumor after radiofrequency ablation of liver metastasis with dual-modality PET/CT: initial results. Eur Radiol. 2006;16:80–7.
19. Mazzaferro V, Chun YS, Poon RTP, et al. Liver transplantation for the treatment of small hepatocellular carcinomas in patients with cirrhosis. N Engl J Med. 1996;11:693–9.
20. Dromain C, de Baerre T, Elias D, et al. Hepatic tumors treated with percutaneous radio-frequency ablation: CT and MR imaging follow-up. Radiology. 2002;223:255–62.
21. Livraghi T, Solbiati L, Meloni MF, et al. Treatment of focal liver tumors with percutaneous radiofrequency ablation: complications encountered in a multicenter study. Radiology. 2003;226:441–51.
22. Rhim H, Yoon KH, Cho Y, et al. Major complications after radio-frequency thermal ablation of hepatic tumors: spectrum of imaging findings. Radiographics. 2003;23:123–36.
23. Uppot RN, Silverman SG, Zagoria RJ, Tuncali K, Childs DD, Gervais DA. Image-guided percutaneous ablation of renal cell carcinoma: a primer of how we do it. AJR Am J Roentgenol. 2009;192:1558–70.
24. Frank I, Blute ML, Cheville JC, Lohse CM, Weaver AL, Zinke H. Solid renal tumors: an analysis of pathological features related to tumor size. J Urol. 2003;170:2217–20.
25. Matin SF, Ahrar K, Cadeddu JA, et al. Residual and recurrent disease following renal energy ablative therapy: a multi-institutional study. J Urol. 2006;176:1973–7.
26. Cantwell CP, Wah TM, Gervais DA, et al. Protecting the ureter during radiofrequency ablation of renal cell cancer: a pilot study of retrograde pyeloperfusion with cooled dextrose 5% in water. J Vasc Interv Radiol. 2008;19:1034–40.
27. Wah TM, Koenig P, Irving HC, Gervais DA, Mueller PR. Radiofrequency ablation of a central renal tumor: protection of the collecting system with a retrograde cold dextrose pyeloperfusion technique. J Vasc Interv Radiol. 2005;16:1551–5.
28. Zagoria RJ, Traver MA, Werle DM, Perini M, Hayasaka S, Clark PE. Oncologic efficacy of CT-guided percutaneous radiofrequency ablation of renal cell carcinomas. AJR Am J Roentgenol. 2007;189:429–36.
29. Miyakita H, Tukunaga M, Ouda H, et al. Significance of 18 F-fluorodeoxyglucose positron emission tomography (FDG-PET) for detection of renal cell carcinoma and immunohistochemical glucose transporter 1 (GLUT-1) expression in the cancer. Int J Urol. 2002;9:15–8.
30. Kand GE, White Jr RL, Zuger JH, Sasser HC, Teigland CM. Clinical use of fluorodeoxyglucose F 18 positron emission tomography for detection of renal cell carcinoma. J Urol. 2004;171:1806–9.
31. Schirmang TC, Mayo-Smith WW, Dupuy DE, Beland MD, Grand DJ. Kidney neoplasms: renal halo sign after percutaneous radiofrequency ablation – incidence and clinical importance in 101 consecutive patients. Radiology. 2009;253:263–9.
32. Gervais DA, McGovern FJ, Arellano RS, McDougal WS, Mueller PR. Renal cell carcinoma: clinical experience and technical success with radio-frequency ablation of 42 tumors. Radiology. 2003;226:417–24.
33. Javadi S, Matin SF, Tamboli P, Ahrar K. Unexpected atypical findings on CT after radiofrequency ablation of small renal-cell carcinoma and the role of percutaneous biopsy. J Vasc Interv Radiol. 2007;18:1186–91.
34. Gervais DA, Arellano RS, McGovern FJ, McDougal WS, Mueller PR. Radiofrequency ablation of renal cell carcinoma: part 2, Lessons learned with ablation of 100 tumors. AJR Am J Roentgenol. 2005;185:72–80.
35. Lokken RP, Gervais DA, Arellano RS, et al. Inflammatory nodules mimic applicator track seeding after percutaneous ablation of renal tumors. AJR Am J Roentgenol. 2007;189:845–8.
36. Mayo-Smith WW, Dupuy DE, Parikh PM, Pezzullo JA, Cronan JJ. Imaging-guided percutaneous radiofrequency ablation of solid renal masses: techniques and outcomes of 38 treatment sessions in 32 consecutive patients. AJR Am J Roentgenol. 2003;180:1503–8.
37. Beland MD, Wasser EJ, Mayo-Smith WW, Dupuy DE. Primary non-small cell lung cancer: review of frequency, location, and time of recurrence after radiofrequency ablation. Radiology. 2010;254:301–7.
38. American Cancer Society. Cancer facts and figures 2005. Atlanta, GA: American Cancer Society; 2005.
39. Lanuti M, Sharma A, Digumarthy SR, et al. Radiofrequency ablation for treatment of medically inoperable stage I non-small cell lung cancer. J Thorac Cardiovasc Surg. 2009;137:160–6.
40. Soga N, Yamakado K, Gohara H, et al. Percutaneous radiofrequency ablation of unresectable pulmonary metastases from renal cell carcinoma. BJU Int. 2009;104:790–4.
41. Morris DL, Glenn D, King J, et al. Radiofrequency ablation (RFA) of pulmonary colorectal metastases. J Clin Oncol. 2004;22:3732.
42. Bojarski JD, Dupuy DE, Mayo-Smith WW. CT imaging findings of pulmonary neoplasms after treatment with radiofrequency ablation: results in 32 tumors. AJR Am J Roentgenol. 2005;185:466–71.
43. Thanos L, Mylona S, Giannoulakos N, et al. Percutaneous radiofrequency ablation of lung tumors in contact with the aorta: dangerous and difficult but efficient: a report of two cases. Cardiovasc Intervent Radiol. 2008;31:1205–9.
44. Giraud P, Antoine M, Larrouy A, et al. Evaluation of microscopic tumor extension in non-small-cell lung cancer for three-dimensional conformal radiotherapy planning. Int J Radiat Oncol Biol Phys. 2000;48:1015–24.

45. Okuma T, Matsuoka T, Yamamota A, et al. Determinants of local progression after computed tomography-guided percutaneous radiofrequency ablation for unresectable lung tumors: 9-year experience in a single institution. Cardiovasc Intervent Radiol. 2010;33(4):787–93.

46. Laurent F, Philippe M, Latrabe V, Tunon de Lara M, Marthan R. Pneumothoraces and chest tube placement after CT-guided transthoracic lung biopsy using a coaxial technique: incidence and risk factors. AJR Am J Roentgenol. 1999;172:1049–53.

47. Dupuy DE, Goldberg SN. Image-guided radiofrequency tumor ablation: challenges and opportunities – Part II. J Vasc Interv Radiol. 2001;12:1135–48.

48. Okuma T, Matsuoka T, Yamamota A, et al. Assessment of early treatment response after CT-guided radiofrequency ablation of unresectable lung tumours by diffusion-weighted MRI: a pilot study. Br J Radiol. 2009;82:989–94.

49. Anderson EM, Lees WR, Gillams AR. Early indicators of treatment success after percutaneous radiofrequency of pulmonary tumors. Cardiovasc Intervent Radiol. 2009;32:478–83.

50. Steinke K, King J, Glenn D, Morris DL. Pulmonary hemorrhage during percutaneous radiofrequency ablation: a more frequent complication than assumed? Interact Cardiovasc Thorac Surg. 2003;2:462–5.

51. Haga H, Saito T, Okumoto K, et al. Successful percutaneous radiofrequency ablation of adrenal metastasis from hepatocellular carcinoma. J Gastroenterol. 2005;40:1075–6.

52. Spieza S, Garbepglio R, Milone F, et al. Thyroid nodules and related symptoms are stably controlled two years after radiofrequency thermal ablation. Thyroid. 2009;19:219–25.

53. Kinoshita T, Iwamoto E, Tsuda H, Seki K. Radiofrequency ablation as local therapy for early breast carcinomas. Breast Cancer. 2011;18(1):10–7.

Chapter 7
Principles of Embolization

Rony Avritscher and Michael J. Wallace

Introduction

Catheter-directed embolization is one of the fundamental image-guided therapies that have shaped the specialty of interventional radiology. The term embolization refers to the act of delivering an agent or device into a target vessel to produce intentional vascular occlusion. This occlusion may be permanent or temporary depending on the clinical indication and the agent or device utilized. Catheter-directed embolization was first reported in 1972 [1] when autologous blood clot was used to treat a patient with gastrointestinal hemorrhage. The indications for embolization encompass a wide spectrum of clinical situations including tumor devascularization, tissue ablation, organ protection against nontargeted embolization, blood flow redistribution, control of hemorrhage secondary to malignancy, and delivery of therapeutic agents. Embolic agents and devices range from liquid and particulate agents that are flow directed to mechanical devices that are deployed in a precise location. The agents and devices are chosen for their unique properties, the territory or target site being embolized, and the desired endpoint of the therapeutic intervention. Proper preprocedure planning and familiarity with the indications, advantages, and shortcomings of each one of the tools available to the interventionalist is absolutely essential to render optimal care during these complex procedures.

Over the past several decades embolization techniques have served as a platform for other therapies in which the embolic agent is combined with drugs, radiation, genes, and other biologic agents and delivered to a desired target site for therapy. In addition to the remarkable advances in embolization products, there are parallel advances in catheter technologies. Coaxial microcatheter systems that range from 2 to 3 Fr (French) in outer diameter can be delivered through 4–5 Fr standard angiographic catheters to facilitate the technical challenges needed for small-vessel catheterization. An additional advantage of these microcatheter systems is the potential reduction of arterial injuries (dissection and perforation) that can occur with larger catheters. This chapter will focus on the application of categories of embolic material and how they are applied in clinical application.

Basic Principles

The choice of an embolic agent is dependent on the first question that must be applied to the clinical situation at hand. Should the embolization be central (proximal – medium to large vessel) or peripheral (distal – small vessel)? A central or proximal embolization is traditionally considered one that entails the precise deployment of a device (coil, plug, or balloon) to arrest a large or medium-sized vessel. A peripheral or distal embolization is typically considered one that entails the occlusion of small precapillary vascular structures by the injection of a flow-directed agent (particles and liquids).

A central (proximal) occlusion of a vessel near its origin has an effect similar to a surgical ligation with immediate formation of collateral circulation. The more proximal the occlusion, the more abundant is the development of collateral circulation. Proximal embolizations are not the best approach for intraarterial therapy to directly treat neoplasms and vascular malformations. This approach ultimately restricts the ability to re-treat the target lesion from the same artery and

R. Avritscher (✉) • M.J. Wallace
Department of Diagnostic Radiology, The University of Texas M.D. Anderson Cancer Center, Houston, TX, USA
e-mail: rony.avritscher@mdanderson.org

P.R. Mueller and A. Adam (eds.), *Interventional Oncology: A Practical Guide for the Interventional Radiologist*,
DOI 10.1007/978-1-4419-1469-9_7, © Springer Science+Business Media, LLC 2012

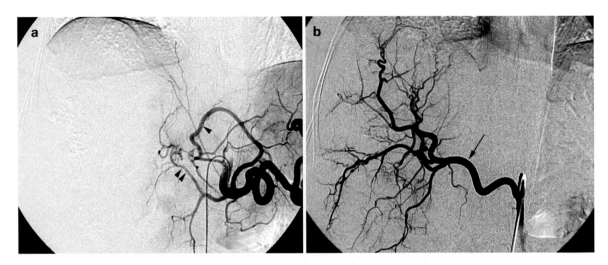

Fig. 7.1 Hepatic arterial redistribution using central/proximal coil embolization in a patient with variant hepatic arterial anatomy undergoing hepatic arterial infusion of chemotherapy. Celiac angiograph (**a**) demonstrates an absent, right and left hepatic artery from the traditional proper hepatic artery distribution. The left hepatic artery (*arrowhead*) arises from a shared artery with the left gastric arteries (gastrohepatic trunk). The proper hepatic artery (*arrowheads*) is attenuated in size and supplies the central portion of the liver with an artery, often called the "middle hepatic" artery. Superior mesenteric angiography (**b**) demonstrates a replaced right hepatic artery (*arrow*) arising from the superior mesenteric artery supplying the right lobe of the liver. After coil embolization of the proper hepatic artery and the left hepatic artery with coils angiography via the replaced right hepatic artery demonstrates immediate reconstitution of arterial supply to the embolized portions of the liver (*shaded oval region*)

requires the pursuit of technically challenging collaterals. For the management of patients with bleeding (neoplasm, ulcer, diverticulum, trauma, etc.), central embolic approach is often desirable to sufficiently reduce the arterial pressure at the bleeding site until hemostasis can be achieved but allowing for the subsequent development of a collateral arterial supply to the treated territory. The use of peripheral embolic agents would potentially increase the risk of undesired tissue necrosis.

Proximal embolizations can also be used to redistribute flow from one vessel to another. This is of particular value when variant hepatic arterial anatomy is present and the desire to infuse the entire hepatic circulation is accomplished by embolizing the trunk of the variant arteries. Immediate collateralization often occurs and can be depicted in the follow-up angiography from the vessel in which infusion is intended. An example of this is depicted in Fig. 7.1.

Most of the commercially available embolic materials fit into one of the following categories: deployable devices (coils, plugs, and balloons), sponge material, particulate agents (spherical and nonspherical agents), and liquid agents (polymers, sclerosants, and other agents that precipitate).

When evaluating a product for clinical application the first question that should be entertained is how the agent or device satisfies the question posed in the previous section regarding the location within a vessel or territory for embolization (central vs. peripheral). The next question that should be answered is the permanence of the embolization (temporary vs. permanent). The third question that should be answered is that whether the level of occlusion requires a precision within the target vessel (push/deploy vs. inject). The answers to these questions will help narrow down the appropriate embolic material that best suites the clinical application.

Permanent occlusions of medium to large vessels are commonly accomplished with the deployment of a vascular device such as coils or vascular plugs. Embolization coils are one of the more common categories of embolic materials and are available in a wide range of shapes, sizes, and mechanisms of deployment. A newer generation of coils with detachment mechanisms is now more readily available and best suited for embolizations in which the site of vessel occlusion requires precise deployment to avoid nontarget vessel occlusion. One example of this added benefit is during gastroduodenal artery embolization prior to radioembolization where embolization of the vessel as close to the gastroduodenal artery (GDA) origin is beneficial to reduce the chance of nontarget therapy to small bowel arterial branches.

Peripheral embolization involves the occlusion of small precapillary vascular structures using flow-directed embolic agents and most commonly in liquid or particulate forms. This deep penetration or peripheral level of occlusion is well suited for embolization of tumors. The more peripheral the embolization is to the tumor, the less the opportunity for collateral circulation and the greater likelihood of tumor necrosis. While tumor necrosis is a desired effect, necrosis of adjacent nontargeted tissue is not.

Embolic Agents

Gelatin Sponge

Gelatin sponge (Gelfoam®, Pfizer, New York, NY) is a white, water-insoluble, porous material prepared from purified pig skin gelatin. The most common application of gelatin sponge is temporary occlusion of bleeding vessels. Gelfoam appears to promote clotting via physical effects by supporting thrombus development. Vascular occlusion with gelatin sponge causes an acute necrotizing arteritis followed by a foreign-body reaction. This inflammatory process eventually leads to breakdown of the gelfoam within 1–3 weeks after embolization with subsequent vascular recanalization [2]. Nonetheless, multiple instances of permanent occlusion after gelatin-sponge embolization have been described [3]. Gelfoam is commonly used for the treatment of hepatic tumors usually combined with chemotherapy drugs; preoperative embolization of renal cell carcinoma and hypervascular bone metastases; as well as in the palliative treatment of bleeding from a variety of sites. Transcatheter delivery of gelfoam can be achieved is two basic preparations that dramatically change the level of occlusion and the desired angiographic endpoint. It can be delivered as a uniform solution by mixing gelatin in powder form (~50 μm) with contrast that can be administered in a similar manner to other particulate agents producing distal small-artery occlusion. These small particles can cause capillary occlusion and severe ischemia, and are not optimal for use in the mesenteric arterial system supplying bowel. An alternative method of preparation includes cutting the sheets of gelatin sponge into small strips (torpedoes) or cubes (2–6 mm) that can be deposited through a catheter to achieve a more proximal occlusion compared to the powder form. Pieces can be made small enough to inject through larger-sized microcatheters to occlude small arteries but are more commonly delivered through 4 and 5 Fr catheters to occlude medium-sized arteries like the gastroduodenal artery.

Particulate Agents

Particulate agents are essentially broken down into spherical and nonspherical products that are available in a multitude of common sizing range options (40–1,200 μm).

Nonspherical Agents

Polyvinyl alcohol (PVA) particles (Ivalon, Fabco, New London, CT) are polymers formed by reticulation and foaming of polyvinyl alcohol with formaldehyde. Nonspherical PVA particles are subsequently fragmented into different size range sieves. PVA is hydrophobic and nonabsorbable and is considered an agent that produces permanent occlusion. Animal studies have, however, demonstrated that recanalization can occur with PVA and other traditionally "permanent" embolic agents [4]. PVA particles cause flow cessation via mechanical occlusion and thrombus formation followed by a foreign-body reaction that can persist for months or even years. Nonspherical particle label sizes are not reliable, since the sizes reflect sieve pore and not particle diameter. In addition, particles tend to aggregate in clumps that can reach up to ten times individual particle sizes resulting in potential microcatheter occlusion and a more proximal level of embolization than would be anticipated by the size of individual PVA particles.

Spherical Agents

Spherical PVA microspheres (Contour SE; Target Therapeutics, Boston Scientific, Freemont, California) have recently emerged to address the limitation described for nonspherical PVA (Ivalon). They are available in the following size ranges 100–300, 500–700, 700–900, and 900–1,200 μm. Spherical PVA offers a more consistent size particle and produces a more precise and predictable level of vessel penetration upon delivery relating to the reduction in aggregation and clumping as compared to nonspherical PVA.

Tris-acryl gelatin microspheres (Embosphere; Biosphere Medical, Rockland, Massachusetts) are pliable acrylic polymer matrix crosslinked with a bovine gelatin overcoating. They are hydrophilic and nonresorbable particles available in the following size ranges 40–120, 100–300, 500–700, and 700–900 μm. They can be much more precisely separated by size ranges. Calibration accuracy is improved 10- to 100-fold compared to nonspherical particles. The microporous polymer is coated with collagen, which promotes cell adhesion. The particles cause a moderate giant cell and polymorphonuclear inflammatory reaction.

Due to their hydrophilic nature, the particles are easily suspended in saline and iodinated contrast and do not aggregate. Their pliable features allow delivery through microcatheters smaller than the calibrated size of the particle. These agents are ideal for situations, when precise control over the exact size of embolized vascular diameter is necessary, thus reducing the extent of nontargeted tissue damage.

Hydrogel-based microspheres are more recent additions to the category of particulate agents. Bead Block (Biocompatibles, Farhan, UK) is a hydrogel microspheres produced from polyvinyl alcohol (100–300, 500–700, and 700–900 μm) and Embozene (CeloNova Biosciences, Newnan, Georgia) is based on a hydrogel core with a poly(bis[trifluoroethoxy]phosphazene) nanocoat approximately 30 nm in thickness (40, 100, 250, 500, 700, and 900 μm). Embozene, unlike many of the alternative agents, provides a tighter calibration of microspheres with a tolerance of ±5%.

Liquid Agents

Liquid agents available for use include a range of materials from tissue adhesives (cyanoacrylates), sclerosants (absolute alcohol, sodium tetradecyl sulfate), procoagulants (thrombin), and contrast (Ethiodol, Hot Contrast). Liquid agents in general are often more challenging to handle and frequently require specialized or advanced training, compared to particles or devices, to master and control the product effectively so that complications are minimized.

Glue is a liquid, nonradiopaque, permanent embolic agent that can be used to produce fast occlusion of small and large vessels. There are several different polymers that can be used as biological glue. The most commonly utilized are the cyanoacrylates, due to their low viscosity. N-2-butyl-cyanoacrylate (NBCA) is approved by the Food and Drug Administration (FDA) for the presurgical devascularization of cerebral arteriovenous malformations. In the interventional oncology setting, the main application for peripheral embolotherapy using biological glue includes the control of hemorrhagic complications and redistribution of flow, but there are sporadic reports of its use for tumor embolization, especially in the preoperative setting [5, 6] and for use in portal vein embolization [7]. This agent is particularly useful when embolizing a hepatic pseudoaneurysm, in which access to both the afferent and efferent vessels is difficult or not feasible. Manipulation of the embolic agent must be meticulous, since immediate polymerization of NBCA is induced by contact with anionic substances, such as blood or saline. This feature requires that preparation of the glue on a separate tray and cleansing of all catheters and syringes with a 5% dextrose solution (D5W). NBCA is subsequently loaded into a 1-cc syringe. In preparation for delivery, NBCA is mixed with iodized oil (Ethiodol). This step ensures opacification of the agent and slows polymerization time by increasing contact surface between glue and blood. Addition of tantalum powder to enhance visibility is optional. The ratio of the Ethiodol–NBCA mixture is customized to the velocity of flow. The higher the iodized oil ratio, the longer the solution will take to polymerize. Ratios tend to range from 1:1 (rapid flow) to 4:1 (slow flow).

Absolute (dehydrated) ethanol is a liquid sclerosing embolic agent that acts by causing immediate blood protein denaturation and clot formation, while damaging endothelial cells and exposing subendothelial tissue [8]. Ethanol is not radiopaque and highly diffusible, thus creating substantial risk of nontargeted embolization. These risks may be mitigated by mixing ethanol with iodized oil for better angiographic visualization or by delivering the embolic agent using balloon occlusion catheters, to control inflow. In the setting of interventional oncology, ethanol embolization has been described in the treatment of large renal cell carcinomas [9] (Fig. 7.2). Efficacy and depth of tissue penetration are related to the concentration of the ethanol, volume infused, and time of contact with vascular bed [10]. Injury to the subendothelial and neighboring tissues increases with velocity of the injection. Ellman et al. demonstrated that ethanol infusions slower than 5 ml/min causes extensive embolization due to prolonged contact with the vessel wall with minimal, associated perivascular damage [8].The maximum tolerated dose of intravascular absolute ethanol (at least 95%) is 1 ml/kg. Usual doses range between 0.5 and 1 ml/kg. In addition, risk of systemic toxicity increases with volumes greater than 60 ml.

Ethiodol (iodized oil), an iodinated ester derived from poppy-seed oil, revolutionized transcatheter hepatic arterial chemoembolization. The iodized oil functions as a distal embolic agent reaching the sinusoids, as well as a vehicle for chemotherapeutic agents [11]. The use of Ethiodol produces a more homogeneous mixture of the chemoembolic agents and prolongs contact with the tumoral tissues.

In addition, iodized oil is well suited for chemoembolization because of its preferential tumoral uptake by hepatocellular carcinoma (HCC) and certain hepatic hypervascular metastases. These findings are partially explained using the concept of enhanced permeability and retention suggested by Maeda et al. [12].The increased permeability observed in newly formed tumoral vessels coupled with a lack of lymphatics in the neoplasm, result in retention of molecules of higher molecular weight (greater than 30,000 Da) within the tumor interstitium for a more prolonged period. This retention may explain, in part, the accumulation of iodized oil or the increase in concentration of polymer conjugates of chemotherapeutic agents in neoplasms.

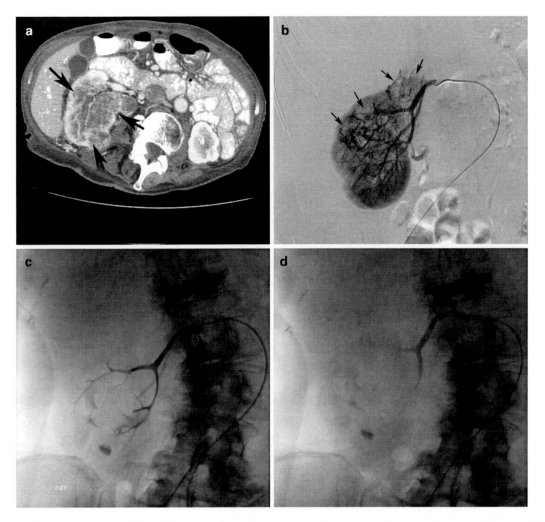

Fig. 7.2 Preoperative transcatheter arterial embolization of the right renal artery using absolute ethanol performed in a 78-year-old female with right renal cell carcinoma. (**a**) Computed tomography (CT) scan obtained prior to the embolization shows a large hypervascular mass arising from the right renal parenchyma and extending into the ipsilateral renal vein and inferior vena cava (*arrows*). (**b**) Anteroposterior selective right renal angiogram using a 5-Fr Cobra 2 catheter demonstrates a large hypervascular mass in the upper pole of the right kidney extending into the inferior vena cava (*arrows*). (**c**) Anteroposterior image of the right renal artery during infusion of absolute ethanol mixed with iodized oil through a 5-Fr balloon occlusion catheter. Note the balloon in the main right renal artery (*arrow*). (**d**) Anteroposterior selective right renal angiogram after embolization showing marked devascularization of the right kidney and renal vein tumor

Mechanical Devices

Coils are one of the most commonly used devices in interventional radiology. They are made of stainless steel or platinum and covered with fibers. These fibers cause an intense inflammatory reaction that leads to vascular occlusion. The metallic coils range in size from 0.018 in. (microcoils) to the standard 0.035–0.038 in. sizes. Coils are permanent embolic agents with level of occlusion dependant on coil size. These devices are typically used for proximal vessel embolization that range from 1–2 to 12–15 mm. They are routinely used in interventional oncology to embolize gastrointestinal branches prior to liver-directed therapy, in order to prevent gastric and duodenal complications relating to hepatic artery chemotherapy administration or hepatic artery radioembolization. In addition, coils can be used to control hemorrhagic complications. Embolization coils can be broken down into two basic categories based on the mechanism of delivery: nondetachable and detachable. Traditional coils are not attached to a delivery device but are pushed or injected through the lumen of an appropriately sized catheter or microcatheter. Once the coil has exited the tip of the catheter, there is no means of retrieving the device other than using snare-like devices to capture the coil. Detachable devices first developed for neuro applications are now more commonly being used in the periphery. These devices are pushed with a delivery system that tethers the coil to the delivery system and when the coil is satisfactorily positioned, the coil is released by various detachment mechanisms.

The advantages of using detachable coils in difficult locations is quite clear, but the substantial difference in cost with these advanced type coils has limited its more widespread use. Coils sizing is based on the target vessel size and typically oversized to the measured diameter of the vascular lumen to be occluded.

Summary

To be proficient in transarterial embolization, one must fully understand the advantages and disadvantages of the various embolic agents and materials available for clinical practice. It is also important to understand the basic principles of embolization that include the level or depth of penetration of the planned occlusion so that the appropriate embolic agent or device can be applied to the appropriate vascular territory to assure the best chance for both technical and clinical success.

References

1. Rosch J, Dotter CT, Brown MJ. Selective arterial embolization. A new method for control of acute gastrointestinal bleeding. Radiology. 1972;102(2):303–6.
2. Barth KH, Strandberg JD, White Jr RI. Long term follow-up of transcatheter embolization with autologous clot, oxycel and gelfoam in domestic swine. Invest Radiol. 1977;12(3):273–80.
3. Jander HP, Russinovich NA. Transcatheter gelfoam embolization in abdominal, retroperitoneal, and pelvic hemorrhage. Radiology. 1980;136(2):337–44.
4. Laurent A, Wassef M, Namur J, Martal J, Labarre D, Pelage JP. Recanalization and particle exclusion after embolization of uterine arteries in sheep: a long-term study. Fertil Steril. 2009;91(3):884–92.
5. Gupta AK, Purkayastha S, Bodhey NK, Kapilamoorthy TR, Kesavadas C. Preoperative embolization of hypervascular head and neck tumours. Australas Radiol. 2007;51(5):446–52.
6. Mindea SA, Eddleman CS, Hage ZA, Batjer HH, Ondra SL, Bendok BR. Endovascular embolization of a recurrent cervical giant cell neoplasm using N-butyl 2-cyanoacrylate. J Clin Neurosci. 2009;16(3):452–4.
7. Denys A, Lacombe C, Schneider F, et al. Portal vein embolization with N-butyl cyanoacrylate before partial hepatectomy in patients with hepatocellular carcinoma and underlying cirrhosis or advanced fibrosis. J Vasc Interv Radiol. 2005;16(12):1667–74.
8. Ellman BA, Parkhill BJ, Marcus PB, Curry TS, Peters PC. Renal ablation with absolute ethanol. Mechanism of action. Invest Radiol. 1984;19(5):416–23.
9. Imai S, Kajihara Y, Nishishita S, Hayashi T. Effect of ethanol induced occlusion of the renal artery in rabbit kidney implanted with VX2 carcinoma. Acta Radiol. 1989;30(5):535–9.
10. Konya A, Van Pelt CS, Wright KC. Ethiodized oil-ethanol capillary embolization in rabbit kidneys: temporal histopathologic findings. Radiology. 2004;232(1):147–53.
11. Kan Z. Dynamic study of iodized oil in the liver and blood supply to hepatic tumors. An experimental investigation in several animal species. Acta Radiol Suppl. 1996;408:1–25.
12. Maeda H, Seymour LW, Miyamoto Y. Conjugates of anticancer agents and polymers: advantages of macromolecular therapeutics in vivo. Bioconjug Chem. 1992;3(5):351–62.

Part II
Liver

Chapter 8
Nonradiological Treatment for Liver Tumors

Shiva Jayaraman and Yuman Fong

Introduction

Historically, liver resection was associated with high operative morbidity as well as high perioperative mortality rates [1]. There was a routine need for blood transfusion due to high operative blood loss. Advances in surgical techniques, an increased understanding of the importance of low central venous pressure anesthesia to minimize bleeding, and improved perioperative care have resulted in reduced morbidity and very low operative mortality rates even with extensive liver resections [2, 3].

Surgical Indications

In general, resection is avoided in benign diagnoses such as focal nodular hyperplasia (FNH), hemangioma, and simple hepatic cysts unless patients are significantly symptomatic [4]. Hepatic adenomas are premalignant liver tumors. Patients with adenomas should be offered operative resection to prevent rupture [5] and to avoid malignant transformation. In patients who have small tumors and take oral contraception, an expectant approach with discontinuation of the oral contraception pill can be employed; however, if the adenomata persist, resection is advised [6]. Other benign diseases include complications of gallstone or inflammatory diseases of the liver; in this clinical situation, patients may develop complex strictures with unilateral liver atrophy which will necessitate surgical removal of the affected liver lobe. Only the minimum amount of normal liver tissue should be removed in benign disease.

The most common indications for liver resection are malignant diseases. These can broadly be divided into three categories: primary liver cancers, secondary liver tumors, and tumors of the gallbladder and extrahepatic biliary tree. Malignancy requires that tumors are completely removed with an adequate margin of normal liver tissue. One centimeter is generally accepted as a sufficient margin [7, 8]; however, margins of less than 1 cm may be accepted if the tumor is located near the hepatic inflow pedicles or the hepatic venous outflow and may not compromise survival [7, 9, 10] (Table 8.1).

Cirrhotic patients pose unique challenges for liver resection, and one must heed certain precautions while considering resection in these patients [11]. Portal hypertension and hepatic fibrosis can lead to increased operative blood loss. Similarly, impaired liver function may result in a diminished ability for the remnant liver to regenerate, resulting in liver failure. Therefore, nonoperative strategies may require consideration in patients with severe cirrhosis [12].

Surgical Management and Technical Considerations

The basic principles of liver resection stipulate that the future liver remnant (FLR) should have adequate hepatic arterial and portal venous inflow, adequate biliary drainage, as well as adequate hepatic venous outflow. The FLR should also be of sufficient volume to preserve liver function and allow regeneration. A healthy, noncirrhotic liver can tolerate resection

S. Jayaraman (✉) • Y. Fong
Department of Surgery, Memorial Sloan-Kettering Cancer Center, New York, NY, USA
e-mail: jayars@stjoe.on.ca

P.R. Mueller and A. Adam (eds.), *Interventional Oncology: A Practical Guide for the Interventional Radiologist*,
DOI 10.1007/978-1-4419-1469-9_8, © Springer Science+Business Media, LLC 2012

Table 8.1 Solid liver masses

Benign	
Epithelial	Adenoma
	Focal nodular hyperplasia
	Nodular regenerative hyperplasia
Mesenchymal	Hemangioma
	Angiomyolipoma
Biliary	Adenoma
	Hamartoma
Malignant	
Primary	Hepatocellular carcinoma
	Intrahepatic cholangiocarcinoma
Secondary	Colorectal cancer
	Noncolorectal cancer metastases
	Neuroendocrine

of up to 80% of its volume [13]. Diseased livers will only tolerate smaller resections. To preserve hepatic function and to increase the volume of the FLR, portal vein embolization of the side to be resected may induce hypertrophy of the FLR [14] and diminish the chances of postoperative liver failure [15].

Surgical resection is planned according to tumor location using the Couinaud hepatic anatomic classification system (Fig. 8.1a) [16]. Depending on the location of tumor(s) the appropriate type of resection is selected. The most commonly performed major resections of the liver are the right hepatectomy, left hepatectomy, extended right hepatectomy, left lateral-section resection, and extended left hepatectomy (Fig. 8.1b).

Hepatocellular Carcinoma

Hepatocellular carcinoma (HCC) is the most common primary malignant tumor of the liver [17]. As previously mentioned, the extent of cirrhosis and portal hypertension in the background liver is of utmost importance in selecting patients for surgery. There are several methods whereby the liver function can be assessed; however, the Child-Pugh [18, 19] classification is the technique that the authors use to assess liver function and help predict operative mortality.

If a patient is a suitable operative candidate based on their liver function, the goals of surgery are to resect the tumor with an adequate margin and to preserve enough functional hepatic parenchyma. Liver resection is the standard of care for patients with solitary tumors with preserved hepatic function. Unfortunately, only a small minority of patients are eligible for resection due to multifocal disease, metastases, or poor liver function [17, 20]. However, in highly selected, noncirrhotic patients 5-year survival rate after resection has been reported to be greater than 70%. Overall 5-year survival rates of greater than 40% are also possible even with extensive resections [21, 22].

Liver transplantation is offered to patients who are not candidates for resection using very specific criteria. Indeed, according to the Milan criteria, patients who are not the candidates for resection with a solitary tumor less than 5 cm or with three or fewer tumors less than 3 cm are best treated with liver transplantation [23, 24]. This may be provided via traditional orthotopic donors or living-related donor programs. In order to pursue this strategy, it is imperative to rule out extrahepatic disease as well as vascular invasion. If patients are expected to wait greater than 6 months for a donor organ, percutaneous ablative techniques, described in other chapters, may be employed [25, 26]. The seminal study of 48 patients using this approach yielded a 4-year survival rate of 75% with a 4-year recurrence-free survival of 83% [23].

Unfortunately, no systemic therapy has lead to reproducible response rates that show beneficial effect of systemic chemotherapy on survival rates. Increasing knowledge of molecular structure of HCC has led to novel, targeted therapies such as sorafenib. In vitro studies have shown that this drug inhibits vascular endothelial growth factor 1 (VEGFR-1), VEGFR-2, VEGFR-3, and platelet-derived growth factor receptor beta PDGFR-β, thus inhibiting angiogenesis and tumor growth [27]. In a randomized trial comparing sorafenib to placebo, it showed modest improvement in median overall survival of 10.7 from 7.9 months. It also increased the 1-year survival rate to 44% compared to 33% for placebo in patients with advanced HCC. It was also associated with significantly more toxicity, particularly hand-foot syndrome [28]. As a result, it may be considered in patients with advanced HCC; however, its role compared to other strategies such as chemoembolization or bland embolization has yet to be elucidated. The authors' approach to the management of HCC is shown in Fig. 8.2.

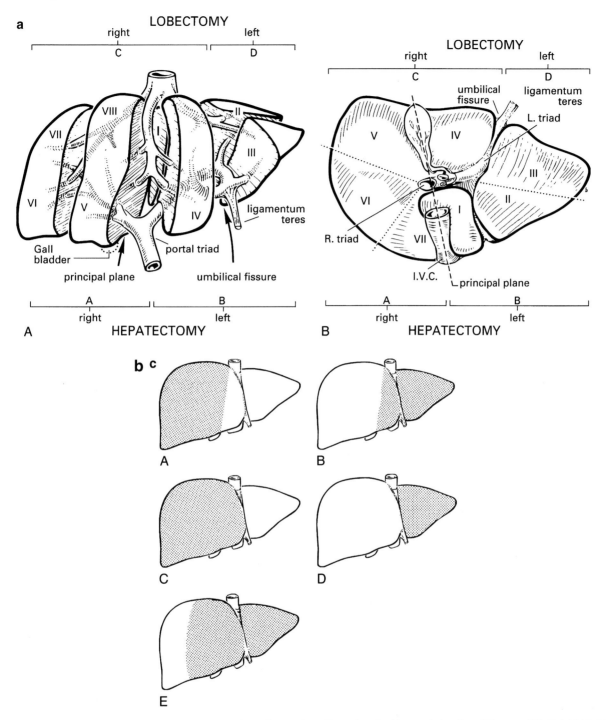

Fig. 8.1 (**a**) Couinaud segments and (**b**) commonly performed operations (Reproduced with permission from Blumgart LH, Belghiti J. Liver Resection for benign disease and for liver and biliary tumors. In: Blumgart LH. Surgery of the liver, biliary tract, and pancreas. Philadelphia: Saunders Elsevier; 2007:1341–1416)

Metastatic Colorectal Cancer

Partial hepatectomy is the only chance for cure and prolonged survival in patients with resectable liver metastasis from colorectal cancer. Patients who are not candidates for resection have an abysmal prognosis with a median survival of only 5–10 months and extremely low rates of 2- and 5-year survival [29]. In order for patients to be considered candidates for

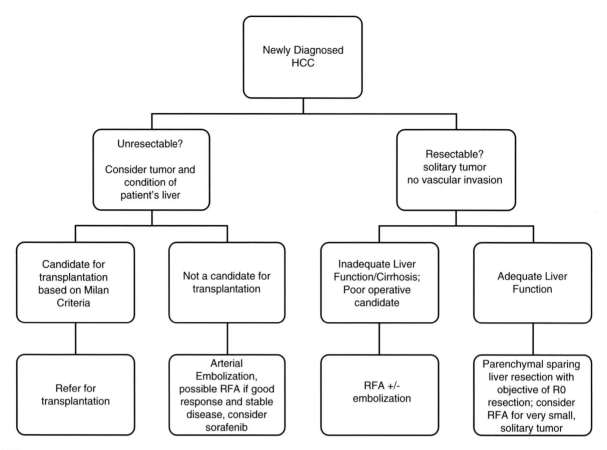

Fig. 8.2 Author's approach to hepatocellular carcinoma (HCC)

surgical resection, they must not have any extrahepatic disease. However, selected patients with stable extrahepatic disease are candidates for resection [30], which can be confirmed with computed tomography (CT) or positron emission tomography (PET) scanning. As with patients with HCC, patients must also have a sufficient FLR, which is especially pertinent in metastatic colorectal cancer, as many of these patients have received neoadjuvant chemotherapy, which can affect liver function. There are two pillars of therapy that promote long-term survival in metastatic colorectal cancer to the liver: surgery and perioperative chemotherapy.

When performing resection of liver metastases, patients having proper anatomic resections have better operative outcomes and lower rates of margin positivity compared to wedge resections where a small, nonanatomic cuff of liver is removed from the area around tumors [31]. Anatomic resections in the form of segmental resections or more extensive hepatectomies can be combined with radiofrequency ablation to eliminate tumors affecting both the left and right sides of the liver.

Fong et al. have proposed and validated a prognostic scoring system to predict survival in patients undergoing resection for metastatic colorectal cancer [32]. The Fong score is composed of five features, each of which is given a score of 0 or 1 for each positive criterion. They are a node primary tumor, disease-free interval less than 12 months between colon resection and appearance of metastases, size of largest liver lesion greater than 5 cm, more than one tumor, and carcinoembryonic antigen CEA level of greater than 200 ng/dL. Table 8.2 summarizes the relationship between clinical risk score and survival after liver resection for metastatic colorectal cancer.

Neoadjuvant chemotherapy delivered before surgery has been proposed as a means of potentially improving long-term survival and increasing the likelihood of tumor resectability [33]. Unfortunately, to date, there has been no randomized trial assessing the role of preoperative chemotherapy to placebo. The only trial that partially assesses this problem was recently published by Nordlinger et al. [34]. Their study demonstrates that administering chemotherapy as an adjunct to surgery improves progression-free survival, but it did not assess the timing of chemotherapy before or after a potentially curative resection, because the control group was randomized to surgery alone and did not receive any chemotherapy. In the modern era of chemotherapy, multiple regimens are available. At the author's institution, an approach combining adjuvant systemic

Table 8.2 Correlation between Fong score and survival after liver resection

Score	5-Year survival (%)	Median survival (months)
0	60	74
1	44	51
2	40	47
3	20	33
4	25	20
5	14	22

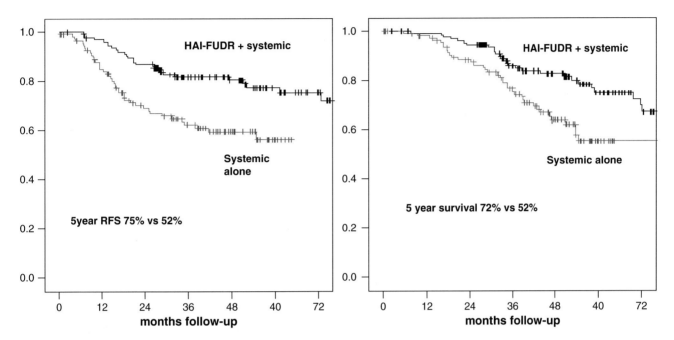

Fig. 8.3 Comparison of survival curves for different adjuvant chemotherapy regimens in metastatic colorectal cancer to the liver (Courtesy of House MG, Kemeny N, Jarnigin W, et al. Comparison of adjuvant systemic chemotherapy with or without hepatic arterial infusional chemotherapy after hepatic resection for metastatic colorectal cancer. In: Proceedings from the American Society of Clinical Oncology Gastrointestinal Cancers Symposium; 2009 Jan 15–17; San Francisco, California. Abstract 383)

and hepatic arterial pump chemotherapy is preferred. A comparison of survival using this approach versus other contemporary regimens is shown in Fig. 8.3. In cases where liver tumors are unresectable, a combined approach using systemic therapy can convert 15% of patients to resectable, whereas intraarterial chemotherapy can result in a 47% conversion to resection in all patients with the possibility of a 57% conversion rate in chemotherapy naïve patients [35, 36].

Summary

Liver resection remains the standard of care for primary and metastatic colorectal tumors of the liver. New systemic and local therapies may enhance long-term survival and offers the opportunity for improved outcomes in these patients.

References

1. Pawlik TM, Scoggins CR, Thomas MB, Vauthey JN. Advances in the surgical management of liver malignancies. Cancer J. 2004;10(2):74–87.
2. Blumgart LH. Resection of the liver. J Am CollSurg. 2005;201(4):492–4.
3. Fong Y, Blumgart LH, Cohen AM. Surgical treatment of colorectal metastases to the liver. CA Cancer J Clin. 1995;45(1):50–62.

4. Charny CK, Jarnagin WR, Schwartz LH, et al. Management of 155 patients with benign liver tumours. Br J Surg. 2001;88(6):808–13.
5. Colli A, Fraquelli M, Massironi S, et al. Elective surgery for benign liver tumours. *Cochrane Database Syst Rev* 2007(1):CD005164.
6. Nagorney DM. Benign hepatic tumors: focal nodular hyperplasia and hepatocellular adenoma. World J Surg. 1995;19(1):13–8.
7. Vandeweyer D, Neo EL, Chen JW, et al. Influence of resection margin on survival in hepatic resections for colorectal liver metastases. HPB (Oxford). 2009;11(6):499–504.
8. Are C, Gonen M, Zazzali K, et al. The impact of margins on outcome after hepatic resection for colorectal metastasis. Ann Surg. 2007;246(2):295–300.
9. Muratore A, Ribero D, Zimmitti G, Mellano A, Langella S, Capussotti L. Resection margin and recurrence-free survival after liver resection of colorectal metastases. Ann Surg Oncol. 2010;17(5):1324–9.
10. Zorzi D, Mullen JT, Abdalla EK, et al. Comparison between hepatic wedge resection and anatomic resection for colorectal liver metastases. J Gastrointest Surg. 2006;10(1):86–94.
11. Esnaola N, Vauthey JN, Lauwers G. Liver fibrosis increases the risk of intrahepatic recurrence after hepatectomy for hepatocellular carcinoma. Br J Surg. 2002;89(7):939–40. author reply 940.
12. Bilimoria MM, Lauwers GY, Doherty DA, et al. Underlying liver disease, not tumor factors, predicts long-term survival after resection of hepatocellular carcinoma. Arch Surg. 2001;136(5):528–35.
13. Blumgart LH, Leach KG, Karran SJ. Observations on liver regeneration after right hepatic lobectomy. Gut. 1971;12(11):922–8.
14. Makuuchi M, Thai BL, Takayasu K, et al. Preoperative portal embolization to increase safety of major hepatectomy for hilar bile duct carcinoma: a preliminary report. Surgery. 1990;107(5):521–7.
15. Covey AM, Tuorto S, Brody LA, et al. Safety and efficacy of preoperative portal vein embolization with polyvinyl alcohol in 58 patients with liver metastases. AJR Am J Roentgenol. 2005;185(6):1620–6.
16. Couinaud C. Anatomic principles of left and right regulated hepatectomy: technics. J Chir (Paris). 1954;70(12):933–66.
17. Bruix J, Sherman M, Llovet JM, et al. Clinical management of hepatocellular carcinoma. Conclusions of the Barcelona-2000 EASL Conference. European Association for the Study of the Liver. J Hepatol. 2001;35(3):421–30.
18. Child CG, Turcotte JG. Surgery and portal hypertension. Major Probl Clin Surg. 1964;1:1–85.
19. Pugh RN, Murray-Lyon IM, Dawson JL, et al. Transection of the oesophagus for bleeding oesophageal varices. Br J Surg. 1973;60(8):646–9.
20. Ribero D, Abdalla EK, Thomas MB, Vauthey JN. Liver resection in the treatment of hepatocellular carcinoma. Expert Rev Anticancer Ther. 2006;6(4):567–79.
21. Poon RT, Fan ST, Lo CM, et al. Long-term survival and pattern of recurrence after resection of small hepatocellular carcinoma in patients with preserved liver function: implications for a strategy of salvage transplantation. Ann Surg. 2002;235(3):373–82.
22. Cherqui D, Laurent A, Mocellin N, et al. Liver resection for transplantable hepatocellular carcinoma: long-term survival and role of secondary liver transplantation. Ann Surg. 2009;250(5):738–46.
23. Mazzaferro V, Regalia E, Doci R, et al. Liver transplantation for the treatment of small hepatocellular carcinomas in patients with cirrhosis. N Engl J Med. 1996;334(11):693–9.
24. Mazzaferro V, Llovet JM, Miceli R, et al. Predicting survival after liver transplantation in patients with hepatocellular carcinoma beyond the Milan criteria: a retrospective, exploratory analysis. Lancet Oncol. 2009;10(1):35–43.
25. Llovet JM, Bruix J, Fuster J, et al. Liver transplantation for small hepatocellular carcinoma: the tumor-node-metastasis classification does not have prognostic power. Hepatology. 1998;27(6):1572–7.
26. Fuster J, Charco R, Llovet JM, Bruix J, García-Valdecasas JC. Liver transplantation in hepatocellular carcinoma. Transpl Int. 2005;18(3):278–82.
27. Llovet JM, Bruix J. Molecular targeted therapies in hepatocellular carcinoma. Hepatology. 2008;48(4):1312–27.
28. Llovet JM, Ricci S, Mazzaferro V, et al. Sorafenib in advanced hepatocellular carcinoma. N Engl J Med. 2008;359(4):378–90.
29. Taylor R, Fong Y. Surgical treatment of hepatic metastases from colorectal cancer. In: Blumgart LH, editor. Surgery of the liver, biliary tract, and pancreas, vol. 2. Philadelphia: Saunders; 2007. p. 1178–9.
30. Carpizo DR, Are C, Jarnagin W, et al. Liver resection for metastatic colorectal cancer in patients with concurrent extrahepatic disease: results in 127 patients treated at a single center. Ann Surg Oncol. 2009;16(8):2138–46.
31. DeMatteo RP, Palese C, Jarnagin WR, Sun RL, Blumgart LH, Fong Y. Anatomic segmental hepatic resection is superior to wedge resection as an oncologic operation for colorectal liver metastases. J Gastrointest Surg. 2000;4(2):178–84.
32. Fong Y, Fortner J, Sun RL, et al. Clinical score for predicting recurrence after hepatic resection for metastatic colorectal cancer: analysis of 1001 consecutive cases. Ann Surg. 1999;230(3):309–18. discussion 318–21.
33. Allen PJ, Kemeny N, Jarnagin W, et al. Importance of response to neoadjuvant chemotherapy in patients undergoing resection of synchronous colorectal liver metastases. J Gastrointest Surg. 2003;7(1):109–15. discussion 116–7.
34. Nordlinger B, Sorbye H, Glimelius B, et al. Perioperative chemotherapy with FOLFOX4 and surgery versus surgery alone for resectable liver metastases from colorectal cancer (EORTC Intergroup trial 40983): a randomised controlled trial. Lancet. 2008;371(9617):1007–16.
35. Kemeny NE, Melendez FD, Capanu M, et al. Conversion to resectability using hepatic artery infusion plus systemic chemotherapy for the treatment of unresectable liver metastases from colorectal carcinoma. J Clin Oncol. 2009;27(21):3465–71.
36. House MG, Kemeny N, Jarnigin W, et al. Comparison of adjuvant systemic chemotherapy with or without hepatic arterial infusional chemotherapy after hepatic resection for metastatic colorectal cancer. In: Proceedings from the American Society of Clinical Oncology Gastrointestinal Cancers Symposium; 2009 Jan 15–17; San Francisco, California. Abstract 383.

Chapter 9
Principles of Liver Embolization

Michael J. Wallace and Rony Avritscher

Introduction

The basic principles of embolization can be used in a variety of applications in patients with hepatic malignancies. These applications range from tumor devascularization, organ protection against nontargeted embolization, blood flow redistribution, treatment of acute hemorrhage, and delivery of therapeutic agents [1]. Tumor devascularization is traditionally accomplished using particulate agents to occlude the peripheral small precapillary arterial branches and produce tumor ischemia that yields growth arrest and tissue necrosis.

Hepatic arterial embolization may be performed using embolic agents alone or in combination with chemotherapeutic or radiotherapeutic agents. Embolization in this setting can then be considered as a platform for delivering a payload rather than simply a means of vessel occlusion. In the context of hepatic embolization, the application of central occlusions can be valuable to protect extrahepatic arterial territories from nontarget therapy, when radioembolization or hepatic artery chemotherapy infusions are utilized. Central or proximal hepatic artery embolization can also be utilized for redistributing the hepatic arterial blood flow to allow for hepatic arterial chemotherapeutic infusion to the entire liver via a single infusion point. This is most often applied when variant anatomy is present and the potential hepatic arterial supply arises from the superior mesenteric or left gastric artery. Embolization for redirection of hepatic blood flow can also be applied in the portal venous system to divert blood flow from one portion of the liver to another to stimulate hepatic hypertrophy. Portal venous embolization (PVE) has emerged as a safe and viable means of preoperatively causing hypertrophy of the intended future remnant that would remain after hepatectomy. The use of PVE has ultimately led to a reduction in perioperative morbidity and mortality and increased the number of patients considered for surgical resection [2]. Redistribution of flow for PVE is different than redistribution of flow in the hepatic arterial system. Occlusion in PVE is peripheral, and the flow is diverted away from one territory to another. This is in contrast to occlusion in hepatic arterial redistribution where the occlusion is more central and intrahepatic collaterals are desired to reconstitute blood flow to the embolized territory via an alternative pathway.

Hepatic Arterial Embolization

Hepatic arterial embolization was first used to treat liver tumors in the early 1970s [3]. The rationale for the transarterial approach was based on the understanding that liver neoplasms derived most of their nutrient supply from the hepatic arterial system, in contrast to the nontumor bearing liver that derived most of its nutrient supply from the portal venous system [4, 5]. Historically, a wide range of embolic agents have been used for hepatic tumor embolization demonstrating varying degrees of success [6–8]. The most common agents currently utilized in clinical practice include absorbable gelatin sponge particles and powder, and a wide variety of spherical and nonspherical particulate agents that are described in more detail in Chap. 7. Hepatic tumors that are hypervascular in nature tend to respond more favorably to embolization than tumors that are modestly vascular or hypovascular in appearance. This is usually demonstrated on preembolization computed tomography where a multiphase contrast-enhanced examination offers important planning information.

M.J. Wallace (✉) • R. Avritscher
Department of Diagnostic Radiology, The University of Texas M.D. Anderson Cancer Center, Houston, TX, USA
e-mail: mwallace@mdanderson.org

P.R. Mueller and A. Adam (eds.), *Interventional Oncology: A Practical Guide for the Interventional Radiologist*,
DOI 10.1007/978-1-4419-1469-9_9, © Springer Science+Business Media, LLC 2012

Complications related to "bland" hepatic tumor embolization typically include a postembolization syndrome that consists of fever, nausea, fatigue, white blood cell count, and liver enzyme elevation [9]. Liver necrosis, hepatic abscess or biloma formation, and liver failure are recognized, but less common serious complications of liver embolization. Complications resulting from nontargeted embolization include cholecystitis, pancreatitis, and gastrointestinal ulcer development. Gastrointestinal and pancreatic complications are often avoidable and usually occur when extrahepatic arteries are not recognized during preembolization angiography. Nontarget pulmonary complications like pulmonary hypertension and respiratory failure can occur when the embolic agents pass into the hepatic venous system via unrecognized arterial-venous shunts. There is a relative paucity of large patient series that addresses complications of bland hepatic embolization. Eriksson et al. in 1998 [10] reported a serious complication rate of 10% in a series of 41 patients undergoing gel-foam powder embolization for neuroendocrine hepatic metastasis. In a similar patient population, Brown et al. in 1999 [11] reported an overall complication rate of 17% and a mortality rate of 6%. More recently, Maluccio et al. in 2008 [12] reported a series of 322 patients who underwent small-particle (40–120 μm) hepatic bland embolization for treatment of hepatocellular carcinoma. Complications occurred in 11.9% with a 30-day mortality rate of 2.5%.

In current practice, hepatic artery embolization for the treatment of hepatic tumors has been plagued with controversy regarding the value of adding a chemotherapeutic agent to the embolization regimen (chemoembolization). Despite these controversies, bland embolization is often utilized in patients with multiple nonresectable, hormonally active neuroendocrine hepatic metastasis [10, 11]. There are also advocates for bland embolization in the treatment of hepatocellular carcinoma [12]. A more complete discussion based on the disease type is included later in this chapter.

Hepatic Arterial Chemoembolization

Arterial chemoembolization reflects the combination of two treatment paradigms that result in the intraarterial delivery of a chemotherapeutic agent mixed with an embolic agent directly to the tumor bed within the liver. The rationale behind chemoembolization is based on the theory that tumor ischemia caused by embolization of the dominant arterial supply has a synergistic effect with the chemotherapeutic drugs. This technique has been the mainstay of interventional radiology for transarterial local–regional hepatic therapy since it was originally introduced by Yamada in 1977 [13]. The introduction of Ethiodol (iodized oil), an iodinated ester derived from poppy-seed oil, greatly advanced this technique. Ethiodol is well suited for chemoembolization because of its preferential tumoral uptake by hepatocellular carcinoma (HCC) and certain hepatic metastases; it acts simultaneously as an embolic agent and a vehicle for the chemotherapeutic drugs [14, 15]. These findings are partially explained by the concept of "enhanced permeability and retention" suggested by Maeda et al. [15]. Newly formed tumor vessels are more permeable. This increased permeability coupled with a lack of lymphatics in the neoplasm, result in retention of molecules of higher molecular weight within the tumor interstitium for a more prolonged period. This retention may explain, in part, the accumulation of iodized oil and the increase in concentration of polymer conjugates of chemotherapeutic agents in neoplasms.

There are a wide variety of chemoembolization regimens currently being used in clinical practice. One of the more common chemotherapeutic agents for hepatic chemoembolization is doxorubicin, and it is often combined with cisplatin and mitomycin C. These chemotherapeutic agents are often mixed with iodized oil and slowly injected into the hepatic artery branches that supply the tumor (Fig. 9.1). Additional embolization with gel foam or other particulate agents is routinely used to enhance the ischemic effect on the tumor. More recently embolization particles with drug-loading capabilities have emerged in clinical practice and have gained interest from the interventional community [16–18]. These are biocompatible, nonresorbable hydrogel particles that can be loaded with a variety of chemotherapic agents, such as doxorubicin and irinotecan. Pharmacokinetic studies with doxorubicin-loaded beads demonstrated a significant reduction in systemic exposure to doxorubicin in the drug-eluting bead group compared to the conventional chemoembolization group [19, 20]. Based on these favorable pharmacokinetics, it is believed that higher intralesional drug concentrations will result in concomitant lower systemic toxicity and longer dwell times between the chemotherapeutic agent and the tumor. Preclinical and clinical studies have demonstrated higher and prolonged retention of doxorubicin within tumors after treatment with drug-eluting bead [19]. In the phase I portion of the phase I/II study reported by Poon et al. [19] there was no dose-limiting toxicity observed for up to 150 mg doxorubicin administered in the form of doxorubicin-loaded beads. Pharmacokinetics showed low-peak plasma doxorubicin concentration and no systemic toxicity.

In general, tumors that are hypervascular in nature are best suited for chemoembolization or other transarterial therapies (bland embolization, radioembolization). Chemoembolization has been proven in randomized control trials to improve survival compared to supportive care and is currently the front line therapy for patients with hepatocellular carcinoma that are not amenable to resection or local ablation [21, 22]. Chemoembolization also plays a role in palliative

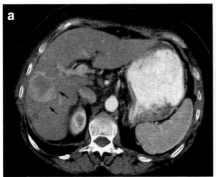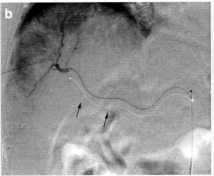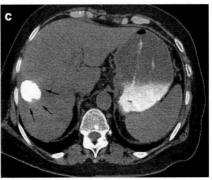

Fig. 9.1 Transarterial hepatic chemoembolization using doxorubicin, cisplatin, mitomycin C, and iodized oil in a 64-year-old male with hepatocellular carcinoma. (**a**) Computed tomography (CT) scan obtained prior to the intervention shows a hypervascular mass in the right hepatic lobe (*arrows*). (**b**) Anteroposterior image of the right hepatic artery branch angiogram during infusion of chemoembolic agent through a 3-French microcatheter (*arrows*). (**c**) CT scan obtained 6 weeks after treatment demonstrates homogeneous accumulation of iodized oil within the right hepatic mass (*arrows*)

therapies, including hepatic metastasis from neuroendocrine metastasis [10, 11, 23–29] and other metastasis such as melanoma [30–34]. Less common applications of chemoembolization include cholangiocarcinoma [35–37] and metastasis from colorectal carcinoma [38], renal cell carcinoma [39], breast carcinoma [40], gastrointestinal stromal tumor [41], and medullary thyroid carcinoma [42].

With chemoembolization, there is an increased local effect on the target tumor, and there is an expectation of an increase in local toxicity. Based on the Society of Interventional Radiology Quality improvement guidelines [43] overall complications can be expected in 10% of patients undergoing chemoembolization. Liver failure has been reported to occur in 2.3% of patients, and prolonged postembolization syndrome has been reported to occur after approximately 4.6% of procedures [43]. Other complications associated with chemoembolization occur in less than 1% of patients.

Sakamoto et al. [44] in 1998 reported an incidence of 102 (4.4%) complications in 2,300 chemoembolization procedures for hepatic neoplasms. Of those related to the chemotherapeutic agents, 63 (1.8%) produced injury to the liver including acute liver failure, liver abscess, intrahepatic biloma formation, liver infarction, and multiple intrahepatic aneurisms. Injury to extrahepatic structures, probably secondary to inadvertent chemoembolization of adjacent arteries, occurred in 28 sessions (0.09%) including severe cholecystitis, gallbladder and splenic infarction, gastrointestinal mucosal lesions (ulcer, especially along the lesser curvature of the stomach, from inadvertent right gastric chemoembolization), pulmonary embolism or infarction, tumor rupture, and variceal bleeding. In 39 (1.7%) adverse events the complications were secondary to catheter or guide wire trauma leading to iatrogenic dissection, occlusion, or vascular perforation.

Song et al. [45] in 2001 reported the incidence and predisposing factors for the development of postembolization liver abscess. In their series of 2,439 patients, a total of 6,255 chemoembolization procedures were performed. A total of 15 abscesses occurred in 14 patients (0.2%) with an associated mortality rate of 13.3% (2/14). Abscesses developed in 3/987 (0.03%) with portal vein obstruction, 3/114 (2.6%) with metastatic tumors, 1/49 (1.8%) with simple biliary obstruction, 4/55 (7.4%) with complex biliary abnormalities at risk for ascending infection, 2/18 (11.1%) for malignant gastrointestinal mucosal lesions, and 9/2,108 (0.4%) for protocols including additional embolization with gelatin sponge particles [45]. Several recent reports utilizing intensive periprocedural regimens that include antibiotics and bowel preparation have demonstrated a significant reduction in hepatic complications after chemoembolization in patients with complex biliary abnormalities [46, 47].

Hepatic Arterial Radioembolization

Radioembolization with yttrium-90 (^{90}Y) microspheres is a technique in which particles incorporating the isotope ^{90}Y are instilled through a catheter directly into the hepatic arteries. Yttrium-90 is a beta emitter with a short half-life. The concept of radioembolization is similar to that of chemoembolization in that the injected particles are selectively distributed into the arterial bed of hypervascular tumors. This distribution is possible because the blood flow within the tumor is several times greater than the flow in the surrounding liver parenchyma. As a consequence, a much higher dose of radiation can be delivered to the target lesion(s) relatively sparing the higher doses to the remaining liver. This is in contrast to external beam

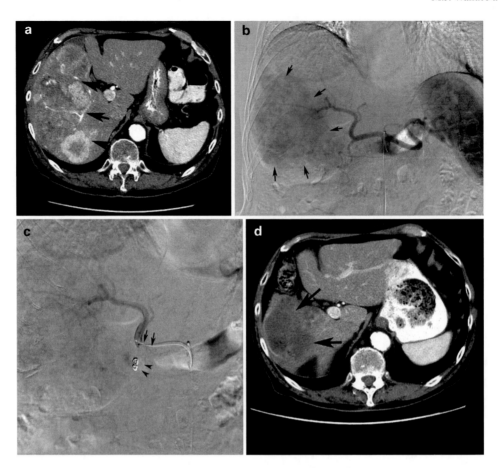

Fig. 9.2 Radioembolotherapy using Yttrium-90 resin microspheres in a 79-year-old male with newly diagnosed multinodular hepatocellular carcinoma. (**a**) CT scan obtained prior to the intervention shows large heterogeneous hypervascular multinodular mass in the right hepatic lobe (*arrows*). Additional lesions (not shown) were also present in the left lobe. (**b**) Anteroposterior selective celiac angiogram using a 5-French Sos 2 catheter demonstrates a large hypervascular mass in the right hepatic lobe (*arrows*). (**c**) Close-up of an anteroposterior image of the proper hepatic artery angiogram during infusion of Ytrrium-90 resin microspheres through a 3-French microcatheter (*arrows*). Metallic coils are noted within the gastroduodenal artery (*arrowheads*). (**d**) CT scan obtained 6 months after initial treatment demonstrates marked improvement with pronounced reduction in size and enhancement of the multinodular large right-hepatic mass (*arrows*)

radiation where both tumor and adjacent nontumor bearing liver receive an equal dose, greatly limiting the use of this technique for the treatment of liver tumors. There are two yttrium-90 radioembolization products available for clinical use. TheraSphere® beads (Nordion Inc., Ottawa, Ontario, Canada) (glass microspheres) are Food and Drug Administration (FDA) approved for neoadjuvant treatment of unresectable HCC in patients with portal vein thrombosis or as a bridge to transplantation. SIR-Spheres® (Sirtex Medical, Wilmington, Massachusetts) (resin microspheres) are approved for the treatment of metastatic colorectal cancer to the liver with concomitant use of floxuridine. Knowledge of the vascular anatomic variants in the celiac axis and superior mesenteric artery is critical to safely administering this therapy to avoid nontargeted embolization of the radioactive microspheres, which can have devastating consequences. Multiple studies have demonstrated the safety of radioembolization with yttrium-90 for the treatment of unresectable HCC [48] (Fig. 9.2), metastasis from colorectal cancer [49, 50], and neuroendocrine cancer [45, 51]. Other less common diseases treated with radioembolization and reported as a distinct patient population include breast metastasis [52, 53] and cholangiocarcinoma [54].

Radioembolization and chemoembolization are associated with a similar spectrum of toxicities except for three unique radiation-induced adverse events. These events include radiation pneumonitis, gastroduodenal ulcerations, and radiation-induced liver disease; and they are essentially preventable. Radiation pneumonitis is related to the embolization of radioactive microspheres into the terminal pulmonary arterial branches that reach the lung via shunts within the hepatic tumor. These potential shunts can be identified prior to radioembolization using Tc 99m macroaggregated albumin (MAA) as a surrogate injected into the hepatic artery during the planning arteriogram. Once injected, a quantitative analysis of their distribution, that mimics the ultimate microsphere distribution and shunt fraction, can be obtained scintigraphically. Radiation exposure to the lung exceeding 30 Gy ^{90}Y will lead to clinically apparent treatment-recalcitrant radiation pneumonitis. The incidence of this devastating adverse event is well below 1% [27, 48]. Radiation-related gastroduodenal injury can occur from the deposition of yttrium-90 microspheres into the gastrointestinal submucosal arterioles via nontarget delivery. The reported incidence is <5%, when proper precautions are instituted during preadministration angiography, where extrahepatic branches are meticulously sought after and embolized [55]. Radiation-induced liver disease is a form-fruste of hepatic venoocclusive disease with a reported incidence after radioembolization ranging between 0 and 4% [55].

Portal Vein Embolization

For patients with primary and secondary hepatic tumors, the best chance for cure or long-term survival rests in the ability to undergo surgical resection. As the number of major and extended hepatectomies increases to meet the needs of surgical resection, portal vein embolization has become a key intervention to address the increasing perioperative risks of hepatic dysfunction and hepatic insufficiency associated with extensive resection of functional liver parenchyma. The volume and function of residual liver after resection impacts the incidence of postoperative complications despite the risk of hepatic insufficiency being multifactorial [56–59]. When the portal vein is occluded, hepatocyte growth factors (hepatopoietin A, insulin, and glucagon) are shunted into the liver segments supplied by nonembolized vessels [60]. These growth factors are mostly supplied through the portal vein, not through the hepatic artery, and ultimately result is atrophy of the embolized segments and hypertrophy of the unembolized future liver remnant (FLR). Thus, the role of this preoperative maneuver is to induce hypertrophy in the portion of the liver anticipated to remain in situ after resection to reduce the risk of major morbidity and mortality and to broaden the candidacy of patients with marginal remnant volumes that would be amenable to resection. Makuuchi et al. [61] in 1990 were the first to publish their experience with preoperative PVE to induce hypertrophy of the left liver prior to right hepatectomy.

There is substantial variability of the reported rates of FLR hypertrophy in the literature. This is in part due to the marked differences in patient populations, the technique of computed tomography (CT) volumetry utilized to measure/calculate the remnant volume, the timing of the imaging follow-up utilized to evaluate the postembolization hypertrophy, and the embolization technique. The FLR is calculated by measuring the remnant on CT and standardizing the volume calculation by using a total estimated liver volume (TELV) that takes into account the body surface area. This ultimately produces a standardized value FLR/TELV [62] that can be used to compare the FLR before and after PVE. Based on previous reports, patients with "normal" livers have significantly lower perioperative complications when the FLR/TELV is above 20% [62]. Patients with substantial exposure to chemotherapy or those with chronic liver disease require higher FLR volumes of 30–40% [58, 59]. The majority of the reported rates of hypertrophy range from 8 to 14% [2, 63]. The degree of hypertrophy (DH) is also an important predictor of perioperative complications and can be used in combination with the FLR to assess the risk [2]. Patients with either <20% FLR or <5% DH have a significantly higher complication rate compared to patients with >20% FLR and >5% DH. Kinetics of FLR hypertrophy demonstrates a plateau period that typically begins 3 weeks following PVE, thus imaging for the assessment of growth should not occur before this time period.

At this point it is not clear whether the type of embolic material can impact degree of hypertrophy. Common agents used for PVE include n-butyl cyanoacrylate, gel foam, and particles (spherical and nonspherical). When embolization particles are used as a primary small-vessel occlusive agent, coils are often used as a secondary line of occlusion in the larger more proximal major portal vein branches. When evaluating the various published reports of PVE efficacy, it is important to not simply look at the amount of hypertrophy but also evaluate the patients who did not undergo surgical resection. Roughly 5% of PVE patients do not ultimately go on to resection because of inadequate hypertrophy. Disease progression or comorbidities are other reasons for patients not ultimately undergoing surgery.

One controversial point with regards to PVE is the inclusion of segment IV as part of the embolization territory. Advocates of segment IV embolization typically include segment IV as part of an extended right PVE when tumor is present in segment IV or that a portion of segment IV will be resected due to particular lesion location with the goal of an R0 resection. The embolization of segment IV reduces the risk of tumor progression related to the increased flow and growth factor stimulation that would potentially occur in the unembolized segment. Though the inclusion of segment IV as part of the embolization territory increases procedure time and complexity, it has not been associated with a higher complication rate [2].

Major complications relating to the portal vein embolization that ultimately lead to major morbidity or unresectability are rare. Based on all published series containing more than ten patients, the overall complication rate can range between 8 and 13% [2, 64]. Di Stefano et al. [64] in 2005 reported an overall complication rate of 12.8% in a series of 188 patients undergoing portal vein embolization. These included 12 complications and 12 incidental imaging findings. Complications included portal thrombosis within the FLR ($n=1$); nontarget embolization into the FLR necessitating a rescue intervention

($n=2$); hemoperitoneum ($n=1$); rupture of a metastasis in the gallbladder ($n=1$); transitory hemobilia ($n=1$); and transient liver failure ($n=6$). Other incidental events identified on follow-up imaging included small nontarget embolization in the FLR ($n=10$) and subcapsular hematoma ($n=2$). In their series, there was a statistically significantly higher incidence of complications in patients with cirrhosis (5/30; 16%) compared to those without cirrhosis (1/157; 0.6%). Only one liver resection was cancelled due to a complication of portal vein embolization, and another three were cancelled due to inadequate hypertrophy after portal vein embolization. Ribero et al. [2] in 2007 reported a complication rate of 8.9% in a series of 112 patients. Complications included partial portal vein thrombosis ($n=4$), complete portal thrombosis ($n=1$), nontarget coil migration ($n=1$), subcapsular hematoma ($n=1$), portal hypertension with variceal hemorrhage ($n=1$).

Hepatic Neoplasms

Primary and secondary hepatic neoplasms are some of the most common tumors worldwide. In Western countries, hepatic metastases are the most common malignant hepatic neoplasms, whereas in worldwide, hepatocellular carcinoma is the most common primary visceral malignancy in adults.

Hepatocellular Carcinoma

Transcatheter arterial chemoembolization has been used to treat, in addition to unresectable HCC, cholangiocarcinomas and hepatic metastases and has been used in conjunction with liver resection or tumor ablation. There are a number of treatment options for patients with hepatocellular carcinoma. These options depend on the extent of disease, the morphologic characteristics on pretherapy intervention, the underlying status of the liver, and the performance status of the patient. A host of scoring systems has been developed to take these factors into account, and algorithms have been created to balance the oncologic factors with the liver disease factors. In general, patients with very low-volume disease can potentially be cured by transplantation, resection, or ablation (≤3 cm). When patients do not meet the inclusion criteria for these curative options, chemoembolization can be entertained as the next best option for treatment. Chemoembolization has the best chance for response when the disease can be approached subselectively in contrast to a lobar administration. Intermediate (5–10 cm) and large (>10 cm) lesions that are morphologically well demarcated can be effectively treated with chemoembolization, when the number of lesions is limited (~4). Chemoembolization can still provide survival benefit in patients where tumors are large in number, infiltrative/ill-defined, or demonstrate portal vein invasion; but in these difficult scenarios radioembolization may also be considered a valuable option with similar response and survival expectations. To date, there are no randomized control trials comparing the two transarterial therapies, thus no definitive conclusions regarding superiority of one therapy can be made.

With regard to chemoembolization, two randomized studies have reported survival benefit when compared to best supportive care [21, 22]. Lo et al. [22] in 2002 demonstrated a survival benefit for patients with unresectable hepatocellular carcinoma ($n=80$) treated with chemoembolization (iodized oil, cisplatin, and gel foam) compared to a control group treated with symptomatic therapy alone. Survival at 1, 2, and 3 years in the chemoembolization group was significantly (=0.006) better (57%, 31%, and 26%), than the control group (32%, 11%, and 3%), respectively. Llovet et al. [21] in 2002 compared chemoembolization (doxorubicin and gel foam, $n=40$) and bland embolization (gel foam, $n=37$) to a control population ($n=35$) that received supportive care in a series of 112 patients. Chemoembolization demonstrated a survival benefit compared to conservative therapy, and the study was discontinued before any conclusion on the benefits of bland embolization could be made. The 1- and 2-year survival rates, respectively, for chemoembolization were 82% and 63%, for bland embolization were 75% and 50%, and for conservative therapy were 63% and 27%. There is continued controversy regarding the use of chemoembolization vs. bland embolization for treating hepatocellular carcinoma as well as other hypervascular hepatic metastasis. In the absence of randomized controlled trials comparing the two interventions, it is difficult to summarize the literature effectively with retrospective case series using a host of different chemotherapeutic and embolization agents, not to mention the wide variation with regard to technique among operators.

In the past several years, drug-eluting embolization particles have emerged and begun to make a presence in the treatment of hepatic tumors. One attraction to this new group of agents is the ability to improve upon regimen standardization for chemoembolization. After initial investigations demonstrated its favorable pharmacokinetics and safety profile, drug-eluting particles were compared to conventional chemoembolization. In a multicenter randomized controlled trial reported in 2010, Lammer et al. [17] compared conventional chemoembolization (doxorubicin–oil emulsion followed by gelfoam sponge) to drug-eluting bead chemoembolization (300–500 μm vial followed by 500–700 μm vial up to 150 mg doxorubicin) in a series of 212 patients with Child-Pugh A/B cirrhosis and large and/or multinodular, unresectable, N0, M0 HCCs. The primary endpoint was tumor response from the European Association for Study of the Liver (EASL) criteria at 6 months. The drug-eluting bead group showed higher rates of complete response, objective response, and disease control compared with the conventional chemoembolization group (27% vs. 22%, 52% vs. 44%, and 63% vs. 52%, respectively). The hypothesis of superiority was not met (one-sided $P=0.11$). Patients with Child-Pugh B, Eastern Cooperative Oncology Group (ECOG) 1, bilobar disease, and recurrent disease showed a significant increase in objective response ($P=0.038$) compared to conventional chemoembolization. Drug-eluting bead was associated with improved tolerability, with a significant reduction in serious liver toxicity ($P<0.001$) and a significantly lower rate of doxorubicin-related side effects ($P=0.0001$). Dhanasekaran et al. [18] reported a series of 73 patients in which consecutive patients who underwent conventional chemoembolization ($n=26$) were compared to patients who underwent drug-eluting bead chemoembolization ($n=47$) and demonstrated a statistically significant longer median survival ($P=0.03$) in the drug-eluting bead group (610 days) compared to the conventional group (284 days).

Regarding chemoembolization vs. bland embolization, Malagari et al. [16] recently reported their results from a randomized comparison between doxorubicin drug-eluting beads ($n=41$) and bland embolization ($n=43$). The size of embolization particles was consistent (100–300 and 300–500 μm) between both treatment arms. Complete response was seen in 11 patients (26.8%) in the drug-eluting bead group and in 6 patients (14%) in the bland embolization group; a partial response was achieved in 19 patients (46.3%) and 18 (41.9%) patients in the drug-eluting bead and bland embolization groups, respectively. Time to progression (TTP) was longer for the drug-eluting bead group (42.4 ± 9.5 and 36.2 ± 9.0 weeks), at a statistically significant level ($P=0.008$). It is difficult to compare this study with other studies in which bland embolization was utilized due to the differences in size and type of embolic agents used. This study used particles >100 μm in size in contrast to many investigators that advocate bland embolization with smaller particles [12].

Maluccio et al. [12] in 2008 published their experience using transcatheter arterial embolization for the treatment of hepatocellular carcinoma. The group analyzed 766 procedures performed in 322 patients. Embolizations were carried out solely using small 50 μm polyvinyl alcohol (PVA) or 40–120 μm tri-acryl gelatin microspheres. The median survival was 21 months with 1-, 2-, and 3-year overall survival of 66%, 46%, and 33%, respectively.

Salem et al. [65] prospectively evaluated 291 hepatocellular carcinoma patients with a total of 526 treatments. Using the World Health Organization (WHO) criteria, the authors observed response rate of 42% and the TTP of 7.9 months. In patients with mild underlying liver disease (Child-Pugh class A), median survival was 17.2 months and for those with moderate disease (Child-Pugh B), it was 7.7 months. In another recent study, Lewandowski et al. [66] compared radioembolization to chemoembolization for downstaging of hepatocellular carcinoma prior to liver transplant. The authors enrolled a total of 86 patients, of those 43 underwent chemoembolization and the other 43, radioembolization. Partial response rates favored radioembolization over chemoembolization (61% vs. 37%). Time to tumor progression was similar in both groups (18.2 months), and the overall survival tended to favor radioembolization over chemoembolization (35.7 vs. 18.7 months).

Neuroendocrine Metastasis

The goal of treatment in the setting of neuroendocrine hepatic metastasis is to reduce tumor bulk and hormone secretion. Symptomatic and biochemical responses after hepatic embolization/chemoembolization range from 40 to 80% and 50 to 60%, respectively, with an associated 5-year postembolization survival range of 50–60% [67]. Moertel et al. in 1994 chronicled a 10-year experience in 111 patients with neuroendocrine hepatic metastases. In their series, hepatic occlusion was performed surgically, and 71 patients received subsequent alternating chemotherapy regimens (dacarbazine + doxorubicin, alternating with streptozotocin + 5-fluorouracil). Patients who underwent vascular occlusion alone demonstrated objective regression in 60% compared to 80% in patients who also received chemotherapy in addition to vascular occlusion. Median survival times for patients with islet cell metastasis and carcinoid metastasis were 37 and 49 months, respectively [28]. Bloomston et al. in 2007 [24] reported a series of 122 patients with metastatic carcinoid tumor that underwent chemoembolization. Radiologic tumor response was demonstrated in 82% and stabilization of disease was identified in 12%, with a median duration of 19 months. Symptom improvement was recorded in 92% of patients with a median duration of 13 months. The median overall survival was 33.3 months after chemoembolization.

There are conflicting reports as to the best transarterial therapy for neuroendocrine hepatic metastasis. There are advocates that support the use of bland embolization for carcinoid metastasis [25, 26] and those that support chemoembolization for all neuroendocrine hepatic metastasis [29]. To add an additional wrinkle, radioembolization has recently emerged as a viable alternative to both bland embolization and chemoembolization [48, 68, 69].

Gupta et al. in 2003 [26] reported on 81 patients with carcinoid syndrome who were treated with either bland embolization (50 patients) or chemoembolization (31 patients). Imaging was available for evaluation of a response in 69 patients with partial response observed in 46 patients (67%), minimal response in 6 patients (8.7%), stable disease in 11 (16%), and progression of tumor in 6 (8.7%). The median response duration was 17 months in patients with a partial response. A reduction of tumor-related symptoms occurred in 63%, with a median progression-free survival of 19 months and a median overall survival time of 31 months. In a subsequent study by Gupta et al. in 2005 [25], patients with carcinoid metastasis (n=69) were compared with pancreatic islet cell metastasis (n=54). Patients with carcinoid compared to islet cell tumors had a higher response rate (66.7% vs. 35.2%, respectively; P=0.0001) and a longer progression-free survival (22.7 vs. 16.1 months, respectively; P=0.046). Patients who were treated with bland embolization had a higher response rate than patients who were treated with chemoembolization (P=0.004). Patients with islet cell carcinoma who underwent chemoembolization had a prolonged overall survival (31.5 vs. 18.2 months) and improved response (50% vs. 25%) compared with patients who were treated with bland embolization, but these results were not statistically different. They concluded that patients with carcinoid tumors had better outcomes than patients with islet cell carcinomas and that the addition of intraarterial chemotherapy (chemoembolization) did not improve the outcome of patients with carcinoid tumors. Chemoembolization did, however, appear to benefit patients with islet cell carcinomas.

Ruutiainen et al. in 2007 [29] reported on a series of 67 patients who underwent 219 interventions that included bland embolization (n=23) and chemoembolization (n=44) as the primary therapy. The 30-day mortality rate was 1.4% with common terminology criteria for adverse events (CTCAEv3) Grade 3 or higher toxicity after 25% of chemoembolization procedures and 22% of bland embolization procedures. Rates of freedom from progression at 1, 2, and 3 years, respectively, were 49%, 49%, and 35% after chemoembolization, and 0%, 0%, and 0% after bland embolization (log-rank test, P=0.16). Among the subgroup with carcinoid tumors, the respective proportions without progression were 65%, 65%, and 52% after chemoembolization, and 0%, 0%, and 0% after bland embolization (log-rank test, P=0.08). Patients treated with chemoembolization and bland embolization experienced symptomatic relief for means of 15 and 7.5 months, respectively (P=0.14). Survival rates at 1, 3, and 5 years after therapy were 86%, 67%, and 50%, respectively, after chemoembolization and 68%, 46%, and 33%, respectively, after bland embolization (log-rank test, P=0.18). Based on their data, they concluded that chemoembolization was not associated with a higher degree of toxicity than bland embolization and that chemoembolization demonstrated trends toward improvement in time to tumor progression, symptom control, and survival.

Kennedy et al. [48] in 2008 reported on 148 patients with neuroendocrine hepatic metastasis treated with radioembolization. The regimen was well tolerated with the most common side effect of fatigue in 6.5% of patients. Imaging response demonstrated a complete response in 2.7%, a partial response in 60.5%, and a stable disease in 22.7% with tumor progression identified in 4.9%. The median survival is 70 months.

Ocular Melanoma

Ocular melanoma can arise from various structures within the eye and accounts for 70% of all primary malignancies of the eye. At the time of diagnosis, metastases are uncommon but appear in 19–35% of patients within 5 years. Unlike cutaneous melanoma, metastases from uveal melanoma is most commonly found within the liver in more than 50% of patients [70], followed by lungs, bone, and skin. Metastatic uveal melanoma has a poor prognosis with a mortality rate of >50% within 5 months. Median survival rates related to patients undergoing chemoembolization range from 6.7% to 14.5% [30–34]. Patients who demonstrate a response following chemotherapy can have median survival approaching 22 months, in contrast to those that do not respond having median survival below 6 months [32].

Bedikian et al. [30] reported 201 cases of uveal melanoma with hepatic involvement that were treated over a period of two decades. Cisplatin-based chemoembolization regimens yielded a 36% rate of response compared to systemic therapies that only produced a 1% response rate [30]. Patel et al. [32] presented their experience in 28 patients who underwent Ethiodol–gelatin sponge chemoembolization with 1,3-bis(2-chloroethyl)-1-nitrosourea (BCNU). The mean survival for all patients was 208 days (range 4–829). Patients with <20% (n=5), 20–50% (n=12), and >50% (n=11) liver replacement by tumor survived a mean of 471, 199, and 107 days, respectively, demonstrating the influence of tumor burden on survival. Gupta et al. [31] reported on 125 patients who underwent chemoembolization for ocular and cutaneous hepatic metastasis. Partial response was demonstrated in 12 (11%), minor responses were demonstrated in 17 (16%), stable disease was demonstrated in 68 (65%), and disease progression was demonstrated in 8 (8%). The median overall survival and progression-free survival durations were 6.7 and 3.8 months, respectively. Sharma et al. [33] reported their experience with chemoembolization in 20 patients with liver-dominant metastasis from both ocular and cutaneous melanoma. The median overall survival was 271 days with 13/20 demonstrating disease progression. The median progression-free survival was 185 days.

Gastrointestinal Stromal Tumor

There are only a limited number of studies in the literature addressing the use of transcatheter therapy metastatic sarcomas. Maluccio et al. [71] reported on a series of 24 patients with metastatic sarcoma treated with bland hepatic arterial embolization, including 16 patients with gastrointestinal stromal tumor (GIST). No chemotherapy or iodized oil was used in combination with the embolic material. The overall survival was 62% at 1 year, 41% at 2 years, and 29% at 3 years, with an overall median survival of 24 months. The seven patients who remained alive >4 years after the initial embolization had metastatic GIST. Most of the patients included in this study were enrolled before the advent of imatinib. There are four studies investigating the use of chemoembolization for locoregional therapy of liver-dominant metastatic GIST. In the initial report in 1991, Mavligit et al. [72] reported tumor regression on two patients with gastrointestinal leiomyosarcoma after transcatheter hepatic arterial chemoembolization (TACE) with cisplatin and PVA, followed by hepatic arterial infusion of vinblastine. Later, in 1995, Mavligit et al. [73] reported a series of 14 patients with gastrointestinal leiomyosarcoma metastatic to the liver treated with TACE using the combination of cisplatin and PVA, followed by arterial infusion of vinblastine. The authors reported a 70% radiologic response rate with an overall median survival of 12 months after an average of two procedures. In 2001, Rajan et al. [74] published their experience with TACE for the treatment of 16 patients with metastatic sarcomas, including 11 GISTs. The authors used a combination of cisplatin, doxorubicin, mitomycin C, iodized oil, and PVA. 13% of the patients demonstrated radiologic response and 69% stable disease. The overall survival from time of embolization was 67% at 1 year, 50% at 2 years, and 40% at 3 years, with a median survival time of 13 months. The largest series to date, from Kobayashi et al. [41], published in 2006, reported on 85 patients with metastatic GIST treated with TACE. Partial response was identified in 12 patients (14%), stable disease was identified in 63 patients (74%), and disease progression was encountered in 10 patients (12%). Progression-free survival (liver) rates were 31.2%, 8.2%, and 5.4% at 1, 2, and 3 years, respectively; the median progression free survival time was 8.2 months. The median overall survival time was 17.2 months.

Colorectal Metastasis

Colorectal carcinoma patients with liver dominant disease that did not respond to systemic chemotherapy are candidates for palliative transcatheter chemotherapy. Vogl et al. [75] prospectively evaluated the use of chemoembolization in 463 patients with liver metastases of colorectal cancer. The authors observed partial response in 14.7% of patients, stable disease in 48.2%, and progressive disease in 37.1%. A recently published study by Albert et al. [38] analyzed 245 treatments in 121 patients with unresectable colorectal liver metastases after failure of second-line systemic therapy using a combination of cisplatin, doxorubicin, mitomycin C, Ethiodol, and polyvinyl alcohol. The study showed partial response in 2% of the patients, 41% stable disease, and 57% disease progression. Survival was significantly better when chemoembolization was performed after first- or second-line systemic therapy (11–12 months) than after third- to fifth-line therapies (6 months).

Radioembolization has emerged as a viable transarterial therapy for patients with unresectable or unablatable hepatic metastasis from colorectal cancer. Mulcahy et al. [76] in 2009 reported a series of 72 patients with unresectable colorectal hepatic metastasis treated with radioembolization. The tumor response rate was 40.3%. The median time to hepatic progression was 15.4 months. Overall survival from the first Y90 treatment was 14.5 months, and from the date of initial hepatic metastases was 34.6 months. Chua et al. [50] reported on 133 patients and demonstrated a complete response in 2 patients (1%), partial in 43 patients (31%), stable in 44 patients (31%), and disease progression in 51 patients (37%). Combining chemotherapy with radioembolization was associated with a favorable treatment response ($P=0.007$). The median overall survival was 9 (95% CI, 6.4–11.3) months with a 1-, 2-, and 3-year survival rate of 42%, 22%, and 20%, respectively.

Gray et al. [77] reported on the first Phase III clinical trial comparing 36 patients treated with radioembolization combined with intrahepatic floxuridine vs. 34 patients who received intrahepatic floxuridine alone. Response (complete + partial) in the radioembolization group (44%) was significantly better than the response in the infusion only (18%) ($P=0.01$). In addition there was a significant prolongation in median time to disease progression, as well as a significant survival benefit for patients who underwent radioembolization.

More recently Hendlisz et al. [78] reported their results from a phase III clinical trial of protracted intravenous chemotherapy (fluorouracil) infusion with or without radioembolization for liver-limited metastatic colorectal carcinoma in a series of 44 patients. Twenty-one patients received the combination therapy, and 23 patients received intravenous fluorouracil alone. Median time to liver progression was 5.5 months in the combination group compared to 2.1 in the infusion-only group. Time to progression also favored the combination therapy group (4.5 vs. 2.1 months).

References

1. Sun JH, Wang LG, Bao HW, et al. Emergency embolization in the treatment of ruptured hepatocellular carcinoma following transcatheter arterial chemoembolization. Hepatogastroenterology. 2010;57(99–100):616–9.
2. Ribero D, Abdalla EK, Madoff DC, Donadon M, Loyer EM, Vauthey JN. Portal vein embolization before major hepatectomy and its effects on regeneration, resectability and outcome. Br J Surg. 2007;94(11):1386–94.
3. Allison DJ, Modlin IM, Jenkins WJ. Treatment of carcinoid liver metastases by hepatic-artery embolisation. Lancet. 1977;2(8052–8053):1323–5.
4. Ackerman NB. Alteration of intra-hepatic circulation due to increased tumour growth. Proc. VIII Cong. Eur. Soc. Exp. Surg. 1972:182.
5. Taylor I, Bennett R, Sherriff S. The blood supply of colorectal liver metastases. Br J Cancer. 1978;38(6):749–56.
6. Chuang VP, Wallace S. Hepatic artery embolization in the treatment of hepatic neoplasms. Radiology. 1981;140(1):51–8.
7. Chuang VP, Wallace S, Soo CS, Charnsangavej C, Bowers T. Therapeutic Ivalon embolization of hepatic tumors. AJR Am J Roentgenol. 1982;138(2):289–94.
8. Wallace S, Charnsangavej C, Carrasco CH, Bechtel W. Ethanol for hepatic artery embolization. Radiology. 1984;152(3):821–2.
9. Hemingway AP, Allison DJ. Complications of embolization: analysis of 410 procedures. Radiology. 1988;166(3):669–72.
10. Eriksson BK, Larsson EG, Skogseid BM, Löfberg AM, Lörelius LE, Oberg KE. Liver embolizations of patients with malignant neuroendocrine gastrointestinal tumors. Cancer. 1998;83(11):2293–301.
11. Brown KT, Koh BY, Brody LA, et al. Particle embolization of hepatic neuroendocrine metastases for control of pain and hormonal symptoms. J Vasc Interv Radiol. 1999;10(4):397–403.
12. Maluccio MA, Covey AM, Porat LB, et al. Transcatheter arterial embolization with only particles for the treatment of unresectable hepatocellular carcinoma. J Vasc Interv Radiol. 2008;19(6):862–9.
13. Yamada R, Nakatsuka H, Nakamura K, et al. Hepatic artery embolization in 32 patients with unresectable hepatoma. Osaka City Med J. 1980;26(2):81–96.
14. Kan Z. Dynamic study of iodized oil in the liver and blood supply to hepatic tumors. An experimental investigation in several animal species. Acta Radiol Suppl. 1996;408:1–25.
15. Maeda H, Seymour LW, Miyamoto Y. Conjugates of anticancer agents and polymers: advantages of macromolecular therapeutics in vivo. Bioconjug Chem. 1992;3(5):351–62.
16. Malagari K, Pomoni M, Kelekis A, et al. Prospective randomized comparison of chemoembolization with doxorubicin-eluting beads and bland embolization with BeadBlock for hepatocellular carcinoma. Cardiovasc Intervent Radiol. 2010;33(3):541–51.
17. Lammer J, Malagari K, Vogl T, et al. Prospective randomized study of doxorubicin-eluting-bead embolization in the treatment of hepatocellular carcinoma: results of the PRECISION V study. Cardiovasc Intervent Radiol. 2010;33(1):41–52.
18. Dhanasekaran R, Kooby DA, Staley CA, Kauh JS, Khanna V, Kim HS. Comparison of conventional transarterial chemoembolization (TACE) and chemoembolization with doxorubicin drug eluting beads (DEB) for unresectable hepatocellular carcinoma (HCC). J Surg Oncol. 2010;101(6):476–80.
19. Poon RT, Tso WK, Pang RW, et al. A phase I/II trial of chemoembolization for hepatocellular carcinoma using a novel intra-arterial drug-eluting bead. Clin Gastroenterol Hepatol. 2007;5(9):1100–8.
20. Varela M, Real MI, Burrel M, et al. Chemoembolization of hepatocellular carcinoma with drug eluting beads: efficacy and doxorubicin pharmacokinetics. J Hepatol. 2007;46(3):474–81.
21. Llovet JM, Real MI, Montaña X, et al. Arterial embolisation or chemoembolisation versus symptomatic treatment in patients with unresectable hepatocellular carcinoma: a randomised controlled trial. Lancet. 2002;359(9319):1734–9.
22. Lo CM, Ngan H, Tso WK, et al. Randomized controlled trial of transarterial lipiodol chemoembolization for unresectable hepatocellular carcinoma. Hepatology. 2002;35(5):1164–71.
23. Ajani JA, Carrasco CH, Charnsangavej C, Samaan NA, Levin B, Wallace S. Islet cell tumors metastatic to the liver: effective palliation by sequential hepatic artery embolization. Ann Intern Med. 1988;108(3):340–4.
24. Bloomston M, Al-Saif O, Klemanski D, et al. Hepatic artery chemoembolization in 122 patients with metastatic carcinoid tumor: lessons learned. J Gastrointest Surg. 2007;11(3):264–71.
25. Gupta S, Johnson MM, Murthy R, et al. Hepatic arterial embolization and chemoembolization for the treatment of patients with metastatic neuroendocrine tumors: variables affecting response rates and survival. Cancer. 2005;104(8):1590–602.
26. Gupta S, Yao JC, Ahrar K, et al. Hepatic artery embolization and chemoembolization for treatment of patients with metastatic carcinoid tumors: the M.D. Anderson experience. Cancer J. 2003;9(4):261–7.
27. Leung TW, Lau WY, Ho SK, et al. Radiation pneumonitis after selective internal radiation treatment with intraarterial 90yttrium-microspheres for inoperable hepatic tumors. Int J Radiat Oncol Biol Phys. 1995;33(4):919–24.
28. Moertel CG, Johnson CM, McKusick MA, et al. The management of patients with advanced carcinoid tumors and islet cell carcinomas. Ann Intern Med. 1994;120(4):302–9.
29. Ruutiainen AT et al. Chemoembolization and bland embolization of neuroendocrine tumor metastases to the liver. J Vasc Interv Radiol. 2007;18(7):847–55.
30. Bedikian AY, Legha SS, Mavligit G, et al. Treatment of uveal melanoma metastatic to the liver: a review of the MD. Anderson Cancer Center experience and prognostic factors. Cancer. 1995;76(9):1665–70.
31. Gupta S, Bedikian AY, Ahrar J, et al. Hepatic artery chemoembolization in patients with ocular melanoma metastatic to the liver: response, survival, and prognostic factors. Am J Clin Oncol. 2010;33(5):474–80.
32. Patel K, Sullivan K, Berd D, et al. Chemoembolization of the hepatic artery with BCNU for metastatic uveal melanoma: results of a phase II study. Melanoma Res. 2005;15(4):297–304.
33. Sharma KV, Gould JE, Harbour JW, et al. Hepatic arterial chemoembolization for management of metastatic melanoma. AJR Am J Roentgenol. 2008;190(1):99–104.

34. Agarwala SS, Panikkar R, Kirkwood JM. Phase I/II randomized trial of intrahepatic arterial infusion chemotherapy with cisplatin and chemoembolization with cisplatin and polyvinyl sponge in patients with ocular melanoma metastatic to the liver. Melanoma Res. 2004;14(3):217–22.

35. Poggi G, Amatu A, Montagna B, et al. OEM-TACE: a new therapeutic approach in unresectable intrahepatic cholangiocarcinoma. Cardiovasc Intervent Radiol. 2009;32(6):1187–92.

36. Gusani NJ, Balaa FK, Steel JK, et al. Treatment of unresectable cholangiocarcinoma with gemcitabine-based transcatheter arterial chemoembolization (TACE): a single-institution experience. J Gastrointest Surg. 2008;12(1):129–37.

37. Aliberti C, Benea G, Tilli M, Fiorentini G. Chemoembolization (TACE) of unresectable intrahepatic cholangiocarcinoma with slow-release doxorubicin-eluting beads: preliminary results. Cardiovasc Intervent Radiol. 2008;31(5):883–8.

38. Albert M, Kiefer MV, Sun W, et al. Chemoembolization of colorectal liver metastases with cisplatin, doxorubicin, mitomycin C, ethiodol, and polyvinyl alcohol. Cancer. 2011;117(2):343–52.

39. Nabil M, Gruber T, Yakoub D, Ackermann H, Zangos S, Vogl TJ. Repetitive transarterial chemoembolization (TACE) of liver metastases from renal cell carcinoma: local control and survival results. Eur Radiol. 2008;18(7):1456–63.

40. Yayoi E, Furukawa J, Sekimoto M, et al. A comparison of intra-arterial chemoembolization and infusion chemotherapy for liver metastases of breast cancer. Gan To Kagaku Ryoho. 1995;22(11):1519–22.

41. Kobayashi K, Gupta S, Trent JC, et al. Hepatic artery chemoembolization for 110 gastrointestinal stromal tumors: response, survival, and prognostic factors. Cancer. 2006;107(12):2833–41.

42. Fromigué J, De Baere T, Baudin E, Dromain C, Leboulleux S, Schlumberger M. Chemoembolization for liver metastases from medullary thyroid carcinoma. J Clin Endocrinol Metab. 2006;91(7):2496–9.

43. Brown DB, Cardella JF, Sacks D, et al. Quality improvement guidelines for transhepatic arterial chemoembolization, embolization, and chemotherapeutic infusion for hepatic malignancy. J Vasc Interv Radiol. 2006;17(2 Pt 1):225–32.

44. Sakamoto I, Aso N, Nagaoki K, et al. Complications associated with transcatheter arterial embolization for hepatic tumors. Radiographics. 1998;18(3):605–19.

45. Song SY, Chung JW, Han JK, et al. Liver abscess after transcatheter oily chemoembolization for hepatic tumors: incidence, predisposing factors, and clinical outcome. J Vasc Interv Radiol. 2001;12(3):313–20.

46. Geschwind JF, Kaushik S, Ramsey DE, et al. Influence of a new prophylactic antibiotic therapy on the incidence of liver abscesses after chemoembolization treatment of liver tumors. J Vasc Interv Radiol. 2002;13(11):1163–6.

47. Patel S, Tuite CM, Mondschein JI, Soulen MC. Effectiveness of an aggressive antibiotic regimen for chemoembolization in patients with previous biliary intervention. J Vasc Interv Radiol. 2006;17(12):1931–4.

48. Kennedy AS, Dezarn WA, McNeillie P, et al. Radioembolization for unresectable neuroendocrine hepatic metastases using resin 90Y-microspheres: early results in 148 patients. Am J Clin Oncol. 2008;31(3):271–9.

49. Stubbs RS, Cannan RJ, Mitchell AW. Selective internal radiation therapy (SIRT) with 90Yttrium microspheres for extensive colorectal liver metastases. Hepatogastroenterology. 2001;48(38):333–7.

50. Chua TC, Bester L, Saxena A, Morris DL. Radioembolization and systemic chemotherapy improves response and survival for unresectable colorectal liver metastases. J Cancer Res Clin Oncol. 2011;137(5):865–73.

51. Cao CQ, Yan TD, Bester L, Liauw W, Morris DL. Radioembolization with yttrium microspheres for neuroendocrine tumour liver metastases. Br J Surg. 2010;97(4):537–43.

52. Jakobs TF, Hoffmann RT, Fischer T, et al. Radioembolization in patients with hepatic metastases from breast cancer. J Vasc Interv Radiol. 2008;19(5):683–90.

53. Bangash AK, Atassi B, Kaklamani V, et al. 90Y radioembolization of metastatic breast cancer to the liver: toxicity, imaging response, survival. J Vasc Interv Radiol. 2007;18(5):621–8.

54. Saxena A, Bester L, Chua TC, Chu FC, Morris DL. Yttrium-90 radiotherapy for unresectable intrahepatic cholangiocarcinoma: a preliminary assessment of this novel treatment option. Ann Surg Oncol. 2010;17(2):484–91.

55. Riaz A, Lewandowski RJ, Kulik LM, et al. Complications following radioembolization with yttrium-90 microspheres: a comprehensive literature review. J Vasc Interv Radiol. 2009;20(9):1121–30. quiz 1131.

56. Nagino M, Kamiya J, Nishio H, Ebata T, Arai T, Nimura Y. Two hundred forty consecutive portal vein embolizations before extended hepatectomy for biliary cancer: surgical outcome and long-term follow-up. Ann Surg. 2006;243(3):364–72.

57. Shoup M, Gonen M, D'Angelica M, et al. Volumetric analysis predicts hepatic dysfunction in patients undergoing major liver resection. J Gastrointest Surg. 2003;7(3):325–30.

58. Kubota K, Makuuchi M, Kusaka K, et al. Measurement of liver volume and hepatic functional reserve as a guide to decision-making in resectional surgery for hepatic tumors. Hepatology. 1997;26(5):1176–81.

59. Azoulay D, Castaing D, Krissat J, et al. Percutaneous portal vein embolization increases the feasibility and safety of major liver resection for hepatocellular carcinoma in injured liver. Ann Surg. 2000;232(5):665–72.

60. Yokoyama Y, Nagino M, Nimura Y. Mechanisms of hepatic regeneration following portal vein embolization and partial hepatectomy: a review. World J Surg. 2007;31(2):367–74.

61. Makuuchi M, Thai BL, Takayasu K, et al. Preoperative portal embolization to increase safety of major hepatectomy for hilar bile duct carcinoma: a preliminary report. Surgery. 1990;107(5):521–7.

62. Vauthey JN, Abdalla EK, Doherty DA, et al. Body surface area and body weight predict total liver volume in Western adults. Liver Transpl. 2002;8(3):233–40.

63. Makuuchi M, Kosuge T, Lygidakis NJ. New possibilities for major liver surgery in patients with Klatskin tumors or primary hepatocellular carcinoma – an old problem revisited. Hepatogastroenterology. 1991;38(4):329–36.

64. Di Stefano DR, de Baere T, Denys A, et al. Preoperative percutaneous portal vein embolization: evaluation of adverse events in 188 patients. Radiology. 2005;234(2):625–30.

65. Salem R, Lewandowski RJ, Mulcahy MF, et al. Radioembolization for hepatocellular carcinoma using Yttrium-90 microspheres: a comprehensive report of long-term outcomes. Gastroenterology. 2010;138(1):52–64.

66. Lewandowski RJ, Kulik LM, Riaz A, et al. A comparative analysis of transarterial downstaging for hepatocellular carcinoma: chemoembolization versus radioembolization. Am J Transplant. 2009;9(8):1920–8.
67. Ramage JK, Davies AH, Ardill J, et al. Guidelines for the management of gastroenteropancreatic neuroendocrine (including carcinoid) tumours. Gut. 2005;54 Suppl 4:1–16.
68. King J, Quinn R, Glenn DM, et al. Radioembolization with selective internal radiation microspheres for neuroendocrine liver metastases. Cancer. 2008;113(5):921–9.
69. Saxena A, Chua TC, Bester L, Kokandi A, Morris DL. Factors predicting response and survival after yttrium-90 radioembolization of unresectable neuroendocrine tumor liver metastases: a critical appraisal of 48 cases. Ann Surg. 2010;251(5):910–6.
70. Kath R, Hayungs J, Bornfeld N, Sauerwein W, Höffken K, Seeber S. Prognosis and treatment of disseminated uveal melanoma. Cancer. 1993;72(7):2219–23.
71. Maluccio MA, Covey AM, Schubert J, et al. Treatment of metastatic sarcoma to the liver with bland embolization. Cancer. 2006;107(7):1617–23.
72. Mavligit GM, Zukiwski AA, Salem PA, Lamki L, Wallace S. Regression of hepatic metastases from gastrointestinal leiomyosarcoma after hepatic arterial chemoembolization. Cancer. 1991;68(2):321–3.
73. Mavligit GM, Zukwiski AA, Ellis LM, Chuang VP, Wallace S. Gastrointestinal leiomyosarcoma metastatic to the liver. Durable tumor regression by hepatic chemoembolization infusion with cisplatin and vinblastine. Cancer. 1995;75(8):2083–8.
74. Rajan DK, Soulen MC, Clark TW, et al. Sarcomas metastatic to the liver: response and survival after cisplatin, doxorubicin, mitomycin-C, Ethiodol, and polyvinyl alcohol chemoembolization. J Vasc Interv Radiol. 2001;12(2):187–93.
75. Vogl TJ, Gruber T, Balzer JO, Eichler K, Hammerstingl R, Zangos S. Repeated transarterial chemoembolization in the treatment of liver metastases of colorectal cancer: prospective study. Radiology. 2009;250(1):281–9.
76. Mulcahy MF, Lewandowski RJ, Ibrahim SM, et al. Radioembolization of colorectal hepatic metastases using yttrium-90 microspheres. Cancer. 2009;115(9):1849–58.
77. Gray B, Van Hazel G, Hope M, et al. Randomised trial of SIR-Spheres plus chemotherapy vs. chemotherapy alone for treating patients with liver metastases from primary large bowel cancer. Ann Oncol. 2001;12(12):1711–20.
78. Hendlisz A, Van den Eynde M, Peeters M, et al. Phase III trial comparing protracted intravenous fluorouracil infusion alone or with yttrium-90 resin microspheres radioembolization for liver-limited metastatic colorectal cancer refractory to standard chemotherapy. J Clin Oncol. 2010;28(23):3687–94.

Chapter 10
Radiofrequency Ablation and Microwave Ablation for Liver Tumors

Riccardo Lencioni and Laura Crocetti

Introduction

The development of image-guided percutaneous techniques for local tumor ablation has been one of the major advances in the treatment of liver malignancies. Among these methods, radiofrequency (RF) ablation is currently established as the primary ablative modality at most institutions. RF ablation is accepted as the best therapeutic choice for patients with early stage hepatocellular carcinoma (HCC) when liver transplantation or surgical resection is not a suitable option [1, 2]. In addition, RF ablation is considered a viable alternative to surgery in patients with limited hepatic metastatic disease, especially from colorectal cancer, in patients deemed ineligible for surgical resection, because of the extent and location of the disease or concurrent medical conditions [2]. Microwave (MW) ablation is a new, promising technique that seems to offer many of the advantages of RF ablation while possibly overcoming some of the limitations [3]. The following is a practical guide for performing image-guided thermal ablation of liver tumors.

Indications

There is substantial published evidence that supports the application of RF ablation in the treatment of primary and secondary liver tumors [1, 2]. As yet, there are no substantial data relating to the use of MW ablation for the same purpose. However, experimental studies suggest that MW ablation shares many of the advantages of RF ablation, while overcoming some of its limitations. In this chapter, the terminology "thermal ablation" encompasses RF and MW ablation.

1. *Hepatocellular carcinoma.* RF ablation is the therapy of choice in very-early and early HCC as classified in the Barcelona Clinic Liver Cancer (BCLC) classification (Table 10.1), when patients are not candidates for either liver resection or transplantation. Patients are required to have a single tumor smaller than 5 cm or as many as three nodules smaller than 3 cm each, no evidence of vascular invasion or extrahepatic spread, performance status test of 0, and liver cirrhosis in Child-Pugh class A or B.

2. *Liver metastases*:

    (a) *Primary tumor histotype.* Thermal ablation is generally indicated for nonsurgical patients with a small number of colorectal cancer metastases limited to the liver. Selected patients with combined hepatic and pulmonary colorectal metastases, however, may qualify for percutaneous treatment provided that the extrahepatic disease is deemed curable. In patients with hepatic metastases from other primary cancers, promising initial results have been reported in the treatment of breast and endocrine tumors [2].

    (b) *Number of lesions.* The number of lesions should not be considered an absolute contraindication to ablation if successful treatment of all metastatic deposits can be accomplished. Nevertheless, most centers preferentially treat patients with five or fewer lesions [2].

R. Lencioni (✉) • L. Crocetti
Division of Diagnostic Imaging and Intervention, Department of Liver Transplants, Hepatology, and Infectious Diseases,
Pisa University School of Medicine, Pisa, Italy
e-mail: riccardo.lencioni@med.unipi.it

P.R. Mueller and A. Adam (eds.), *Interventional Oncology: A Practical Guide for the Interventional Radiologist*,
DOI 10.1007/978-1-4419-1469-9_10, © Springer Science+Business Media, LLC 2012

Table 10.1 Barcelona Clinic Liver Cancer (BCLC) classification in patients diagnosed with hepatocellular carcinoma (HCC)

Very-early stage:	PS 0, Child-Pugh A, single HCC <2 cm
Early stage:	PS 0, Child-Pugh A–B, single HCC or three nodules <3 cm
Intermediate stage:	PS 0, Child-Pugh A–B, multinodular HCC
Advanced stage:	PS 1–2, Child-Pugh A–B, portal neoplastic invasion, nodal metastases, distant metastases
Terminal stage:	PS >2, Child-Pugh C

PS performance status

(c) *Tumor size*. The target tumor should not exceed 3 cm in the longest axis to achieve best rates of complete ablation with most of the currently available RF devices [2]. One of the potential advantages of MW ablation would be the ability of creating larger zones of ablation. This could increase the maximum diameter of the treatable tumors with high rates of complete ablation.

Contraindications

Absolute contraindications for thermal ablation are [2]:

1. Tumor located <1 cm away from the common bile duct due to risk of delayed occlusion of the biliary tree.
2. Intrahepatic bile duct dilation.
3. Anterior exophytic location of the tumor, due to the risk of tumor seeding.
4. Untreatable/unmanageable coagulopathy.

Relative contraindications for thermal ablation are [2]:

1. Bilioenteric anastomosis, because of the risk of hepatic abscesses.
2. Superficial lesions, because of a higher risk of complications.
3. Superficial lesions that are adjacent to any part of the gastrointestinal tract, because of the risk of thermal injury of the gastric or bowel wall (consider hydro/gas dissection).
4. Tumors located in the vicinity of the gallbladder, due to the risk of iatrogenic cholecystitis.

Preprocedure Preparation

1. *Evaluate* patient records, history, physical examination, and prior imaging studies to determine the indication and the feasibility of thermal ablation.
2. *Preprocedural imaging*.

   (a) The appropriate tumor staging protocol must be used. In patients with HCC, the detection of a mass by ultrasound (US) is usually followed by multidetector spiral computed tomography (CT) or dynamic magnetic resonance (MR), following the recommendations of the American Association for the Study of Liver Diseases (AASLD) [1]. In patients with liver metastases, the tumor staging protocol should include abdominal US and CT or MR of the abdomen. Chest CT and positron emission tomography (PET) or PET–CT may be required to exclude or confirm the presence of extrahepatic disease [4].

   (b) Pretreatment imaging must carefully define the location of each lesion in relation to surrounding structures. Tumors on the surface of the liver can be considered for thermal ablation, but their treatment may be associated with a higher risk of complications and requires substantial expertise. Thermal ablation of superficial lesions that are adjacent to any part of the gastrointestinal tract must be avoided because of the risk of thermal injury of the gastric or bowel wall. The use of special techniques, such as intraperitoneal injection of dextrose to displace the bowel, can be considered in such instances. Treatment of lesions adjacent to the hepatic hilum carries the risk of thermal biliary stricture. In experienced hands, thermal ablation of tumors located in the vicinity of the gallbladder has been shown to be feasible but is often associated with transient iatrogenic cholecystitis. Thermal ablation of lesions adjacent to hepatic vessels is not contraindicated, as the flowing blood usually protects the vascular wall from thermal injury.

I:	A normal healthy patient
II:	A patient with mild systemic disease
III:	A patient with severe systemic disease
IV:	A patient with severe systemic disease that is a constant threat to life
V:	A moribund patient who is not expected to survive without the operation
VI:	A declared brain-dead patient whose organs are being removed for donor purposes

However, in such cases, there is a risk of incomplete treatment of the neoplastic tissue close to the vessel because of the heat loss by convection [2].

3. *Preprocedural testing.* Laboratory tests should include:

  (a) Measurement of serum tumor markers, such as alpha-fetoprotein for HCC and carcinoembryonic antigen for colorectal metastases [4].
  (b) Evaluation of patient's coagulation status. This includes measurement of the complete blood count, including platelet count, prothrombin time (PT), and international normalized ratio (INR). In some institutions the activated partial thromboplastin time and/or cutaneous bleeding time are also measured. A PT ratio (normal time/patient's time) >50% and a platelet count higher than 50,000 per microliter are required to keep the risk of bleeding at an acceptable level [2].

4. *Management of medications.* An important issue surrounds management of antiplatelet medications, such as aspirin, ticlopidine, clopidogrel, IIb/IIIa receptor antagonists, and nonsteroidal anti-inflammatory drugs, and/or anticoagulant drugs such as warfarin, before and after the ablation procedure. According to the AASLD, antiplatelet medications should be discontinued approximately 10 days before liver biopsy. Antiplatelet therapy may be restarted 48–72 h after liver biopsy. Even anticoagulant medications should be discontinued prior to liver biopsy. Warfarin should generally be discontinued at least 5 days before the procedure. Heparin and related products should be discontinued 12–24 h prior to biopsy. Warfarin may be restarted the day following liver biopsy [5].

Procedure

1. *Anesthesiology care.* Thermal ablation is usually performed under intravenous sedation and local anesthesia with standard monitoring of cardiac rhythm, blood pressure, and oxygen saturation. In some centers general anesthesia with tracheal intubation is used. The American Society of Anesthesiologists' (ASA) score (Table 10.2) can be used to assess the patient's physical status prior to thermal ablation; patients up to ASA III score can be treated [2].
2. *Technical principles: RF ablation.* RF ablation produces thermal injury to tissue through electromagnetic energy deposition. The patient is part of a closed-loop circuit, which includes the RF generator, the needle electrode, and one or more dispersive electrode (grounding pads). An alternating electric field is created within the tissues of the patient. Because of the relatively high electrical resistance of tissue in comparison with the metal electrodes, there is marked agitation of the ions present in the target tissue that surrounds the electrode, since the tissue ions attempt to follow the changes in direction of alternating electric current. The agitation results in frictional heat around the electrode. The discrepancy between the small surface area of the needle electrode and the large area of the ground pads causes the generated heat to be focused and concentrated around the needle electrode [4]. The thermal damage caused by RF heating is dependent on both the tissue temperature achieved and the duration of heating. Heating of tissue at 50–55°C for 4–6 min produces irreversible cellular damage. At temperatures between 60 and 100°C near immediate coagulation of tissue is induced, with irreversible damage to mitochondrial and cytosolic enzymes within the cells. At temperatures exceeding 100–110°C, tissue vaporizes and carbonizes. For adequate destruction of tumor tissue, the entire target volume must be subjected to cytotoxic temperatures. Thus, an essential objective of ablative therapy is the achievement and maintenance of a 50–100°C temperature throughout the entire target volume for at least 4–6 min. However, the relatively slow thermal conduction from the electrode surface through the tissues necessitates an increase in the duration of application to 10–20 min. To accomplish the increase of energy deposition into tissues, the RF output of all commercially available generators has been increased to 150–250 W. However, the tissue temperature should not exceed 100–110°C to avoid carbonization, since this results in significant gas production that both serves as an insulator and retards the ability to effectively establish a RF field [4]. Another important factor that affects the success of RF thermal ablation is the heat loss through convection by means of blood circulation, the so-called heat-sink effect, which may prevent RF ablation of all the viable tumor tissue. To achieve rates of local tumor recurrence with RF ablation that are comparable to those obtained with hepatic resection,

physicians should produce a 360°, 0.5- to 1-cm-thick tumor-free margin around each tumor. This cuff will ensure the eradication of all microscopic tumor extensions around the periphery of a mass. Therefore, the target diameter of the ablated area ideally should be 1–2 cm larger than the diameter of the tumor being treated [4]. RF generators are run by automate programs, designed to modulate the released power relying on direct temperature measurement or on electrical measurement of tissue impedance, to avoid overheating and carbonization. At the end of the procedure coagulation of the needle track is performed to prevent tumor seeding [4]. To minimize heat loss as a result of the heat-sink effect, various methods of reducing blood flow during ablation therapy have been tried. Total portal inflow occlusion (the Pringle maneuver) has been used at open laparotomy and at laparoscopy. Angiographic balloon catheter occlusion of the hepatic artery or embolization of the tumor-feeding artery has also been shown to be useful in hypervascular tumors [6]. In the setting of HCC, combining thermal ablation with other therapies, such as chemoembolization or transarterial administration of drug-eluting beads, has produced very promising results in pilot studies [7]. There is ongoing research in the methods of combining chemotherapeutic regimens (both agent and route of administration) with RF ablation.

3. *Types of RF electrode*. One or several electrodes have to be inserted directly into the tumor to deliver RF energy. Electrodes can be monopolar or bipolar, and various designs are available (multitined expandable, internally cooled, perfused) [2].

   (a) Monopolar electrode: there is a single active electrode, with the current dissipated by one or several grounding pads.
   (b) Bipolar electrode: there are two active electrode applicators, which have to be placed in close proximity to each other.
   (c) Multitined expandable electrode: multiple electrode tines that protrude from a larger needle cannula following expansion. They permit the deposition of this energy over a larger volume and ensure more uniform heating of the tumor.
   (d) Internally cooled electrode: the electrode has an internal lumen which is cooled by saline without coming into direct contact with the tissues of the patient. Such electrodes minimize carbonization and gas formation around the needle tip by eliminating excess heat near the electrode.
   (e) Perfused electrode: the tip of the electrode has small apertures which allow fluid (usually saline) to come into contact with the tissue, thus increasing tissue conductivity and allowing greater deposition of RF energy.

4. *Technical principles: MW ablation*. MW ablation is the term used for all electromagnetic methods of inducing tumor destruction by using devices with frequencies greater in the range of 900–2,450 kHz. The passage of microwaves into cells or other materials containing water results in the rotation of individual molecules. Water molecules are polar; that is, the electric charges on the molecules are not symmetric. The alignment and the charges on the atoms are such that the hydrogen side of the molecule has a positive charge, and the oxygen side has a negative charge [3]. Electromagnetic radiation has electric charge as well; the "wave" representation is actually the electric charge on the wave as it flips between positive and negative. When an oscillating electric charge from radiation interacts with a water molecule, it causes the molecule to flip. MW radiation can be tuned to the optimal frequency for maximum water dipole oscillation to maximize this interaction. As a result of the radiation hitting the molecules, the electrical charge on the water molecule flips back and forth 2–5 billion times a second depending on the frequency of the MW energy. The vigorous movement of water molecules raises the temperature of water. Therefore, electromagnetic microwaves heat matter by agitating water molecules in the surrounding tissue, producing friction and heat, thus inducing cellular death via coagulation necrosis [3]. The main advantages of MW technology, when compared with existing thermoablative technologies, include consistently higher intratumoral temperatures, larger tumor ablation volumes, faster ablation times, and an improved convection profile. During RF ablation, tissue perfusion and thermal conduction contribute more towards tissue cooling and heating compared to MW ablation. This is mainly due to the longer session times necessary with RF ablation, as tissue temperatures are significantly lower compared to MW ablation. The reduced influence of thermal conduction and perfusion due to shorter session times may in part explain why in vivo studies, MW coagulation zones are less affected by tissue perfusion compared to RF [8]. The region of direct heating is not significantly different between MW and RF ablation. One or multiple antennas have to be inserted directly into the tumor to deliver MW energy current. MW irradiation creates an ablation area around the needle in a column or round shape, depending on the type of needle used and the generating power. Several differently designed antennae are available and recent advances in MW engineering have allowed the design of new MW systems with the potential for larger, more controlled ablation zones. In addition, because MW ablation does not rely on an electrical circuit as does RF ablation, multiple applicators can be applied simultaneously [3, 8].

5. *Imaging guidance and monitoring*. Targeting of the lesion can be performed with US, CT, or MR imaging [4] (Fig. 10.1). The guidance system is chosen largely on the basis of operator preference and local availability of dedicated equipment such as fluoro-CT or open MR systems. During the procedure, important aspects to be monitored include how well the tumor is being covered and whether any adjacent normal structures are being affected at the same time. While the

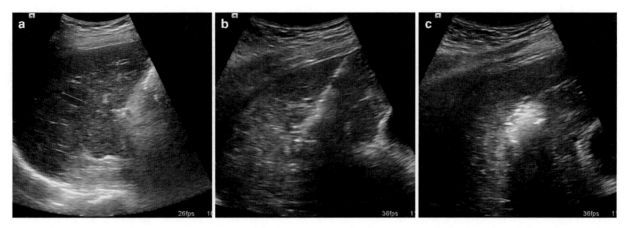

Fig. 10.1 Ultrasound (US)-guided radiofrequency (RF) ablation. (**a**) The tumor is depicted as a small hypoechoic nodule. (**b**) The expandable needle is inserted under US guidance and correct positioning of the needle is confirmed. (**c**) At the end of the procedure, a large hyperechoic cloud covering the tumor as well as a cuff of surrounding liver parenchyma is seen on US

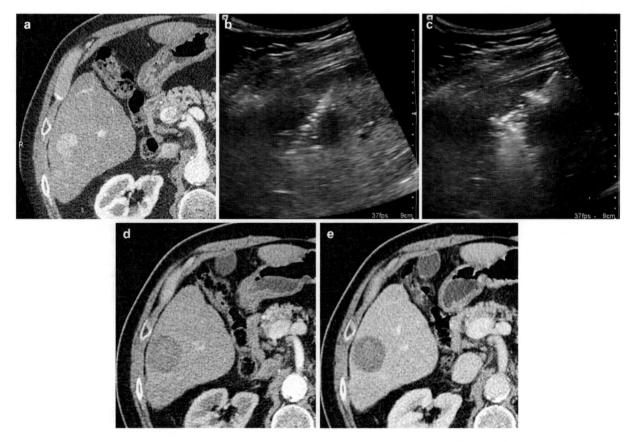

Fig. 10.2 RF ablation of hepatocellular carcinoma (HCC). (**a**) Pretreatment computed tomography (CT) shows the lesion as a small hypervascular nodule in the arterial phase. (**b**, **c**) The tumor is treated with RF ablation under US guidance. On CT images obtained in the arterial (**d**) and the portal venous phase (**e**) 1 month after treatment, the tumor is replaced by a nonenhancing ablation zone that exceeds in size the diameter of the naïve tumor. The findings are consistent with complete response

transient hyperechoic zone that is seen at US within and surrounding a tumor during and immediately after RF ablation can be used as a rough guide to the extent of tumor destruction (Fig. 10.1), MR is currently the only imaging modality with validated techniques for real-time temperature monitoring. Contrast-enhanced US performed after the end of the procedure may allow an initial evaluation of treatment effects. However, contrast-enhanced CT and MR imaging are recognized as the standard modalities to assess treatment outcome [1, 9] (Fig. 10.2).

Postprocedure Management

1. *After thermal ablation* bed rest for 1–2 h is advised; monitoring of vital signs is performed in the recovery room. If vital signs are stable, blood tests are not significantly changed, and no complications are noted, the patient can be discharged the day after the procedure.

2. *Tumor response evaluation.* CT and MR images obtained 4–8 weeks after treatment show successful ablation as a nonenhancing area with or without a peripheral enhancing rim [9, 10] (Fig. 10.2), which appears a relatively concentric, symmetric, and uniform area with smooth inner margins. This is a transient finding that represents a benign physiologic response to thermal injury (initially, reactive hyperemia; subsequently, fibrosis and giant cell reaction). Such rings should be distinguished from irregular peripheral enhancement due to residual tumor. In contrast to benign periablational enhancement, residual unablated tumor often grows in scattered, nodular, or eccentric patterns [10]. Later follow-up imaging studies should be aimed at detecting recurrence of the treated lesion, the development of new hepatic lesions, or the emergence of extrahepatic disease. Evaluation of tumor response should be performed following the criteria recently developed by a panel of experts of the AASLD [9, 11].

Results

1. *Hepatocellular carcinoma.* The therapeutic effect of RF ablation in HCC has been assessed by studies that evaluated tissue histology and by randomized or cohort studies that investigated the long-term survival of treated patients. Histological data from explanted liver specimens in patients who had undergone RF ablation showed that tumor size and the presence of abutting vessels 3 mm or larger in diameter significantly affect the result. Complete tumor necrosis was demonstrated in 83% of tumors <3 cm in size and 88% of tumors in a nonperivascular location [12]. Comparison with percutaneous ethanol injection (PEI) in five randomized trials [13–17] has shown that RF ablation had higher local anticancer effect than PEI, leading to a better local control of the disease (Table 10.3). These data were recently pooled in two independent meta-analyses, and the survival benefit for patients with small HCC submitted to RF ablation was confirmed [18, 19]. Therefore, RF ablation appears as the preferred percutaneous treatment for patients with early stage HCC on the basis of a more consistent local tumor control and better survival outcomes. Recently, the long-term survival outcomes of RF ablation-treated patients were reported (Table 10.4) and enabled the factors influencing patient prognosis to be determined [20–26]. The severity of the underlying cirrhosis and occurrence of new lesions represent the most important prognostic factors. Patients with early stage HCC in Child-Pugh class A had a 5-year survival rate of 51–77%, whereas patients in Child-Pugh class B had a 5-year

Table 10.3 Randomized studies comparing radiofrequency (RF) ablation and percutaneous ethanol injection (PEI) in the treatment of early stage HCC

Author	No. of patients	Tumor size	Complete ablation (%)	Treatment failure (%)[a]	3-Year overall survival	p
Lencioni et al. [13]						
RF	52	1 HCC <5 cm or 3	91	8	81	>0.05
PEI	50	<3 cm	82	34	73	
Lin et al. [14]						
RF	52	1–3 HCC	96	17	74	0.014
PEI	52	<4 cm	88	45	50	
Shiina et al. [15]						
RF	118	1–3 HCC	100	2	80	0.02
PEI	114	<3 cm	100	11	63	
Lin et al. [16]						
RF	62	1–3 HCC	97	16	74	0.031
PEI	62	<3 cm	89	42	51	
Brunello et al. [17]						
RF	70	1–3 HCC	96	34	59	>0.05
PEI	69	<3 cm	66	64	57	

[a]Includes initial treatment failure (incomplete response) and late treatment failure (local recurrence/progression)

Table 10.4 Studies reporting long-term survival outcomes of patients with early stage HCC who underwent percutaneous RF ablation

Author	No. of patients	Survival (%)		
		1 Year	3 Years	5 Years
Tateishi et al. [20]				
Naïve patients[a]	319	95	78	54
Nonnaïve patients[b]	345	92	62	38
Lencioni et al. [21]				
Child A, 1 HCC <5 cm or 3 <3 cm	144	100	76	51
1 HCC <5 cm	116	100	89	61
Child B, 1 HCC <5 cm or 3 <3 cm	43	89	46	31
Cabassa et al. [22]	59	94	65	43
Choi et al. [23]				
Child A, 1 HCC <5 cm or 3 <3 cm	359	NA	78	64
Child B, 1 HCC <5 cm or 3 <3 cm	160	NA	49	38
Takahashi et al. [24]				
Child A, 1 HCC <5 cm or 3 <3 cm	171	99	91	77
Hiraoka et al. [25]				
Child-Pugh A–B	105	NA	88	59
N'Kontchou et al. [26]	235	NA	60	40
Patient fitting BCLC criteria for resection	67	NA	82	76
Unresectable patients	168	NA	49	27

[a]Patients who received radiofrequency ablation as primary treatment
[b]Patients who received radiofrequency ablation for recurrent tumor after previous treatment including resection, ethanol injection, MW ablation, and transarterial embolization
NA not available

survival rate of 31–38%. The incidence of new HCC lesions in a cirrhotic liver approaches 80% 5 years after the first treatment [21]. This limitation applies to all local treatments, including surgical resection. New lesions occurring within 2 years for treatment are related to occult dissemination of the original tumor, while lesions occurring in later periods are often true "de novo" tumors. Only in very-early HCC, with a diameter <2 cm, are there optimal conditions for radical local therapy, as the probability of microvascular invasion and microsatellites is very low. In patient with very-early HCC, the complete response rate approaches 97%, and the 5-year survival rate 68% [27]. In such small tumors, therefore, RF ablation seems to challenge the role of surgical resection, and in many centers RF ablation is offered even in operable patients. The favorable results of RF ablation in HCC patients fitting BCLC criteria for liver resection have been demonstrated by a recent series. Comparing a subgroup of 67 patients who satisfied criteria for resection according to BCLC and unresectable patients, the estimated 3- and 5-year overall survival rates were, respectively, 82% versus 49% and 76% versus 27% [26].

The effect of MW ablation on HCC was assessed by examining the histological changes after treatment [28, 29]. In one study, 89% of 18 small tumors were ablated completely [28]. Coagulative necrosis with faded nuclei and eosinophilic cytoplasm were the predominant findings in the ablated areas. There were also areas in which the tumors maintained their native morphological features as if the area was fixed, but their cellular activity was destroyed as demonstrated by succinic dehydrogenase stain. One study compared MW ablation and PEI in a retrospective evaluation of 90 patients with small HCC [30]. The overall 5-year survival rates for patients with well-differentiated HCC treated with MW ablation and PEI were not significantly different. However, among the patients with moderately or poorly differentiated HCC, overall survival with MW ablation was significantly better than with PEI. In a large series including 234 patients, the 3- and 5-year survival rates were 73% and 57%, respectively [31]. At a multivariate analysis, tumor size, number of nodules, and Child-Pugh classification had a significant effect on survival [32]. Only one randomized trial compared the effectiveness of MW ablation with that of RF ablation [33]. A total of 72 patients with 94 HCC nodules were randomly assigned to RF ablation and MW ablation groups. Unfortunately, in this study, the data were analyzed with respect to lesions and not to patients. Although no statistically significant differences were observed with respect to the efficacy of the two procedures, a tendency favoring RF ablation was recognized with respect to local recurrences and complications rates.

Table 10.5 Studies reporting long-term survival outcomes of patients with colorectal hepatic metastases who underwent percutaneous RF ablation

Author	No. of patients	Survival (%)		
		1 Year	3 Years	5 Years
Solbiati et al. [35]	117	93	46	–
Lencioni et al. [34]	423	86	47	24
Machi et al. [36]	100	90	42	30
Jackobs et al. [37]	68	96	68	–
Sorensen et al. [38]	102	87	46	26[a]
Veltri et al. [39]	122	79	38	22

[a]4-Year survival

2. *Colorectal hepatic metastases.* Many studies have investigated the use of RF ablation in the treatment of limited colorectal hepatic metastases in patients who were excluded from surgery. Early studies reported rates of complete response that did not exceed 60–70% [4, 34]. Subsequently, owing to the advances in RF technique and probably to the treatment of smaller tumors, reported rates of successful local tumor control following RF treatment substantially increased. In recent series, complete response rate to RF ablation was 91–97% [4, 34]. Recently, data on long-term survival of nonsurgical patients with hepatic colorectal metastases who underwent RF ablation have been reported (Table 10.5) [35–39]. In three series including patients with five or fewer lesions, each 5 cm or less in diameter, the 5-year survival rate ranged 24–44% at 5 years [34, 35, 37]. When RF ablation was performed in patients with small (<4 cm), solitary hepatic colorectal metastases, the 5-year survival rate was 40% [40]. These figures are substantially higher than those obtained with any chemotherapy regimens and provide indirect evidence that RF ablation therapy improves survival in patients with limited hepatic metastatic disease. This conclusion is supported by the interim analysis of a randomized controlled trial comparing chemotherapy plus RF ablation versus chemotherapy alone in colorectal cancer metastatic to the liver [41]. The potential role of performing RF ablation during the interval between diagnosis and resection as part of a "test-of-time" management approach was investigated. Among the patients in whom complete tumor ablation was achieved after RF treatment, 98% were spared surgical resection because they remained free of disease or because they developed additional metastases leading to unresectability. No patient in whom RF treatment did not achieve complete tumor ablation became unresectable due to the growth of the treated metastases [42].

Results of MW ablation in large series of patients with liver metastases are scarce. One study reports the long-term survival rate in 74 patients with 149 liver metastases from different primary tumors. The cumulative survival rates of all 74 patients were 91.4% at 1 year, 46.4% at 3 years, and 29% at 5 years. Both univariate and multivariate analysis revealed that tumor grade, number of metastases, tumor size, and local recurrence or new metastasis significantly affected survival [43]. MW ablation has been demonstrated to be able to expand the indication for surgery to treat multiple bilobar colorectal liver metastases, with survival similar to that in less-involved hepatic resection in patients [44].

Complications

1. *RF ablation.* Early major complications associated with RF ablation occur in 2.2–3.1% of patients and include intraperitoneal bleeding, liver abscess, intestinal perforation, pneumo/hemothorax, and bile duct stenosis [45–47]. An uncommon late complication of RF ablation can be tumor seeding along the needle track. In patients with HCC, tumor seeding occurred in 8 (0.5%) of 1,610 cases in a multicenter survey [45] and in 1 (0.5%) of 187 cases in a single-institution series [21]. Lesions with subcapsular location and an invasive tumoral pattern, as shown by a poor differentiation degree, seem to be at higher risk for such a complication [48]. The minor complication rate ranges from 5% to 8.9%. They include pain, fever, asymptomatic pleural effusion, and asymptomatic self-limiting intraperitoneal bleeding [45–47]. The procedure mortality rate is 0.1–0.5%. The most common causes of death are sepsis, hepatic failure, colon perforation, and portal vein thrombosis (particularly in patients submitted to RF ablation with surgical approach and Pringle maneuver) [45–47].

2. *MW ablation.* In a large series of 1,136 patients treated in 3,697 MW ablation sessions, major complications occurred in 30 (2.6%) patients and included liver abscess and empyema, bile duct injury, perforation of the colon, pleural effusion requiring thoracentesis, hemorrhage requiring arterial embolizati on, and skin burn requiring resection. Tumor seeding along the needle track occurred in 0.4% of patients. Minor complications included fever, pain, asymptomatic pleural effusion, gallbladder wall thickening, small stricture of the bile duct, and skin burn requiring no treatment [49].

References

1. Bruix J, Sherman M. Management of hepatocellular carcinoma. Hepatology. 2005;42:1208–36.
2. Crocetti L, DeBaere T, Lencioni R. Quality improvement guidelines for radiofrequency ablation of liver tumours. Cardiovasc Intervent Radiol. 2010;33:11–7.
3. Simon CF, Dupuy DE, Mayo-Smith WW. Microwave ablation: principles and applications. Radiographics. 2005;25:S69–83.
4. Lencioni R, Crocetti L, Pina MC, et al. Percutaneous image-guided radiofrequency ablation of liver tumors. Abdom Imaging. 2009;34:547–56.
5. Rockey DC, Caldwell SH, Goodman ZD, et al. Liver biopsy. Hepatology. 2009;49:1017–44.
6. Rossi S, Garbagnati F, Lencioni R, et al. Percutaneous radio-frequency thermal ablation of nonresectable hepatocellular carcinoma after occlusion of tumor blood supply. Radiology. 2000;217:119–26.
7. Lencioni R, Crocetti L, Petruzzi P, et al. Doxorubicin-eluting bead-enhanced radiofrequency ablation of hepatocellular carcinoma: a pilot clinical study. J Hepatol. 2008;49:217–22.
8. Schramm W, Yang D, Wood BJ, Rattay F, Haemmerich D. Contribution of direct heating, thermal conduction and perfusion during radiofrequency and microwave ablation. Open Biomed Eng J. 2007;19(1):47–52.
9. Llovet JM, Di Bisceglie AM, Bruix J, et al. Panel of Experts in HCC-Design Clinical Trials. Design and endpoints of clinical trials in hepatocellular carcinoma. J Natl Cancer Inst. 2008;100:698–711.
10. Goldberg SN, Charboneau JW, Dodd III GD, et al. Image-guided tumor ablation: proposal for standardization of terms and reporting criteria. Radiology. 2003;228:335–45.
11. Lencioni R, Llovet JM. Modified RECIST (mRECIST) assessment for hepatocellular carcinoma. Semin Liver Dis. 2010;30:52–60.
12. Lu DS, Yu NC, Raman SS, et al. Radiofrequency ablation of hepatocellular carcinoma: treatment success as defined by histologic examination of the explanted liver. Radiology. 2005;234:954–60.
13. Lencioni R, Allgaier HP, Cioni D, et al. Small hepatocellular carcinoma in cirrhosis: randomized comparison of radiofrequency thermal ablation versus percutaneous ethanol injection. Radiology. 2003;228:235–40.
14. Lin SM, Lin CJ, Lin CC, et al. Radiofrequency ablation improves prognosis compared with ethanol injection for hepatocellular carcinoma < or =4 cm. Gastroenterology. 2004;127:1714–23.
15. Shiina S, Teratani T, Obi S, et al. A randomized controlled trial of radiofrequency ablation versus ethanol injection for small hepatocellular carcinoma. Gastroenterology. 2005;129:122–30.
16. Lin SM, Lin CJ, Lin CC, et al. Randomised controlled trial comparing percutaneous radiofrequency thermal ablation, percutaneous ethanol injection, and percutaneous acetic acid injection to treat hepatocellular carcinoma of 3 cm or less. Gut. 2005;54:1151–6.
17. Brunello F, Veltri A, Carucci P, et al. Radiofrequency ablation versus ethanol injection for early hepatocellular carcinoma: a randomized controlled trial. Scand J Gastroenterol. 2008;43:727–35.
18. Orlando A, Leandro G, Olivo M, et al. Radiofrequency thermal ablation vs. percutaneous ethanol injection for small hepatocellular carcinoma in cirrhosis: meta-analysis of randomized controlled trials. Am J Gastroenterol. 2009;104:514–24.
19. Cho YK, Kim JK, Kim MY, et al. Systematic review of randomized trials for hepatocellular carcinoma treated with percutaneous ablation therapies. Hepatology. 2009;49:453–9.
20. Tateishi R, Shiina S, Teratani T, et al. Percutaneous radiofrequency ablation for hepatocellular carcinoma. Cancer. 2005;103:1201–9.
21. Lencioni R, Cioni D, Crocetti L, et al. Early-stage hepatocellular carcinoma in cirrhosis: long-term results of percutaneous image-guided radiofrequency ablation. Radiology. 2005;234:961–7.
22. Cabassa P, Donato F, Simeone F, et al. Radiofrequency ablation of hepatocellular carcinoma: long-term experience with expandable needle electrodes. AJR Am J Roentgenol. 2006;185:S316–21.
23. Choi D, Lim HK, Rhim H, et al. Percutaneous radiofrequency ablation for early-stage hepatocellular carcinoma as a first-line treatment: long-term results and prognostic factors in a large single-institution series. Eur Radiol. 2007;17:684–92.
24. Takahashi S, Kudo M, Chung H, et al. Initial treatment response is essential to improve survival in patients with hepatocellular carcinoma who underwent curative radiofrequency ablation therapy. Oncology. 2007;72:S98–103.
25. Hiraoka A, Horiike N, Yamashita Y, et al. Efficacy of radiofrequency ablation therapy compared to surgical resection in 164 patients in Japan with single hepatocellular carcinoma smaller than 3 cm, along with report of complications. Hepatogastroenterology. 2008;55:2171–4.
26. N'Kontchou G, Mahamoudi A, Aout M, et al. Radiofrequency ablation of hepatocellular carcinoma: long-term results and prognostic factors in 235 Western patients with cirrhosis. Hepatology. 2009;50:1475–83.
27. Livraghi T, Meloni F, Di Stasi M, et al. Sustained complete response and complications rates after radiofrequency ablation of very early hepatocellular carcinoma in cirrhosis: is resection still the treatment of choice? Hepatology. 2008;47:82–9.
28. Yamashiki N, Kato T, Bejarano PA, et al. Histopathological changes after microwave coagulation therapy for patients with hepatocellular carcinoma: review of 15 explanted livers. Am J Gastroenterol. 2003;98:2052–9.
29. Yu NC, Lu DS, Raman SS, et al. Hepatocellular carcinoma: microwave ablation with multiple straight and loop antenna clusters – pilot comparison with pathologic findings. Radiology. 2006;239:269–75.
30. Seki T, Wakabayashi M, Nakagawa T, et al. Percutaneous microwave coagulation therapy for patients with small hepatocellular carcinoma: comparison with percutaneous ethanol injection therapy. Cancer. 1999;85:1694–702.
31. Dong B, Liang P, Yu X, et al. Percutaneous sonographically guided microwave coagulation therapy for hepatocellular carcinoma: results in 234 patients. AJR Am J Roentgenol. 2003;180:1547–54.
32. Liang P, Dong B, Yu X, et al. Prognostic factors for survival in patients with hepatocellular carcinoma after percutaneous microwave ablation. Radiology. 2005;235:299–307.
33. Shibata T, Iimuro Y, Yamamoto Y, et al. Small hepatocellular carcinoma: comparison of radio-frequency ablation and percutaneous microwave coagulation therapy. Radiology. 2002;223:331–7.
34. Lencioni R, Crocetti L, Cioni D, et al. Percutaneous radiofrequency ablation of hepatic colorectal metastases. Technique, indications, results, and new promises. Invest Radiol. 2004;39:589–59.

35. Solbiati L, Livraghi T, Goldberg SN, et al. Percutaneous radio-frequency ablation of hepatic metastases from colorectal cancer: long-term results in 117 patients. Radiology. 2001;221:159–66.
36. Machi J, Oishi AJ, Sumida K, et al. Long-term outcome of radiofrequency ablation for unresectable liver metastases from colorectal cancer: evaluation of prognostic factors and effectiveness in first- and second-line management. Cancer J. 2006;12:318–26.
37. Jackobs TF, Hoffmann RT, Trumm C, et al. Radiofrequency ablation of colorectal liver metastases: mid-term results in 68 patients. Anticancer Res. 2006;26:671–80.
38. Sorensen SM, Mortensen FV, Nielsen DT. Radiofrequency ablation of colorectal liver metastases: long-term survival. Acta Radiol. 2007;48:253–8.
39. Veltri A, Sacchetto P, Tosetti I, et al. Radiofrequency ablation of colorectal liver metastases: small size favorably predicts technique effectiveness and survival. Cardiovasc Intervent Radiol. 2008;31:948–56.
40. Gillams AR, Lees WR. Five-year survival following radiofrequency ablation of small, solitary, hepatic colorectal metastases. J Vasc Interv Radiol. 2008;19:712–7.
41. Ruers T, van Coevorden F, Pierie J, et al. Radiofrequency ablation combined with chemotherapy for unresectable colorectal liver metastases: interim results of a randomised phase II study of the EORTC-NCRI CCSG-ALM Intergroup 40004 (CLOCC). J Clin Oncol. 2008;26 Suppl 20:4012.
42. Livraghi T, Solbiati L, Meloni F, et al. Percutaneous radiofrequency ablation of liver metastases in potential candidates for resection: the "test-of-time approach". Cancer. 2003;97:3027–35.
43. Liang P, Dong B, Yu X, et al. Prognostic factors for percutaneous microwave coagulation therapy of hepatic metastases. AJR Am J Roentgenol. 2003;181:1319–25.
44. Tanaka K, Shimada H, Nagano Y, Endo I, Sekido H, Togo S. Outcome after hepatic resection versus combined resection and microwave ablation for multiple bilobar colorectal metastases to the liver. Surgery. 2006;139:263–73.
45. Livraghi T, Solbiati L, Meloni MF, et al. Treatment of focal liver tumors with percutaneous radio-frequency ablation: complications encountered in a multicentre study. Radiology. 2003;26:441–51.
46. De Baere T, Risse O, Kuoch V, et al. Adverse events during radiofrequency treatment of 582 hepatic tumors. AJR Am J Roentgenol. 2003;181:695–700.
47. Bleicher RJ, Allegra DP, Nora DT, et al. Radiofrequency ablation in 447 complex unresectable liver tumors: lessons learned. Ann Surg Oncol. 2003;10:52–8.
48. Llovet JM, Vilana R, Bru C, et al. Barcelona Clinic Liver Cancer (BCLC) Group. Increased risk of tumor seeding after percutaneous radiofrequency ablation for single hepatocellular carcinoma. Hepatology. 2001;33:1124–9.
49. Liang P, Wang Y, Yu X, Dong B. Malignant liver tumors: treatment with percutaneous microwave ablation – complications among cohort of 1136 patients. Radiology. 2009;251:933–40.

Part III
Kidney

Chapter 11
Nonradiological Treatment for Renal Tumors

Sarah P. Psutka and Brian H. Eisner

Introduction

Renal cell carcinoma (RCC) is the most common, primary renal malignancy, with 39,000 new cases and 12,000 annual deaths annually in the USA [1]. Historically, radical surgery (removal of the kidney in its entirety with surrounding Gerota's fascia, the adrenal gland, and the proximal two-thirds of the ureter) was the treatment of choice for RCC [2]. Recently, technical improvements stemming from a better understanding of the natural history of RCC have altered the approach to localized RCC, shifting treatment towards minimally invasive techniques and nephron-sparing surgery. This chapter reviews the most current trends in the surgical treatment of RCC.

Indications for Surgical Management of Renal Tumors: Localized and Extensive Disease

Surgical Control of Localized Disease

Localized RCC, pathological stage T1–T2, is managed with laparoscopic or open surgery. In recent years, nephron-sparing surgery (i.e., partial nephrectomy) has gained widespread acceptance for small localized renal lesions (i.e., T1a lesions, <4 cm in size). Nephron-sparing surgery is most commonly achieved by creating temporary renal ischemia by clamping of the renal hilar vessels, then enucleating the tumor with a small margin of normal tissue, while preserving the remainder of the renal parenchyma. Multiple studies have demonstrated comparable oncologic outcomes between radical nephrectomy and partial nephrectomy for small (<4 cm) localized renal tumors with 5-year cancer-specific survival rates of 87–100% [3–5]. For T1b (4–7 cm diameter, confined to the kidney) or T2 (>7 cm, confined to the kidney) tumors, larger and more deeply invasive tumors may make this technique more challenging. Partial nephrectomy for renal tumors larger than 4 cm in diameter is considered safe and feasible, with acceptable ischemic times, blood loss, operative times, and hospitalization as well as cancer-specific survival and metastasis-free survival [6–8].

The greatest concern with nephron-sparing surgery is the risk of recurrence of disease within the ipsilateral kidney, which is reported to occur in 4–6% of patients [3–5]. Extended cancer-free survival after partial nephrectomy has been found to be significantly longer in patients with tumors <4 cm than in patients with larger tumors [9]. In patients undergoing partial nephrectomy, improved survival is associated with the following prognostic factors: tumor size, unilateral renal involvement, low pathologic tumor stage, and presence of a solitary tumor. The American Urological Association recently reviewed the management of T1 renal masses and recommended that nephron-sparing surgical options should be offered to all patients with T1 disease where it is feasible based on tumor location on the basis of "compelling data demonstrating an increased risk of chronic kidney disease (CKD) associated with radical nephrectomy and a direct correlation between CKD and morbid cardiovascular events and mortality on a longitudinal basis" [10]. In addition, partial nephrectomy for patients with T1b lesions was recommended for patients with significant extrarenal comorbidities such as diabetes mellitus, poor baseline renal function, or cardiopulmonary disease.

S.P. Psutka (✉) • B.H. Eisner
Department of Urology, Massachusetts General Hospital, Boston, MA, USA
e-mail: spsutka@partners.org

P.R. Mueller and A. Adam (eds.), *Interventional Oncology: A Practical Guide for the Interventional Radiologist*,
DOI 10.1007/978-1-4419-1469-9_11, © Springer Science+Business Media, LLC 2012

In general, T2 lesions (tumors >7 cm) are typically managed with radical nephrectomy, given their size which would require more complicated renal reconstruction if partial nephrectomy is attempted [11], although in many centers, increased experience with partial nephrectomy and laparoscopy or robotic approaches are allowing surgeons to attempt these more complicated nephron-sparing operations to resect larger tumors and multiple tumors in the same kidney [12, 13].

Laparoscopic Versus Open Nephrectomy for Localized RCC

In 1991, Clayman et al. described the first successful laparoscopic nephroureterectomy in an 82-year-old man with low-grade transitional-cell cancer of the renal pelvis [14]. Since then laparoscopic surgery has overtaken open extirpative surgery for renal tumors and is widely practiced for both total nephrectomies and increasingly used for partial nephrectomies. A recent comparison of oncologic outcomes after laparoscopic and open partial nephrectomy demonstrated equivalence in overall and cancer-specific survival at 1 and 7 years for patients undergoing partial nephrectomy for clinical stage T1 (7 cm or less) renal cortical tumors [8]. Similar studies have shown equivalent outcomes for laparoscopic versus open nephrectomy for pT1-2 RCC up to 7 years postoperatively [15].

In a large comparison from the Cleveland Clinic between open ($n = 1,028$) and laparoscopic ($n = 771$) partial nephrectomies, analysis showed that the laparoscopic approach was associated with statistically significant shorter overall operative times, decreased blood loss, and a shorter hospitalization, but longer ischemic times, greater postoperative complications, and an increased requirement for postoperative procedures [16]. These results have been mirrored by other analyses which have confirmed the safety and feasibility for the laparoscopic approach to both total and partial nephrectomy [7, 17, 18]. Other recent meta-analyses of reports in the literature emphasize that complications with laparoscopic partial nephrectomies are most significantly related to the surgeon's experience, and that among high volume surgeons, complication rates are similar between open and laparoscopic procedures [19].

Urologists have, therefore, accepted laparoscopic nephrectomy as the standard of care for T1-3aN0M0 disease. Open surgery is still preferred in cases of major venous or vena caval involvement, local tumor invasion, massive tumor size, or gross lymphadenopathy.

Surgery for Tumor Extending Beyond the Renal Capsule and Metastatic Disease

Patients presenting with locally advanced or metastatic RCC have a poor prognosis [20]. However, extirpative surgery remains a part of the therapeutic armamentarium. In T3 disease, where the renal tumor extends into the adrenal gland, perinephric fat, or renal vein, open and laparoscopic nephrectomy have been evaluated and are widely considered to be acceptable [11, 21]. In comparison to T1 renal tumors, larger, locally invasive and metastatic tumors are associated with greater transfusion requirement (1.5% versus 7.3%, $p < 0.05$) and more postoperative complications ($p = 0.035$) [11]; both open and laparoscopic nephrectomy can be safely performed in these patients and result in equivalent intermediate oncologic outcomes.

Median survival for a patient presenting with T4 RCC (i.e., metastatic disease which has spread outside the kidney and adjacent organs) is a mere 6–12 months when surgery is combined with adjuvant traditional immunosuppressive therapy and is extended to approximately 20–30 months with newer biologically active agents such as the tyrosine kinase inhibitors [22]. Nephrectomy for patients with T4 disease (i.e., cytoreductive nephrectomy) has been shown to slightly increase survival in patients receiving adjuvant therapies such as immunotherapy, and there are rare reports of spontaneous regression of metastases after surgery [23]. Combined analysis of two randomized prospective trials recently demonstrated that in patients with T4 RCC randomized to interferon α-2b alone or interferon α-2b+cytoreductive nephrectomy found a 5.8-month increase in survival months in those treated with surgery [24–26]. However, these patients must be carefully selected, and the survival benefit of several months must be weighed against the morbidity of surgery.

These two randomized studies have demonstrated that cytoreductive nephrectomy for T4 RCC may be considered for patients who have a high-performance status and are fit enough to undergo the surgery. Contraindications include medical comorbidities that increase the risk of anesthesia and surgery, a poor performance status, or high metastatic disease burden [23, 27]. Poor prognosis and an increased risk of death following cytoreductive nephrectomy is correlated with the number of metastatic sites, symptoms at presentation, poor performance status, high tumor grade, and presence of sarcomatoid features [28].

The Case For-and-Against Regional Lymphadenectomy

Approximately 25% of patients with metastatic RCC have clinically evident lymphadenopathy. Lymphadenectomy is typically not performed for low-stage disease (T1–T2). There is some evidence that lymphadenectomy may confer a small survival benefit in patients with micrometastatic involvement of lymph nodes. However, few of these patients had advanced stage disease. A retrospective multicenter analysis from 2008 suggested that in patients with T3 RCC, the higher likelihood of lymph node involvement may render a staging-extended lymphadenectomy worthwhile [29]. The Mayo Clinic group identified five features of RCC that were associated with lymph node metastases: primary tumor stage T3 or T4, nuclear grade 3 or 4, tumor size 10 cm or greater, presence of a sarcomatoid component, and presence of histological tumor necrosis. If patients have none of these features, they have a low likelihood (0.6%) of lymph node (LN) involvement. However, if patients have two or more of these features, there is a 4.4% risk of regional LN involvement. In the case of patients with all five of these features, there is a greater than 50% risk of LN-positive disease. These findings led the authors to conclude that a standard lymphadenectomy is indicated in any patient with two or more risk features, which are determined intraoperatively by frozen section analysis [30]. In an attempt to answer this question conclusively, the European Organisation for Research and Treatment of Cancer (EORTC) performed a multicenter randomized controlled trial (Protocol 30881) in which patients with RCC of all stages were randomized to nephrectomy alone or nephrectomy with an extended lymphadenectomy. This study found that across all patients, there was no significant benefit in mortality, and local or distant progression with lymphadenectomy [31]. Further prospective studies investigating the role of lymphadenectomy in advanced RCC are needed. At this time, the role of lymphadenectomy for higher-stage disease remains controversial, but is performed at many of the large volume centers [32, 33].

Management of Tumor Thrombus

In the case of involvement of the RCC into the renal vein, inferior vena cava (IVC), or right atrium (T3b/c disease), radical nephrectomy with resection of the tumor thrombus remains the only option for cure. RCC involves the renal vein and IVC in 23% and 7% of patients, respectively [34]. Tumor thrombi are generally classified by involvement of the renal vein or infrahepatic, infradiaphragmatic (T3b), or supradiaphragmatic extension (T3c). Involvement of the IVC with tumor thrombus is a well-characterized poor prognostic factor [34, 35]. The significance of the level of thrombus with respect to overall prognosis is controversial [34], but some studies have shown that it may be associated with disease recurrence [35]. In these cases, preoperative staging is most helpful in determining the surgical management of RCC with vascular invasion, which may include cardiopulmonary bypass in advanced cases (Tables 11.1 and 11.2).

Operative Technique

Radical Nephrectomy

The definition of the standard radical nephrectomy historically encompassed the removal of the kidney including Gerota's fascia, the ipsilateral adrenal gland, the proximal two-thirds of the ureter, and a complete regional lymphadenectomy from the crus of the diaphragm to the aortic bifurcation. The rationale for the resection of the kidney by resecting all the tissue encompassed within Gerota's fascia is that capsular invasion with involvement of the perinephric fat occurs in approximately 25% of patients. It is now generally accepted that the ipsilateral adrenal gland does not need to be resected en bloc with the specimen except in the case of extensive involvement of the entire kidney or in the case of upper pole tumors [36, 37].

In general, a nephrectomy can be performed either from a transperitoneal or retroperitoneal approach. There are four possible routes of approach that may be employed: an extraperitoneal flank approach, a dorsal lumbotomy, an abdominal incision such as a subcostal incision, and a thoracoabdominal incision. The extraperitoneal approach is optimal for those patients who have a history of intraabdominal surgery, adhesive disease, or inflammatory disease, which might complicate intraperitoneal dissection. The advantage of the larger incisions and a transperitoneal approach is that the peritoneal cavity can be explored at the same time for evidence of metastatic disease.

Table 11.1 Surgical management options for renal cell carcinoma by pathological stage

Staging	Surgical management options
T: Primary tumor	
TX:	Primary tumor cannot be assessed	
T0:	No evidence of primary tumor	
T1:	Tumor ≤7 cm and confined to the kidney	
T1a:	Tumor ≤4.0 cm and confined to the kidney	Partial nephrectomy, open or laparoscopic approach
T1b:	Tumor >4.0 cm and ≤7.0 cm and confined to the kidney	Partial/radical nephrectomy, open or laparoscopic approach
T2:	Tumor >7.0 cm and confined to the kidney	Partial/radical nephrectomy, open or laparoscopic approach
T2a:	Tumor >7 cm but ≤10 cm and confined to the kidney	Partial nephrectomy, open or laparoscopic approach (if possible; experimental); radical nephrectomy, open or laparoscopic approach
T2b:	Tumor >10 cm and confined to the kidney	
T3:	Tumor extends into the major veins or perinephric tissues but not beyond Gerota's tissue	
T3a:	Tumor extends into the renal vein or perinephric tissues, but not beyond Gerota's fascia	Radical nephrectomy, open or laparoscopic approach
T3b:	Tumor extends into the vena cava below the diaphragm	Open radical nephrectomy, ±adrenalectomy, ±regional lymphadenectomy, vena cava exploration, and caval thrombectomy
T3c:	Tumor extends into the vena cava above the diaphragm or invades the wall of the vena cava	Open radical nephrectomy, ±adrenalectomy, ±regional lymphadenectomy, vena cava exploration, and caval thrombectomy (if tumor thrombus is suprahepatic, cardiac bypass and cardiac standstill is often required for thrombectomy)
T4:	Tumor invades beyond Gerota's fascia (including contiguous extension into the ipsilateral adrenal gland)	Open radical nephrectomy, ±adrenalectomy, ±regional lymphadenectomy, ±vena cava exploration, and caval thrombectomy (if tumor thrombus is suprahepatic, cardiac bypass and cardiac standstill is often required for thrombectomy)
N: Regional lymph nodes	
NX:	Regional lymph nodes cannot be assessed	Regional lymphadenectomy may be performed at the time of surgery
N0:	No regional lymph node metastases	
N1:	Metastasis in regional lymph nodes	
M: Distant metastases	
M0:	No distant metastases	Metastasectomy may be indicated, if cytoreductive nephrectomy is being performed
M1:	Distant metastasis present	

Source: Used with the permission of the American Joint Committee on Cancer (AJCC), Chicago, Illinois. The original source for this material is the AJCC Cancer Staging Manual, Seventh Edition (2010) published by Springer Science and Business Media LLC, "http://www.springer.com"

Table 11.2 Stage-specific 5-year survival for renal cell carcinoma

Group	T Category	N Category	M Category	5-Year survival (%)
Stage I	T1	N0	M0	80–90
	T1a	N0	M0	
	T1b	N0	M0	
Stage II	T2	N0	M0	70–80
Stage III	T1 or T2	N1	M0	40–60
	T3a (perinephric fat or renal vein, confined within Gerota's fascia)	N0 or N1	M0	
	T3b (vena cava below the diaphragm)	N0 or N1	M0	
	T3c (vena cava above the diaphragm or into the wall of the vena cava)	N0 or N1	M0	
Stage IV	T4 (beyond Gerota's fascia, including contiguous extension into ipsilateral adrenal gland)	Any N	M0	0–20
	Any T	Any N	M1	

Source: Used with the permission of the American Joint Committee on Cancer (AJCC), Chicago, Illinois. The original source for this material is the AJCC Cancer Staging Manual, Seventh Edition (2010) published by Springer Science and Business Media LLC, "http://www.springer.com"

The basic principles of a nephrectomy or partial nephrectomy, involve dissection down to the renal hilum to identify and achieve control over the renal artery and vein. This requires medial reflection of the colon and division of the attachments of the kidney to adjacent organs (such as the splenorenal ligament or hepatorenal ligament). During this dissection, care is taken to avoid damage to the spleen, the liver, and the pancreas, all of which may be injured during exposure of the kidney, particularly in larger tumors. After the mobilization of the kidney dissection of the hilum, the kidney is then mobilized outside of Gerota's fascia with a combination of blunt and sharp dissection. The hilar vessels can be ligated with sutures, surgical clips, or vascular staples. Variations in the anatomy of the renal hilum are carefully assessed. Approximately 70% of the population has a single renal artery originating from the abdominal aorta on each side. Accessory renal arteries are seen in approximately 30% such that 23% have two renal arteries, 4% have three renal arteries, and 1% have four or more renal arteries [38, 39]. Following division of any remaining vascular attachments such as the adrenal vessels or any neovasculature feeding the tumor, the ureter is ligated, and the specimen is removed.

The extraperitoneal approach avoids the requirement of reflecting the colon and viscera medially and can avoid complications associated with operating within the peritoneum in patients who may have a history of abdominal surgery or disease resulting in adhesive disease, which can complicate isolation of the kidney. In this case, the hilum is often approached and secured posteriorly within the retroperitoneum, without breaching the posterior boundaries of the peritoneum.

In general, these procedures may be made more complicated if the patient has a history of prior hemorrhage from the renal tumor, prior retroperitoneal surgery, or trauma to the area [40]. Prior trauma or hemorrhage results in perinephric scarring, which obliterates the natural fascial planes, which facilitate a clean dissection with minimal blood loss in their native avascular state. Prior local surgical procedures or renal biopsies, which are increasingly being utilized for preoperative diagnosis of incidentally found and symptomatic renal masses, may result in increased scarring that may complicate resection of a kidney or renal mass.

Partial Nephrectomy

For nephron-sparing surgery, the kidney is approached in much the same way as for a radical nephrectomy; however, complete mobilization of the tumor outside of Gerota's fascia is not necessary. The tumor may be removed by a simple enucleation of the tumor, polar segmental nephrectomy, wedge resection, or transverse resection of the portion of the kidney containing the tumor. Early vascular control is achieved by identifying the renal vessels. The renal artery (and sometimes the renal vein) is then temporarily occluded to permit resection of the tumor-containing portion of the kidney with subsequent closure of the surgical defect. Recent studies have demonstrated conclusively that the degree of renal ischemic damage is proportional to the length of ischemic time, and a goal of 20–30 min of ischemic time is targeted when feasible [41]. For deeper tumors, which invade the collecting system, repair of the collecting system and renal parenchyma is performed [12]. The entire tumor is resected with a small border of normal parenchyma. Intraoperative ultrasound is frequently employed to define the border of the tumor with normal renal parenchyma. In general, the perirenal fat surrounding the tumor is taken with the specimen [42].

Complications of the Surgical Management of Renal Tumors

Complications of the surgical management of renal tumors, either via an open or laparoscopic approach to a radical or partial nephrectomy are related to the preoperative performance status of the patient, medical comorbidities, the choice of approach, incision, and the normal or aberrant relationship of the kidney and/or the tumor to other intraabdominal organs [43].

Summary

The surgical resection of renal cell carcinoma is indicated in the management of both localized tumors and advanced tumors involving local spread and metastatic disease. There are many options available to the surgeon to approach the management of RCC using both open and minimally invasive approaches. Laparoscopic surgery and nephron-sparing techniques have gained widespread acceptance and are commonly used to treat RCC.

References

1. Lipworth L, Tarone RE, McLaughlin JK. The epidemiology of renal cell carcinoma. J Urol. 2006;176(6 Pt 1):2353–8.
2. Schwaibold HE, Stolzenburg JU. Laparoscopic partial nephrectomy. Arch Ital Urol Androl. 2009;81(2):72–5.
3. Butler BP, Novick AC, Miller DP, Campbell SA, Licht MR. Management of small unilateral renal cell carcinomas: radical versus nephron-sparing surgery. Urology. 1995;45(1):34–40. discussion 40–1.
4. Steinbach F, Stockle M, Muller SC, et al. Conservative surgery of renal cell tumors in 140 patients: 21 years of experience. J Urol. 1992;148(1):24–9. discussion 29–30.
5. Morgan WR, Zincke H. Progression and survival after renal-conserving surgery for renal cell carcinoma: experience in 104 patients and extended followup. J Urol. 1990;144(4):852–7. discussion 857–8.
6. Patel MN, Krane LS, Bhandari A, et al. Robotic partial nephrectomy for renal tumors larger than 4 cm. Eur Urol. 2010;57(2):310–6.
7. Makhoul B, De La Taille A, Vordos D, et al. Laparoscopic radical nephrectomy for T1 renal cancer: the gold standard? A comparison of laparoscopic vs open nephrectomy. BJU Int. 2004;93(1):67–70.
8. Lane BR, Gill IS. 7-year oncological outcomes after laparoscopic and open partial nephrectomy. J Urol. 2010;183(2):473–9.
9. Licht MR, Novick AC, Goormastic M. Nephron sparing surgery in incidental versus suspected renal cell carcinoma. J Urol. 1994;152(1):39–42.
10. Campbell SC, Novick AC, Belldegrun A, et al. Guideline for management of the clinical T1 renal mass. J Urol. 2009;182(4):1271–9.
11. Bird VG, Shields JM, Aziz M, Ayyathurai R, De Los Santos R, Roeter DH. Laparoscopic radical nephrectomy for patients with T2 and T3 renal-cell carcinoma: evaluation of perioperative outcomes. J Endourol. 2009;23(9):1527–33.
12. Gill IS, Kamoi K, Aron M, Desai MM. 800 laparoscopic partial nephrectomies: a single surgeon series. J Urol. 2010;183(1):34–41.
13. Flum AS, Wolf Jr JS. Laparoscopic partial nephrectomy for multiple ipsilateral renal tumors using a tailored surgical approach. J Endourol. 2010;24(4):557–61.
14. Clayman RV, Kavoussi LR, Figenshau RS, Chandhoke PS, Albala DM. Laparoscopic nephroureterectomy: initial clinical case report. J Laparoendosc Surg. 1991;1(6):343–9.
15. Luo JH, Zhou FJ, Xie D, et al. Analysis of long-term survival in patients with localized renal cell carcinoma: laparoscopic versus open radical nephrectomy. World J Urol. 2010;28(3):289–93.
16. Gill IS, Kavoussi LR, Lane BR, et al. Comparison of 1,800 laparoscopic and open partial nephrectomies for single renal tumors. J Urol. 2007;178(1):41–6.
17. Novick AC. Laparoscopic and partial nephrectomy. Clin Cancer Res. 2004;10(18 Pt 2):6322S–7.
18. Ganpule AP, Sharma R, Thimmegowda M, Veeramani M, Desai MR. Laparoscopic radical nephrectomy versus open radical nephrectomy in T1-T3 renal tumors: an outcome analysis. Indian J Urol. 2008;24(1):39–43.
19. Breda A, Finelli A, Janetschek G, Porpiglia F, Montorsi F. Complications of laparoscopic surgery for renal masses: prevention, management, and comparison with the open experience. Eur Urol. 2009;55(4):836–50.
20. Dekernion JB, Ramming KP, Smith RB. The natural history of metastatic renal cell carcinoma: a computer analysis. J Urol. 1978;120(2):148–52.
21. Mattar K, Finelli A. Expanding the indications for laparoscopic radical nephrectomy. Curr Opin Urol. 2007;17(2):88–92.
22. Sun M, Lughezzani G, Perrotte P, Karakiewicz PI. Treatment of metastatic renal cell carcinoma. Nat Rev Urol. 2010;7(6):327–38.
23. de Reijke TM, Bellmunt J, van Poppel H, Marreaud S, Aapro M. EORTC-GU group expert opinion on metastatic renal cell cancer. Eur J Cancer. 2009;45(5):765–73.
24. Flanigan RC, Mickisch G, Sylvester R, Tangen C, Van Poppel H, Crawford ED. Cytoreductive nephrectomy in patients with metastatic renal cancer: a combined analysis. J Urol. 2004;171(3):1071–6.
25. Mickisch GH, Garin A, van Poppel H, de Prijck L, Sylvester R. European Organisation for Research and Treatment of Cancer (EORTC) Genitourinary Group. Radical nephrectomy plus interferon-alfa-based immunotherapy compared with interferon alfa alone in metastatic renal-cell carcinoma: a randomised trial. Lancet. 2001;358(9286):966–70.
26. Flanigan RC, Salmon SE, Blumenstein BA, et al. Nephrectomy followed by interferon alfa-2b compared with interferon alfa-2b alone for metastatic renal-cell cancer. N Engl J Med. 2001;345(23):1655–9.
27. Campbell SC, Flanigan RC, Clark JI. Nephrectomy in metastatic renal cell carcinoma. Curr Treat Options Oncol. 2003;4(5):363–72.
28. Kutikov A, Uzzo RG, Caraway A, et al. Use of systemic therapy and factors affecting survival for patients undergoing cytoreductive nephrectomy. BJU Int. 2010;106(2):218–23.
29. Capitanio U, Jeldres C, Patard JJ, et al. Stage-specific effect of nodal metastases on survival in patients with non-metastatic renal cell carcinoma. BJU Int. 2009;103(1):33–7.
30. Leibovich BC, Blute ML. Lymph node dissection in the management of renal cell carcinoma. Urol Clin North Am. 2008;35(4):673–8. viii.
31. Blom JH, van Poppel H, Marechal JM, et al. Radical nephrectomy with and without lymph-node dissection: final results of European Organization for Research and Treatment of Cancer (EORTC) randomized phase 3 trial 30881. Eur Urol. 2009;55(1):28–34.
32. Delacroix Jr SE, Wood CG. The role of lymphadenectomy in renal cell carcinoma. Curr Opin Urol. 2009;19(5):465–72.
33. Margulis V, Wood CG. The role of lymph node dissection in renal cell carcinoma: the pendulum swings back. Cancer J. 2008;14(5):308–14.
34. Wagner B, Patard JJ, Mejean A, et al. Prognostic value of renal vein and inferior vena cava involvement in renal cell carcinoma. Eur Urol. 2009;55(2):452–9.
35. Al Otaibi M, Youssif TA, Alkhaldi A, et al. Renal cell carcinoma with inferior vena caval extension: impact of tumour extent on surgical outcome. BJU Int. 2009;104(10):1467–70.
36. Sagalowsky AI, Kadesky KT, Ewalt DM, Kennedy TJ. Factors influencing adrenal metastasis in renal cell carcinoma. J Urol. 1994;151(5):1181–4.
37. Kobayashi T, Nakamura E, Yamamoto S, et al. Low incidence of ipsilateral adrenal involvement and recurrences in patients with renal cell carcinoma undergoing radical nephrectomy: a retrospective analysis of 393 patients. Urology. 2003;62(1):40–5.

38. Pollak R, Prusak BF, Mozes MF. Anatomic abnormalities of cadaver kidneys procured for purposes of transplantation. Am Surg. 1986;52(5):233–5.
39. Turkvatan A, Ozdemir M, Cumhur T, Olcer T. Multidetector CT angiography of renal vasculature: normal anatomy and variants. Eur Radiol. 2009;19(1):236–44.
40. Hernandez F, Ong AM, Rha KH, Pinto PA, Kavoussi LR. Laparoscopic renal surgery after spontaneous retroperitoneal hemorrhage. J Urol. 2003;170(3):749–51.
41. Becker F, Van Poppel H, Hakenberg OW, et al. Assessing the impact of ischaemia time during partial nephrectomy. Eur Urol. 2009;56(4):625–34.
42. Riggs SB, Larochelle JC, Belldegrun AS. Partial nephrectomy: a contemporary review regarding outcomes and different techniques. Cancer J. 2008;14(5):302–7.
43. McNeil BK, Flanigan RC. Complications of open renal surgery. In: Loughlin KR, editor. Complications of urologic surgery and practice: diagnosis, prevention, and management. New York, NY: Informa Healthcare USA; 2007. p. 65.

Chapter 12
Embolotherapy for Renal Tumors

Rahmi Oklu and Sanjeeva P. Kalva

Introduction

Embolotherapy of renal neoplasms is practiced for various hypervascular tumors including angiomyolipoma, renal cell carcinoma, and metastatic renal cancer. First conceived during 1970s, it was primarily advocated for palliative therapy of symptomatic renal cell carcinomas [1]. Currently, the indications for embolotherapy of malignant renal tumors include, in addition to palliation, preoperative treatment of large renal tumors to reduce intraoperative blood loss, and as an adjunct to radiofrequency ablation to reduce perfusion mediated cooling for a more effective ablation [2, 3]. Embolization of large hypervascular tumors prior to nephrectomy has been shown to significantly reduce the volume of blood transfused during surgery compared to those patients with tumors not embolized or incompletely embolized [2, 4]. In addition, preoperative embolization facilitates surgical dissection. Edema induced by embolization creates a definable plane within the renal parenchyma, and this reduces operative time [4, 5]. In patients with renal cell cancer extending to the renal vein, preoperative embolization may reduce the size of the tumor thrombus making it easier to resect [6, 7]. Though it has not been clinically proven, it is believed that embolization may induce sufficient inflammation, which may accentuate immune response to the tumor [8]. As a palliative measure, embolization helps in the management of pain, hematuria, and paraneoplastic syndromes such as hypercalcemia [9]. In patients with angiomyolipoma, embolotherapy is indicated for treatment of acute bleeding [10]. It helps to avoid nephrectomy and preserves renal function [10]. In addition, prophylactic embolization is often advocated in large angiomyolipomas (size >4 cm) to prevent bleeding and renal dysfunction [11].

Technical Considerations

The technique of embolotherapy is similar to that used for embolization of other organs. The purpose of embolization, angiography findings including the presence of large aneurysms and arteriovenous shunts, and the operator's experience play an important role in the selection of appropriate embolic materials. Several embolic agents have been used including absolute alcohol, polyvinyl alcohol particles, acrylic microspheres, gel foam, n-acetyl cyanoacrylate, and metallic coils. Typically, small particulate materials or liquid embolic agents are used either alone or in combination to achieve distal tumor embolization for purposes of palliation. This technique allows future embolotherapy, if required, as hypervascular tumors may recruit new vessels over time and become symptomatic. Therefore, proximal arterial embolization using metallic coils is not advocated, as it would preclude future access to the arteries supplying the tumor. Proximal arterial occlusion with metallic coils may be applied as an adjunct to distal embolization during preoperative embolization of renal cell carcinomas, as surgery is often performed within 48 h of embolotherapy. In addition, coil occlusion may be applied for treatment of large intratumoral aneurysms and arteriovenous shunts.

R. Oklu • S.P. Kalva (✉)
Division of Vascular Imaging and Interventions, Department of Imaging,
Massachusetts General Hospital, Harvard Medical School, Boston, MA, USA
e-mail: skalva@partners.org

P.R. Mueller and A. Adam (eds.), *Interventional Oncology: A Practical Guide for the Interventional Radiologist*,
DOI 10.1007/978-1-4419-1469-9_12, © Springer Science+Business Media, LLC 2012

Technique

The procedure may be performed with local anesthesia or under conscious sedation. Detailed angiography should be performed before contemplating embolotherapy. Abdominal aortography is performed to assess the arterial supply to the kidneys. Preoperative cross-sectional imaging studies [contrast-enhanced computed tomography (CT) and magnetic resonance (MR)] may provide enough information to proceed with selective renal angiography. The number of the renal arteries, arterial supply to the tumor, and the presence of collateral arterial supply (capsular, adrenal, gonadal, lumbar, and intercostal arteries) to the tumor are assessed on the aortogram. Selective and subselective renal arteriography is performed to further delineate the arterial supply to the tumor. Angiography findings of renal cell carcinoma or of hypervascular metastases include enlarged, tortuous, poorly tapering feeding arteries, neovascularity, and small-to-medium sized aneurysms, arteriovenous shunts, and tumor staining (Fig. 12.1). Angiomyolipomas may exhibit similar findings (Fig. 12.2); however, arteriovenous shunts and parasitization of adjacent vessels are rare.

Embolization is performed either selectively or subselectively depending on whether or not the sparing of the normal parenchyma is clinically relevant. A catheter is placed in the segmental or lobar artery supplying the tumor, and embolization is performed. When ethanol is used as an embolic agent, a balloon occlusion catheter is often used. The balloon is inflated, and small aliquots of ethanol (4–5 ml) are rapidly infused (at a rate of 1–5 ml/s). This allows distal perfusion of

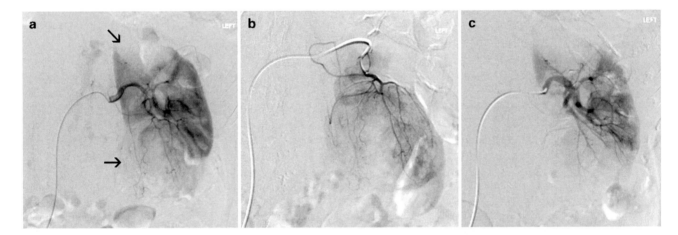

Fig. 12.1 Palliative embolotherapy of renal metastasis for hematuria. Left renal angiography (**a**) shows a large relatively hypervascular mass (*horizontal arrow*) in the lower pole. The filling defect (*oblique arrow*) in the upper pole corresponds to a simple cyst. Selective arteriography (**b**) confirms the abnormal vascularity of the tumor. The tumor was successfully embolized with microparticles. Postembolization left renal angiography (**c**) shows complete devascularization of the tumor with preserved renal parenchyma

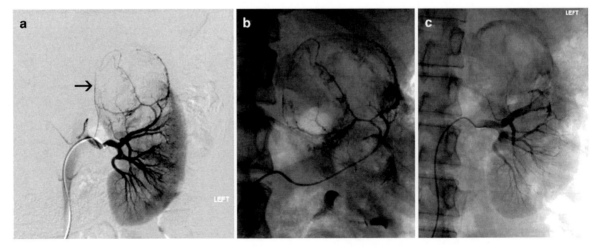

Fig. 12.2 Prophylactic embolization of angiomyolipoma. Left renal angiography (**a**) shows large hypervascular mass with microaneurysms consistent with a diagnosis of angiomyolipoma. Selective arteriography (**b**) confirms the findings. Embolization was performed with microparticles. Postembolization angiography (**c**) confirms complete devascularization of the tumor with preserved renal parenchyma

ethanol and prevents accidental reflux in to the aorta. The balloon is left inflated for 5 min after injection of ethanol. After 5 min, residual alcohol is aspirated, and the balloon deflated. This is repeated till the entire tumor is treated. Ethanol is radiolucent; thus, it is mixed with lipiodol (one part of lipiodol to three parts of ethanol) to make it radio-opaque. When particulate materials are used for embolization, microcatheters may be used to selectively catheterize the segmental arteries supplying the tumor (Figs. 12.1 and 12.2). As mentioned before, various particulate embolic agents are used. Small size of particles (300–500 μm) allows for distal embolization. If large arteriovenous shunts are encountered, large size particles (900–1,200 μm) may be used to avoid the passage of the embolic material to the venous circulation. Even larger arteriovenous shunts warrant occlusion of the feeding vessels with microcoils. When radical nephrectomy is planned, proximal occlusion of the renal arteries with coils is often performed in addition to distal embolization with ethanol or particles.

Following embolization, patients are usually admitted to the hospital for management of pain, nausea, and the tumor lysis syndrome with analgesics, antiemetics, and intravenous fluids. Postembolization syndrome may occur in up to 75% of the cases. It is manifested with low-grade fever, abdominal pain, nausea, and vomiting. Treatment is conservative. Symptoms may spontaneously resolve within 7–10 days. More serious complications of embolization are related to coil migration and nontarget embolization due to reflux of liquid and particulate materials involving the bowel, spinal cord, and the lower extremities. In 121 renal tumor embolizations, Lammer et al. reported a complication rate of 9.9% with a mortality rate of 3.3% [12]. The most common complications encountered in this study were renal failure and nontarget embolization.

Results

Preoperative embolization of renal cell carcinoma results in decreased need for blood transfusion, facilitates resection of large tumors that extend to the veins, and improves survival. In one study, there was significant reduction in the blood transfusion requirement when large hypervascular tumors were embolized preoperatively [4]. Another study stressed the beneficial role of preoperative embolization by facilitating resection when tumors extended to the renal veins [13]. A recent study demonstrated feasibility of laparoscopic partial nephrectomy for renal cell carcinoma without the need for clamping of the hilar vessels when preoperative, selective embolization was applied [14]. The overall 5- and 10-year survival following nephrectomy for renal cell carcinoma were 62% and 47%, respectively, when preoperative embolization was performed. In comparison, a matched group had 35% and 23% 5- and 10-year survival following nephrectomy without preoperative embolization, respectively [15]. For palliation of symptomatic renal cell carcinomas, embolization was successful in reducing symptoms when complete devascularization was achieved [16]. In addition, it had a survival advantage in patients with distal metastases [16]. When embolization was applied prior to ablation, a larger tumor (3.5–9 cm) could be ablated in a single session [17].

Ethanol embolization of symptomatic and asymptomatic angiomyolipomas resulted in significant reduction of symptoms and decreased tumor progression in a study of 34 patients [18]. Another study demonstrated the effectiveness of embolization in the treatment of angiomyolipoma in controlling hemorrhage in the acute setting; however, it had limited value in the long-term management of these tumors [19].

Conclusions

Embolotherapy may be performed with limited morbidity and mortality for hypervascular renal tumors. In addition to palliation, it is often employed prior to resection and radiofrequency ablation. Its role is well established in the management of acute hemorrhage from angiomyolipomas. Its beneficial role as a prophylactic measure to prevent bleeding in the future requires further studies.

References

1. Goldstein HM, Medellin H, Beydoun MT, et al. Transcatheter embolization of renal cell carcinoma. Am J Roentgenol Radium Ther Nucl Med. 1975;123:557–62.
2. Kalman D, Varenhorst E. The role of arterial embolization in renal cell carcinoma. Scand J Urol Nephrol. 1999;33:62–70.
3. Hoffmann RT, Jakobs TF, Kubisch CH, et al. Renal cell carcinoma in patients with a solitary kidney after nephrectomy treated with radiofrequency ablation: mid term results. Eur J Radiol. 2010;73(3):652–6.
4. Bakal CW, Cynamon J, Lakritz PS, Sprayregen S. Value of preoperative renal artery embolization in reducing blood transfusion requirements during nephrectomy for renal cell carcinoma. J Vasc Interv Radiol. 1993;4:727–31.

5. Klimberg I, Hunter P, Hawkins IF, Drylie DM, Wajsman Z. Preoperative angioinfarction of localized renal cell carcinoma using absolute ethanol. J Urol. 1985;133:21–4.

6. Blute ML, Leibovich BC, Lohse CM, Cheville JC, Zincke H. The Mayo Clinic experience with surgical management, complications and outcome for patients with renal cell carcinoma and venous tumour thrombus. BJU Int. 2004;94:33–41.

7. Haferkamp A, Bastian PJ, Jakobi H, et al. Renal cell carcinoma with tumor thrombus extension into the vena cava: prospective long-term followup. J Urol. 2007;177:1703–8.

8. McDermott DF. Immunotherapy of metastatic renal cell carcinoma. Cancer. 2009;115:2298–305.

9. Maxwell NJ, Saleem-Amer N, Rogers E, Kiely D, Sweeney P, Brady AP. Renal artery embolisation in the palliative treatment of renal carcinoma. Br J Radiol. 2007;80:96–102.

10. Hamlin JA, Smith DC, Taylor FC, McKinney JM, Ruckle HC, Hadley HR. Renal angiomyolipomas: long-term follow-up of embolization for acute hemorrhage. Can Assoc Radiol J. 1997;48:191–8.

11. Soulen MC, Faykus Jr MH, Shlansky-Goldberg RD, Wein AJ, Cope C. Elective embolization for prevention of hemorrhage from renal angiomyolipomas. J Vasc Interv Radiol. 1994;5:587–91.

12. Lammer J, Justich E, Schreyer H, Pettek R. Complications of renal tumor embolization. Cardiovasc Intervent Radiol. 1985;8:31–5.

13. Sweeney P, Wood CG, Pisters LL, et al. Surgical management of renal cell carcinoma associated with complex inferior vena caval thrombi. Urol Oncol. 2003;21:327–33.

14. Simone G, Papalia R, Guaglianone S, Forestiere E, Gallucci M. Preoperative superselective transarterial embolization in laparoscopic partial nephrectomy: technique, oncologic, and functional outcomes. J Endourol. 2009;23:1473–8.

15. Zielinski H, Szmigielski S, Petrovich Z. Comparison of preoperative embolization followed by radical nephrectomy with radical nephrectomy alone for renal cell carcinoma. Am J Clin Oncol. 2000;23:6–12.

16. Onishi T, Oishi Y, Suzuki Y, Asano K. Prognostic evaluation of transcatheter arterial embolization for unresectable renal cell carcinoma with distant metastasis. BJU Int. 2001;87:312–5.

17. Yamakado K, Nakatsuka A, Kobayashi S, et al. Radiofrequency ablation combined with renal arterial embolization for the treatment of unresectable renal cell carcinoma larger than 3.5 cm: initial experience. Cardiovasc Intervent Radiol. 2006;29:389–94.

18. Chick CM, Tan BS, Cheng C, et al. Long-term follow-up of the treatment of renal angiomyolipomas after selective arterial embolization with alcohol. BJU Int. 2010;105:390–4.

19. Sooriakumaran P, Gibbs P, Coughlin G, et al. Angiomyolipomata: challenges, solutions, and future prospects based on over 100 cases treated. BJU Int. 2010;105(1):101–6.

Chapter 13
Radiofrequency Ablation, Cryotherapy, and Microwave Ablation for Renal Tumors

J. Louis Hinshaw and Meghan G. Lubner

Introduction

Renal tumor ablation is a technique that has rapidly developed over the last decade. Although some questions remain regarding the long-term efficacy and the most appropriate target patient population, the technique has been shown to have excellent short- and midterm results that are comparable to surgery [1–10]. The purpose of this chapter is to briefly discuss the major factors that determine the role and outcome for radiofrequency (RF), microwave, and cryoablations.

Patient Selection

Although ablation data are promising and image-guided percutaneous ablation is becoming an accepted treatment option for selected cases of renal cell carcinoma, surgical extirpation remains the standard of care in most cases [11]. Patient selection is probably the single most important factor in assuring a successful outcome. The primary considerations can be divided into patient- and tumor-related factors. When selecting patients for ablation, indications such as surgical comorbidities, solitary kidney, renal insufficiency, multiple tumors, or conditions predisposing to multiple tumors are often present (Fig. 13.1). If patients fall into one of these categories, ablation is often a higher consideration, because it is well tolerated, has minimal effect on renal function, and can be repeated as needed. More recently, based upon the success of ablation to date, many groups have become more aggressive with patient selection, choosing younger, healthier patients who would not have been considered candidates for ablation in the past.

Tumor size is a very important consideration when selecting patients for ablation. The optimal tumor size is 4 cm or less. It is generally accepted that smaller tumors are more effectively ablated than larger tumors. A receiver-operating characteristic curve analysis to determine the size for the highest likelihood for complete necrosis showed that using 4 cm as a cutoff will ensure a 90% chance for complete necrosis. Treating cases up to 5.8 cm will allow more patients to be treated but decreases the chance for complete necrosis to 63% [3]. Short-term outcomes in the more aggressive treatment of large masses (>3 cm) have remained favorable [12]. In addition to the problem obtaining adequate local control, larger tumors typically have unfavorable histology or may be of higher grade, which makes surgical excision a more attractive option if possible [13].

Tumor location also plays an important role in patient selection (Fig. 13.2). Although there is conflicting data, central tumors are more likely to be associated with local tumor progression, likely due to central heat-sink effects [3, 10]. One group demonstrated that central masses that obscure calyces may be at a higher risk of bleeding into the collecting system; however, clinically significant injuries to the collecting system, even when treating central masses, were rare and extension of the zone of ablation to a calyx appeared safe [14]. In the past, it was felt that the treatment of anterior tumors was more difficult given the close proximity to vulnerable structures, such as bowel (most commonly colon or duodenum) or ureter, and the difficulty of obtaining percutaneous access. As a result, many of these tumors were treated with an open or laparoscopic technique. However, changes in patient positioning, use of probes for tumor displacement with retraction or leverage

J.L. Hinshaw (✉) • M.G. Lubner
Department of Radiology, University of Wisconsin School of Medicine and Public Health, Madison, WI, USA
e-mail: jhinshaw@uwhealth.org

P.R. Mueller and A. Adam (eds.), *Interventional Oncology: A Practical Guide for the Interventional Radiologist*,
DOI 10.1007/978-1-4419-1469-9_13, © Springer Science+Business Media, LLC 2012

Fig. 13.1 Von Hippel Lindau (VHL). Postcontrast magnetic resonance (MR) image demonstrates bilateral renal cell carcinomas (*arrows*) in this young patient with VHL. Given the presence of multiple tumors, and the risk of developing more, this patient has been successfully treated with percutaneous ablation

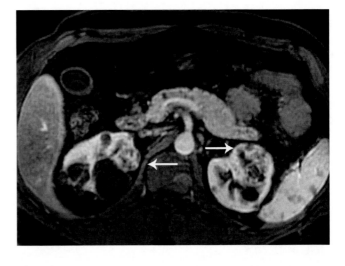

Fig. 13.2 Typical tumor. Postcontrast computed tomography (CT) image demonstrates a small, peripheral posterior solid renal lesion found to represent renal cell carcinoma. This is an ideal tumor for percutaneous ablation

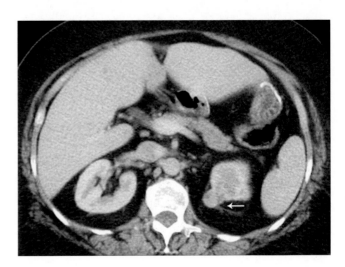

and use of hydrodissection have allowed for more aggressive patient selection and safe treatment of these anterior tumors (Fig. 13.3) [15–21]. Placement of a ureteric stent with pyeloperfusion has been increasingly applied to protect the ureter when treating central or anterior/inferior tumors [20, 22, 23].

The only true contraindications to renal tumor ablation are the location of the tumor such that the ureter cannot be protected/displaced during the procedure and refractory coagulopathy. Relative contraindications include bleeding diatheses, larger tumors, and inability to lie prone or supine for prolonged periods of time.

Modality Selection

Available ablation modalities in the kidney include radiofrequency (RF), microwave, and cryoablations. Currently, limited data is available regarding the use of microwave ablation in the kidney, and although it appears promising, further study is needed [24–26].

The two major modalities used in the kidney are radiofrequency ablation (RFA) and cryoablation. Both tools are efficacious, and in many cases, the decision comes down to institutional resources and experience. However, there are some relative advantages and disadvantages to each modality that warrant further discussion. The clinical outcomes with both techniques are excellent, but the results may be slightly better with cryoablation with a recent meta-analysis of 47 studies and 1,375 kidney lesions showing that cryoablation may require fewer treatment sessions and demonstrates slightly less

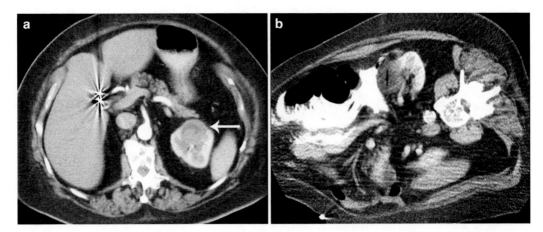

Fig. 13.3 Anterior tumor. (**a**) CT image demonstrates a solid enhancing mass in the anterior upper pole of the left kidney abutting the pancreas (*arrow*). (**b**) Using hydrodissection [5% dextrose in water (D5W) containing dilute contrast], space was created between the tumor and the pancreas and bowel, and the tumor was successfully and safely treated

local tumor progression [27]. In this meta-analysis, cryoablation was more frequently performed laparoscopically (65% of cases). Multiple studies have shown that percutaneous cryoablation is equally efficacious to the laparoscopic approach with fewer complications, lower costs, and shorter hospital stay making the trend in many groups to treat percutaneously whenever possible [5, 7, 28, 29].

Cryoablation is a less painful treatment option than RFA, with one group showing lower pain and sedative medication requirements during procedures performed with cryoablation compared with RF [30]. The iceball generated during cryoablation is well seen with imaging [computed tomography (CT), ultrasound (US), magnetic resonance imaging (MRI)] and correlates with the pathologic zone of necrosis, with complete cell death seen 3 mm inside the edge of the iceball [31, 32]. In addition, each applicator can be controlled individually. These features of cryoablation make it a more precise and customizable modality. In theory, cryoablation is less damaging to the renal collecting system which may be advantageous in the treatment of central tumors [33].

Cryoablation utilizes a dual freeze technique which can be more time consuming than a single RFA cycle (average time of 25 min for cryoablation versus 12–16 min for RF ablation). Cryoablation theoretically has increased risk of bleeding as it lacks the natural cautery effect of RFA, and cracking of the iceball has been described. However, Shock et al. demonstrated only minimal difference in bleeding complications in a porcine hepatic model [34]. Although cryoablation does not require ground pads, it does require pressurized tanks of helium and argon, which can be problematic in earthquake zones. RFA is advantageous in terms of procedural time and costs [11].

Procedural Considerations

Targeting and Monitoring

Ultrasound is the preferred modality for tumor targeting in many groups. It allows excellent soft-tissue differentiation, rapid probe placement, and does not utilize ionizing radiation. In addition, it allows a variety of approaches/angles for tumor access, particularly for tumors located in the superior pole where CT guidance would require either a transpulmonary approach, or an additional intervention such as a protective pneumothorax, which has its own associated morbidity. CT, however, is probably more commonly used in practice and can be helpful as an adjunct to ultrasound. CT is particularly useful for identifying and locating vulnerable adjacent structures, verifying relative positioning of multiple applicators when placed into a large tumor, and ablation zone monitoring with cryoablation. When monitoring cryoablation with US, one is able to identify the leading edge of the iceball and any associated tumor, but the posterior aspects of both the iceball and tumor are obscured by acoustic shadowing. CT allows the entire iceball and any associated tumor margins to be more fully assessed (Fig. 13.4). This increases the safety and efficacy of the procedure.

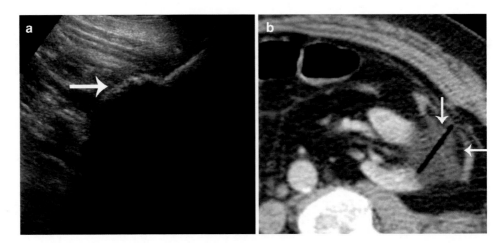

Fig. 13.4 Iceball on imaging. (**a**) Ultrasound (US) demonstrates the hyperechoic anterior border of the iceball with dense posterior acoustic shadowing, redemonstrated as a low attenuation area seen on CT (*arrow*, **b**). This is well seen on the two imaging modalities, as well as on MRI, enabling a precise ablation. In addition, the pathologic zone of necrosis correlates well with the iceball on imaging, with lethal temperatures approximately 3 mm inside the edge of the iceball

Probe Placement

As above, probes can be placed under ultrasound, CT or MRI guidance [35–37]. At the authors' institution, they use ultrasound guidance for real-time probe placement in most cases, and use a combination of US and CT for monitoring the ablation zone. In tumors that are difficult to see with US but are well seen on other cross-sectional imaging, CT or MRI can be used. In addition, fusion platforms have become available that allow fusion of the US image with another study image based on calibration with known landmarks.

Cryoprobes should ideally be placed with the tip at the distal edge of the tumor and spaced 1.0–1.5 cm from each other and from the margin of the tumor [38, 39]. RF probes should be similarly spaced. In a study examining multiple RF electrodes in hepatic tumors, optimal spacing for electrodes was 1–1.4 cm [40]. One group studied the orientation of RF probes with respect to the tumor (parallel or perpendicular to the tumor–kidney interface) and found that this did not affect the number of overlapping ablations performed or the absence of residual tumor [14]. With a cluster RF probes, three needles are mounted roughly 1 cm apart on a single handle, and overlapping ablations can be performed. Multitined expandable electrodes can also be used [41].

Preprocedural and Intraprocedural Adjuncts

With more aggressive tumor selection, measures should be taken to protect vulnerable structures and to prevent complications. Hydrodissection is a useful technique to displace adjacent vulnerable structures such as bowel, ureter, or pancreas [16–19, 21]. With the kidney, the fluid is often injected into the anterior pararenal space. Arellano et al. demonstrated that greater than 10 mm of separation of adjacent structures from the kidney was successful in 53 of 55 cases [16]. For cryoablation, normal saline can be used, but for RFA 5% dextrose in water should be used, because it is iso-osmolar and nonionic, unaffected by RF-induced ionic agitation.

Upper pole renal tumors may be near the adrenal, and ablation of the adrenal gland can produce hypertensive complications [42, 43]. With RF ablation, elevated blood pressures tend to occur as the ablation is being performed, whereas with cryoablation, hypertension develops as the iceball thaws. In these cases, close anesthesia monitoring with an arterial line is extremely helpful and antihypertensives, particularly alpha blockers should be kept on hand. With cryoablation, if hypertension occurs during thawing, a repeat temporary freeze can be performed, while the patient is loaded with alpha blockers.

The ilioinguinal nerve arises from the L1 and L2 nerves and runs on the psoas muscle posterior to the kidney. Ablation zones that extend into the psoas muscle may produce paresthesias or sensory loss extending to the ipsilateral groin [19, 44]. Similarly, when ablation is performed from an intercostal approach, the intercostal nerve just below the rib is at risk. Ablation of these nerves can cause sensory loss and muscular laxity with abdominal bulging in a dermatomal distribution. If the ablation zone may reach the body wall, hydrodissection can be used for protection [19].

Pyeloperfusion, hydrodissection, or both can be used to protect the central collecting system and ureter from injury [16, 20, 22, 45, 46].

Posttreatment infection or urine leak can also occur, and patients with refluxing urostomies may be at higher risk [47]. For most patients, a single dose of antibiotic covering skin flora is utilized prior to the procedure, but those patients at increased risk may benefit from oral antibiotics covering urinary tract organisms for longer periods before and after the procedure.

Postprocedure Management

Many institutions perform renal ablation as an outpatient procedure and discharge the patient to home on the same day. Others keep the patient in-house overnight for observation and symptom control as needed, particularly if the procedure is performed in the afternoon. Prior to discharge to home, the patient should be comfortably ambulating, voiding without significant hematuria, and eating and drinking. Proper hydration is critical for all patients undergoing ablation and should be stressed in the days after an ablation. Most patients can return to baseline activities approximately 1 week after the ablation.

Complications

Reported complications with renal ablation include: hemorrhage (hematuria and perinephric/subcapsular bleeding); damage to the collecting system with associated hydronephrosis and loss of renal function, possibly even leading to renal failure; infection/abscess; damage to the genitofemoral, ilioinguinal, iliohypogastric, or lateral femoral cutaneous nerves (run along the anterior surface of the psoas and quadratus lumborum muscles) resulting in paresthesias and numbness of the trunk and upper leg; and damage to adjacent structures (including colon/duodenum, which can lead to rupture, sepsis, and even death; the adrenal gland, which can lead to hypertensive crisis; and the pancreas, which can result in pancreatitis). These complications tend to be relatively mild, self-limited, and overall, renal ablation is associated with an exceptional safety profile.

One complication specific to cryoablation is tumor lysis syndrome or cryoshock. Because cryoablation does not cauterize vessels in the ablation zone, the necrotic contents of the ablation zone are exposed to the systemic circulation. This can lead to a systemic inflammatory response which can result in severe coagulopathy, thrombocytopenia, disseminated intravascular coagulation, shock, lung injury and multisystem organ failure [48]. This is an uncommon complication, seen in less than 1% of patients, and appears to be related to the volume of tissue cryoablated [49].

Tumor seeding has been described, but is exceedingly rare. The reported rate of seeding from renal biopsies was less than 0.01% [50]. Inflammatory nodules along the applicator track can mimic seeding, so biopsy can be helpful to confirm [51].

Follow-Up Imaging

This subject is somewhat controversial and can be quite variable between institutions. In some cases, a contrast-enhanced CT or MRI is performed at the conclusion of the ablation. This allows early identification of any tumor that has not been completely included within the zone of ablation and immediate retreatment as needed. This scan also serves as a new baseline and can identify any early complications such as bleeding.

Subsequent follow-up imaging can be more variable, but should include a contrast-enhanced CT or MRI within 6 months after the procedure to confirm the complete ablation of the tumor. This is generally followed by imaging at 6–12 month intervals, although the frequency and type of imaging are variable and may change based upon the histology of the treated tumor, renal function, and other patient-related factors. Nodular or crescentic enhancement in the setting of a prior hypervascular tumor is a concern for the residual or recurrent disease. For low attenuation or hypovascular tumor types, residual or recurrent tumor may cause enlargement of or asymmetric changes in a hypoattenuating ablation zone.

Results

Clinical trials to date have been associated with excellent results in general. While surgical resection remains the standard of care for most patients, cryoablation and RFA have emerged as minimally invasive treatments with excellent short- and intermediate-term results [1–10]. Several studies have shown 97–100% technical success and short- and intermediate-term local control in 92–100% of patients [1, 6, 52, 53]. However, there are some important considerations. Endophytic tumors and tumors larger than 5 cm have a significantly reduced complete ablation rate with current techniques. Tumors less than 3 cm in diameter, particularly if exophytic, are generally associated with complete ablation after a single session and larger tumors may require two or more sessions to treat completely. Overall, based upon experience to date, one can expect excellent short- and intermediate-term outcomes. Long-term outcomes are still unknown.

Conclusions

While surgical removal of renal tumors remains the standard of care, thermal-based treatments including RFA and cryoablation are slowly establishing themselves as viable alternatives in select patients. Thermal-based treatments are effective and safe, with protective techniques enabling more aggressive patient selection.

References

1. Atwell TD, Farrell MA, Leibovich BC, et al. Percutaneous renal cryoablation: experience treating 115 tumors. J Urol. 2008;179(6):2136–40. discussion 2140–1.
2. Breen DJ, Rutherford EE, Stedman B, et al. Management of renal tumors by image-guided radiofrequency ablation: experience in 105 tumors. Cardiovasc Intervent Radiol. 2007;30(5):936–42.
3. Gervais DA, Arellano RS, McGovern FJ, McDougal WS, Mueller PR. Radiofrequency ablation of renal cell carcinoma: part 1, Indications, results, and role in patient management over a 6-year period and ablation of 100 tumors. AJR Am J Roentgenol. 2005;185(1):64–71.
4. Gill IS, Remer EM, Hasan WA, et al. Renal cryoablation: outcome at 3 years. J Urol. 2005;173(6):1903–7.
5. Hinshaw JL, Shadid AM, Nakada SY, Hedican SP, Winter 3rd TC, Lee Jr FT. Comparison of percutaneous and laparoscopic cryoablation for the treatment of solid renal masses. AJR Am J Roentgenol. 2008;191(4):1159–68.
6. Littrup PJ, Ahmed A, Aoun HD, et al. CT-guided percutaneous cryotherapy of renal masses. J Vasc Interv Radiol. 2007;18(3):383–92.
7. Malcolm JB, Berry TT, Williams MB, et al. Single center experience with percutaneous and laparoscopic cryoablation of small renal masses. J Endourol. 2009;23(6):907–11.
8. Mayo-Smith WW, Dupuy DE, Parikh PM, Pezzullo JA, Cronan JJ. Imaging-guided percutaneous radiofrequency ablation of solid renal masses: techniques and outcomes of 38 treatment sessions in 32 consecutive patients. AJR Am J Roentgenol. 2003;180(6):1503–8.
9. Park S, Anderson JK, Matsumoto ED, Lotan Y, Josephs S, Cadeddu JA. Radiofrequency ablation of renal tumors: intermediate-term results. J Endourol. 2006;20(8):569–73.
10. Zagoria RJ, Traver MA, Werle DM, Perini M, Hayasaka S, Clarke PE. Oncologic efficacy of CT-guided percutaneous radiofrequency ablation of renal cell carcinomas. AJR Am J Roentgenol. 2007;189(2):429–36.
11. Gontero P, Joniau S, Zitella A, et al. Ablative therapies in the treatment of small renal tumors: how far from standard of care? Urol Oncol. 2010;28(3):251–9.
12. Atwell TD, Farrell MA, Callstrom MR, et al. Percutaneous cryoablation of large renal masses: technical feasibility and short-term outcome. AJR Am J Roentgenol. 2007;188(5):1195–200.
13. Frank I, Blute ML, Cheville JC, Lohse CM, Weaver AL, Zincke H. Solid renal tumors: an analysis of pathological features related to tumor size. J Urol. 2003;170(6 Pt 1):2217–20.
14. Gervais DA, Arellano RS, McGovern FJ, McDougal WS, Mueller PR. Radiofrequency ablation of renal cell carcinoma: part 2, Lessons learned with ablation of 100 tumors. AJR Am J Roentgenol. 2005;185(1):72–80.
15. Allaf ME, Lang E. Bowel separation before percutaneous renal cryoablation. J Urol. 2008;180(2):721.
16. Arellano RS, Garcia RG, Gervais DA, Mueller PR. Percutaneous CT-guided radiofrequency ablation of renal cell carcinoma: efficacy of organ displacement by injection of 5% dextrose in water into the retroperitoneum. AJR Am J Roentgenol. 2009;193(6):1686–90.
17. Farrell MA, Charboneau JW, Callstrom MR, Reading CC, Engen DE, Blute ML. Paranephric water instillation: a technique to prevent bowel injury during percutaneous renal radiofrequency ablation. AJR Am J Roentgenol. 2003;181(5):1315–7.
18. Ginat DT, Saad W, Davies M, Walman D, Erturk E. Bowel displacement for CT-guided tumor radiofrequency ablation: techniques and anatomic considerations. J Endourol. 2009;23(8):1259–64.
19. Lee SJ, Choyke LT, Locklin JK, Wood BJ. Use of hydrodissection to prevent nerve and muscular damage during radiofrequency ablation of kidney tumors. J Vasc Interv Radiol. 2006;17(12):1967–9.
20. Park BK, Kim CK. Complications of image-guided radiofrequency ablation of renal cell carcinoma: causes, imaging features and prevention methods. Eur Radiol. 2009;19(9):2180–90.
21. Park BK, Kim SH, Byun JY, Kim YS, Kwon GY, Jang IS. CT-guided instillation of 5% dextrose in water into the anterior pararenal space before renal radiofrequency ablation in a porcine model: positive and negative effects. J Vasc Interv Radiol. 2007;18(12):1561–9.
22. Cantwell CP, Wah TM, Gervais DA, et al. Protecting the ureter during radiofrequency ablation of renal cell cancer: a pilot study of retrograde pyeloperfusion with cooled dextrose 5% in water. J Vasc Interv Radiol. 2008;19(7):1034–40.
23. Wah TM, Koenig P, Irving HC, Gervais DA, Mueller PR. Radiofrequency ablation of a central renal tumor: protection of the collecting system with a retrograde cold dextrose pyeloperfusion technique. J Vasc Interv Radiol. 2005;16(11):1551–5.

24. Brace CL. Radiofrequency and microwave ablation of the liver, lung, kidney, and bone: what are the differences? Curr Probl Diagn Radiol. 2009;38(3):135–43.

25. Clark PE, Woodruff RD, Zagoria RJ, Hall MC. Microwave ablation of renal parenchymal tumors before nephrectomy: phase I study. AJR Am J Roentgenol. 2007;188(5):1212–4.

26. Laeseke PF, Lee Jr FT, Sampson LA, van der Weide DW, Brace CL. Microwave ablation versus radiofrequency ablation in the kidney: high-power triaxial antennas create larger ablation zones than similarly sized internally cooled electrodes. J Vasc Interv Radiol. 2009;20(9):1224–9.

27. Kunkle DA, Uzzo RG. Cryoablation or radiofrequency ablation of the small renal mass: a meta-analysis. Cancer. 2008;113(10):2671–80.

28. Bandi G, Hedican S, Moon T, Lee FT, Nakada SY. Comparison of postoperative pain, convalescence, and patient satisfaction after laparoscopic and percutaneous ablation of small renal masses. J Endourol. 2008;22(5):963–7.

29. Hui GC, Tuncali K, Tatli S, Morrison PR, Silverman SG. Comparison of percutaneous and surgical approaches to renal tumor ablation: metaanalysis of effectiveness and complication rates. J Vasc Interv Radiol. 2008;19(9):1311–20.

30. Allaf ME, Varkarakis IM, Bhayani SB, Inagaki T, Kavoussi LR, Solomon SB. Pain control requirements for percutaneous ablation of renal tumors: cryoablation versus radiofrequency ablation–initial observations. Radiology. 2005;237(1):366–70.

31. Campbell SC, Krishnaumurthi V, Chow G, Hale J, Myles J, Novick AC. Renal cryosurgery: experimental evaluation of treatment parameters. Urology. 1998;52(1):29–33. discussion 33–4.

32. Chosy SG, Nakada SY, Lee Jr FT, Warner TF. Monitoring renal cryosurgery: predictors of tissue necrosis in swine. J Urol. 1998;159(4):1370–4.

33. Sung GT, Gill IS, Hsu TH, et al. Effect of intentional cryo-injury to the renal collecting system. J Urol. 2003;170(2 Pt 1):619–22.

34. Shock SA, Laeseke PF, Sampson LA, et al. Hepatic hemorrhage caused by percutaneous tumor ablation: radiofrequency ablation versus cryoablation in a porcine model. Radiology. 2005;236(1):125–31.

35. Lewin JS, Nour SG, Connell CF, et al. Phase II clinical trial of interactive MR imaging-guided interstitial radiofrequency thermal ablation of primary kidney tumors: initial experience. Radiology. 2004;232(3):835–45.

36. Silverman SG, Tuncali K, Adams DF, Nawfel RD, Zou KH, Judy PF. CT fluoroscopy-guided abdominal interventions: techniques, results, and radiation exposure. Radiology. 1999;212(3):673–81.

37. Shingleton WB, Sewell Jr PE. Percutaneous renal tumor cryoablation with magnetic resonance imaging guidance. J Urol. 2001;165(3):773–6.

38. Littrup PJ, Jallad B, Vorugu V, et al. Lethal isotherms of cryoablation in a phantom study: effects of heat load, probe size, and number. J Vasc Interv Radiol. 2009;20(10):1343–51.

39. Permpongkosol S, Nicol TL, Khurana H, et al. Thermal maps around two adjacent cryoprobes creating overlapping ablations in porcine liver, lung, and kidney. J Vasc Interv Radiol. 2007;18(2):283–7.

40. Laeseke PF, Frey TM, Brace CL, et al. Multiple-electrode radiofrequency ablation of hepatic malignancies: initial clinical experience. AJR Am J Roentgenol. 2007;188(6):1485–94.

41. del Cura JL, Zabala R, Iriarte JI, Unda M. Treatment of renal tumors by percutaneous ultrasound-guided radiofrequency ablation using a multitined electrode: effectiveness and complications. Eur Urol. 2010;57(3):459–65.

42. Atwell TD, Wass CT, Charboneau JW, Callstrom MR, Farrell MA, Sengupta S. Malignant hypertension during cryoablation of an adrenal gland tumor. J Vasc Interv Radiol. 2006;17(3):573–5.

43. Rhim H, Dodd 3rd GD, Chintapalli KN, et al. Radiofrequency thermal ablation of abdominal tumors: lessons learned from complications. Radiographics. 2004;24(1):41–52.

44. Boss A, Clasen S, Kuczyk M, et al. Thermal damage of the genitofemoral nerve due to radiofrequency ablation of renal cell carcinoma: a potentially avoidable complication. AJR Am J Roentgenol. 2005;185(6):1627–31.

45. Park BK, Kim CK. Mechanical ureteral perforation by a radiofrequency electrode during ablation of a renal tumor. Cardiovasc Intervent Radiol. 2009;32(6):1317–9.

46. Rouviere O, Badet L, Murat FJ, et al. Radiofrequency ablation of renal tumors with an expandable multitined electrode: results, complications, and pilot evaluation of cooled pyeloperfusion for collecting system protection. Cardiovasc Intervent Radiol. 2008;31(3):595–603.

47. Brown DB, Bhayani SB. Persistent urine leak after cryoablation of a renal tumor in a patient with an ileal conduit. J Vasc Interv Radiol. 2007;18(10):1324–7.

48. Glasgow SC, Ramachandran S, Csontos KA, Jia J, Mohanakumar T, Chapman WC. Interleukin-1beta is prominent in the early pulmonary inflammatory response after hepatic injury. Surgery. 2005;138(1):64–70.

49. Seifert JK, Morris DL. World survey on the complications of hepatic and prostate cryotherapy. World J Surg. 1999;23(2):109–13. discussion 113–4.

50. Herts BR, Baker ME. The current role of percutaneous biopsy in the evaluation of renal masses. Semin Urol Oncol. 1995;13(4):254–61.

51. Lokken RP, Gervais DA, Arellano RS, et al. Inflammatory nodules mimic applicator track seeding after percutaneous ablation of renal tumors. AJR Am J Roentgenol. 2007;189(4):845–8.

52. Atwell TD, Farrell MA, Callstrom MR, et al. Percutaneous cryoablation of 40 solid renal tumors with US guidance and CT monitoring: initial experience. Radiology. 2007;243(1):276–83.

53. Gupta A, Allaf ME, Kavoussi LR, et al. Computerized tomography guided percutaneous renal cryoablation with the patient under conscious sedation: initial clinical experience. J Urol. 2006;175(2):447–52. discussion 452–3.

Part IV
Lung

Chapter 14
Nonradiological Treatment for Lung Tumors

Tomas Dvorak and Thomas A. DiPetrillo

Overview of Lung Cancer

Lung cancer is a major public health problem. In the USA, approximately 220,000 patients are diagnosed annually and 160,000 die, far more than from prostate or breast cancer (American Cancer Society 2010 Cancer Statistics). Worldwide, lung cancer is the leading cause of cancer mortality, and the World Health Organization estimates 1.3 million deaths per year. The 5-year survival rate is only approximately 15%, and this survival has not changed dramatically over the past three decades.

Lung cancer is typically divided into two broad groups based on histology: small-cell lung cancer and non-small cell lung cancer. Small-cell lung cancer arises from small "blue" cells with neuroendocrine differentiation characterized by rapid growth and early dissemination. Over 70% of patients present with metastatic disease, and management is primarily with chemotherapy. The small proportions that appear to be confined to the chest (limited-stage disease) are treated with concurrent chemoradiation. There is minimal role for definitive local therapies, including surgery, stereotactic radiotherapy or ablative therapies.

Non-small Cell Lung Cancer

Non-small cell lung cancer (NSCLC) is a composite category consisting of three broad histologies: squamous cell carcinoma, adenocarcinoma, and large-cell carcinoma. They have historically been considered together, because their behavior and outcomes are similar, although emerging evidence suggests they may respond differently to targeted chemotherapy agents [1]. Survival depends dramatically on stage (Table 14.1).

The 5-year overall survival for Stage I is ~50%, but it drops to ~25% for Stage II, ~10% for Stage III, and <5% for Stage IV [2]. Unfortunately, only a quarter of patients present with localized (Stage I) disease; the majority present with locally advanced (Stage III) disease or metastatic (Stage IV) disease, leading to poor overall outcomes for these patients. We will review the management of non-small cell lung cancer in reverse order, starting with metastatic disease and ultimately leading on to Stage I disease.

Metastatic disease (Stage IV) is primarily managed with systemic chemotherapy or symptom palliation. Recently updated guidelines from American Society of Clinical Oncology (ASCO) recommend that any two-agent combination (doublet) containing a platinum compound is a reasonable first-line therapy [3]. Considerable research efforts are under way to evaluate the role of targeted agents, such as epidermal growth factor receptor inhibitors (e.g., erlotinib) or angiogenesis inhibitors (e.g., bevacizumab). Radiation therapy is used for palliative treatment of metastases to prevent or delay pain, neurologic symptoms, and improve quality-of-life.

T. Dvorak (✉)
Department of Radiation Oncology, MD Anderson Cancer Center Orlando, Orlando, FL, USA
e-mail: td39@columbia.edu

T.A. DiPetrillo
Department of Radiation Oncology, Rhode Island Hospital, Providence, RI, USA

P.R. Mueller and A. Adam (eds.), *Interventional Oncology: A Practical Guide for the Interventional Radiologist*,
DOI 10.1007/978-1-4419-1469-9_14, © Springer Science+Business Media, LLC 2012

Table 14.1 AJCC staging and median survival

Stage	Clinical TNM	Brief description	Median survival
Stage IA	T1a N0	≤2 cm Diameter, ≤lobar bronchus	5.0 years
	T1b N0	2–3 cm Diameter, ≤lobar bronchus	
Stage IB	T2a N0	3–5 cm Diameter, ≤main bronchus, or invades visceral pleura	3.6 years
Stage IIA	T2b N0	5–7 cm Diameter, ≤main bronchus, or invades visceral pleura	2.8 years
	T1a–T2a N1	Ipsilateral hilar node disease	
Stage IIB	T3 N0	>7 cm Diameter, <2 cm from carina, invades extrapleural structures	1.5 years
	T2b N1	Ipsilateral hilar node disease	
Stage IIIA	T4 N0–N1	Invades other organs, N0–N1 disease	1.2 years
	T1–T3 N2	Ipsilateral mediastinal node disease	
Stage IIIB	T4 N2	Ipsilateral mediastinal node disease	10 months
	T1–T4 N3	Contralateral mediastinal node disease	
Stage IV	M1	Metastatic disease	6 months

Locally advanced disease (Stage III) consists of two anatomically distinct disease subsets. Stage IIIB is primarily defined by contralateral mediastinal lymph node disease (N3) and is managed with systemic chemotherapy or definitive chemoradiation. A typical U.S. protocol would include thoracic radiation to 66–74 Gy, with concurrent chemotherapy most commonly consisting of either carboplatin with taxotere or cisplatin with etoposide. Stage IIIA is primarily defined by ipsilateral mediastinal lymph node disease (N2), and its management is somewhat controversial. The American College of Chest Physicians (ACCP) considers primary concurrent chemoradiation using comparable protocols to Stage IIIB to be the standard of care [4]. On the other hand, the National Comprehensive Cancer Network (NCCN) guidelines [5] allow neoadjuvant chemotherapy or neoadjuvant chemoradiation followed by surgical resection as appropriate management.

Localized (Stage II) disease consists of either large tumors (>5 cm) with or without chest wall involvement or disease in the ipsilateral hilar lymph nodes (N1). Primary therapy is surgical resection, followed by adjuvant chemotherapy [6] or, to a lesser extent, external-beam radiotherapy. For interventional oncologists, Stage I currently holds the most interest, since the definitive treatment is primarily local. Stage I tumors are either solitary small intraparenchymal lesions (T1N0) or somewhat larger tumors, which may be more centrally located (T2N0).

Stage I NSCLC

Watchful Waiting

Since lung cancer screening efforts appear to identify more Stage I tumors, it is important to understand the natural history of Stage I NSCLC. In prostate cancer, a reasonable treatment strategy is to manage some low-risk patients expectantly with active surveillance to avoid the toxicity of therapy, because most patients with early low-risk prostate cancer die of competing mortalities and not of prostate cancer [7]. Would it be reasonable to consider such expectant management in NSCLC? Retrospective review of the California Cancer Registry between 1989 and 2003 identified more than 19,000 patients with Stage I NSCLC, of whom 1,432 were not treated with surgery, radiation, or chemotherapy [8]. Median survival for the entire cohort was 9 months. Stratification by T-stage revealed poor outcome even in the most favorable T1 patients, who had a median survival of 13 months, whereas T2 patients had a median survival of 8 months. Approximately 32% patients refused surgery; the median survival of this presumably healthier cohort was only 14 months. The 5-year overall survival for all subgroups was <10%, and >80% of these patients died of their disease rather than of competing causes. The authors of the study concluded that long-term survival with untreated Stage I lung cancer is uncommon and that most of these patients will die of lung cancer. Therefore, watchful waiting as a treatment strategy for these patients is generally not successful, and Stage I patients should be offered definitive treatment.

Surgery

Most Stage I patients are offered surgery, dating to a randomized trial performed in the 1950s at the Hammersmith Hospital in UK [9]. Prior to that, most retrospective studies suggested comparable outcomes between radical surgery and radical radiation therapy. Fifty-eight patients, who had no clinical or radiographic involvement of the mediastinum on chest X-ray and were able to undergo pneumonectomy, were randomized to undergo either surgery or radiation therapy. Surgery was pneumonectomy or lobectomy, with hilar and mediastinal lymph node dissection. Radiation therapy was 45 Gy over 4 weeks to visible tumor with 2 cm margin, and to hilar and mediastinal lymph nodes. At 1 year, radiation therapy was superior, with 64% survival compared to 43% survival in the surgical arm. This was partly due to the fact that of the 30 patients randomized to the surgical arm, 13 (43%) were either technically inoperable or refused surgery, and those who underwent surgery experienced a 10% operative mortality. By year 2, survival in the surgical arm was superior (27% vs. 14%) and remained so through the 4-year follow-up (23% vs. 7%). By histology, the 4-year survival was dramatically better in the surgical arm with squamous cell histology (30% vs. 6%), but was no different with anaplastic (small-cell) histology (10% in both arms). The authors concluded that for squamous cell tumors, the results of surgical resection were significantly better than radiation therapy.

Today, practice guidelines from national societies [4, 5, 10] recommend surgery as the primary treatment option for operable Stage I patients. Efforts to spare lung function with a limited (sublobar) resection have been promising in single-institution series [11]; the North American Lung Cancer Study Group carried out a randomized trial (LCSG 821) comparing limited resection (segmentectomy or a wedge resection) with lobectomy for the definitive treatment of patients with Stage I disease in 1980s. A total of 247 patients were eligible for analysis. Limited resection was associated with 30% increase in death rate and 50% increase in death due to lung cancer, both statistically significant. Patients undergoing limited resection had a 75% increase in recurrence rate, which was attributable to the tripling of local failure from 6% with lobectomy to 17% with limited resection, which is also statistically significant [12]. After a reanalysis of the data, most of the outcomes except for local recurrence lost statistical significance, though the authors felt that their original conclusions about inferiority of sublobar approaches was still valid [13]. Full lobectomy remained the standard of care.

After development of video-assisted thoracoscopic surgery (VATS) in the 1990s and several good long-term retrospective results in intentionally limited resection for small tumors in Japan [14, 15], Japanese investigators felt that the question of limited resection remained unanswered. A meta-analysis of the literature found 14 studies, including 1 randomized trial (LCSG 821 discussed above), 1 matched-pair analysis, and 12 retrospective studies [16]. In total, 1,887 patients with lobectomy were compared to 903 patients with limited resection. There was no difference in overall survival at 1 year (0.7% difference), 3 years (1.9% difference), or 5 years (3.6% difference), although there was significant patient heterogeneity among the different studies. The authors ultimately felt that limited resection is inferior to lobectomy, but that there are subsets of NSCLCs that can be resected completely by a limited resection. A more recent meta-analysis performed by Greek investigators identified three new studies published since the Japanese analysis. The authors concluded that while wedge resection was not comparable to lobectomy, a more extensive segmental resection was comparable to lobectomy for small peripheral tumors [17]. A SEER data analysis suggested that lobectomy confers a significant survival benefit for younger patients, but that patients ≥71 years have a similar survival regardless of the type of surgery used [18]. In the USA, investigators at the Cancer and Leukemia Group B (CALGB) felt that improved imaging and surgical techniques, combined with the advantages of limited resection in terms of preserved pulmonary function, decreased hospitalization, and improved resectability of second primaries would merit a new comparison between limited resection and lobectomy. CALGB 140503 is a noninferiority trial comparing sublobar resection with lobectomy in small (≤2 cm) peripheral Stage IA tumors, with disease-free survival as the primary outcome. This trial is expected to complete accrual of 1,297 patients by 2012. Today, lobectomy or pneumonectomy is considered the anatomically appropriate resection, depending on technical considerations. Median 5-year survival is approximately 65% overall [12], although there is a significant correlation with size. Highly selected series report survival rates as high as 95% for peripheral tumors <15 mm in diameter [19].

Surgery Plus Brachytherapy

Unfortunately, only two-thirds of Stage I patients actually undergo anatomically correct resection [National Cancer Database, American College of Surgeons]. Many patients are not good surgical candidates because of poor pulmonary function or other medical comorbidities. For these patients, it is important to balance the tumor control benefit of

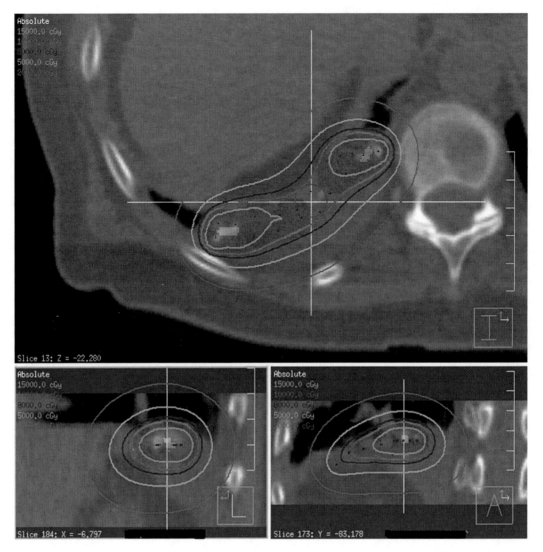

Fig. 14.1 This image represents the postresection placement of Iodine-125 seeds embedded in suture material adjacent to the surgical margin. Such placement results in a localized delivery of radiation to the high-risk region following sublobar resection

definitive surgery with the risk of perioperative and postoperative morbidity and mortality. According to the British Thoracic Society, for thoracic-trained surgeons performing resections at a high-volume institution, surgical mortality should be <4% for lobectomy and <9% for pneumonectomy [20]. The ACCP published guidelines for the physiologic evaluation of patients being considered for resection [21]. If FEV1 < 1.5 L or <80%, further analysis using DLCO, percent predicted FEV1, and VO$_2$ max is recommended. For these patients, current ACCP and NCCN guidelines suggest a subtotal resection, accepting the increased risk of local recurrence seen in LCSG 821. Most of the recurrences in the limited resection arm occurred in the proximal bronchial margin along the suture line, thus efforts are under way to use localized radiation in the form of brachytherapy strands sutured into the staple line after a wedge or segmental resection (Fig. 14.1). Initial exploratory data in 33 patients showed only 6% local recurrence, which is comparable to full lobectomy failure rate [22]. These results were corroborated using an alternative brachytherapy technique in a larger single-institution series, with 2% local failure rate in the sublobar surgery + brachytherapy cohort, compared with 18% rate in the sublobar surgery alone cohort [23]. The promising local control and lack of any significant toxicity led to the opening of the American College of Surgeons Oncology Group (ACOSOG) Z-4032 Phase III trial, which randomly assigns patients with tumors <3 cm to sublobar resection alone or to sublobar resection with an intraoperative brachytherapy implant at the resection margin.

Radiation Therapy

For patients who are not surgical candidates, the primary treatment approach is radiation therapy. Radiation was historically delivered with conventional external-beam techniques (EBRT); more recently stereotactic body radiation therapy (SBRT) and proton therapy have become available. Unfortunately, conventional RT outcomes are less than satisfactory. A meta-analysis of 18 conventional radiation studies published between 1988 and 2000 showed an average 5-year overall survival of 21% and disease-specific survival of only 25% [24]. In fact, an argument has been made based on SEER data analysis that conventional radiation therapy does not cure Stage I patients, but only delays disease progression, with comparable 5-year cancer-specific survival to supportive care [25]. Patterns of failure analysis after conventional radiation revealed initial local recurrence in ~30%, nodal recurrence in 2%, and initial distal failure in 17% of patients [24]. The high rate of local failure meant that higher radiation doses were necessary to control the disease. Analysis of a University of Michigan dose-escalation trial suggested that using conventional doses of 60–66 Gy, probability of tumor control was only 20–30% and that doses in excess of 120–130 Gy using standard fraction size were probably required [26]. The Radiation Therapy Oncology Group (RTOG) performed a dose-escalation study for Stage I–III tumors. The maximum tolerated dose for the group with favorable radiation parameters, which contained 53% Stage I tumors, was 83.8 Gy. Dose-limiting toxicity included development of tracheoesophageal fistula and hemoptysis [27]. In conclusion, the dose necessary to eradicate these tumors could not be safely delivered with conventional radiation fields due to the high amount of radiation given to nearby normal tissues such as lung parenchyma, mediastinum, and esophagus.

Several developments over the past two decades have allowed more tolerable escalation of the radiation dose. The first development was improved visualization of the tumor with CT- or PET/CT-guided treatment planning, and the realization that it may not be necessary to electively treat the regional lymphatic drainage in the hilum and mediastinum. A Dutch prospective study treating only "postage stamp" fields surrounding the primary tumor showed local control of 94% and a significantly improved 3-year disease-free survival (76%) and overall survival (42%) compared with historical controls [28]. The second development was improved precision in the delivery of radiation with proton therapy or alternatively, intensity modulated radiation therapy (IMRT), and image-guidance. The third development was improved radiobiological understanding of tumor control, which suggested that fewer large fractions (>5 Gy) might have a higher biological impact than more conventional (1.8–2 Gy) fractions. Early evidence of this approach came from a Loma Linda University series of 326 Stage I patients treated between 1994 and 1998 with proton therapy. Radiation was delivered in ten fractions of 5.1 Gy each. The 2-year local control was 87%, and 2-year disease-free survival was 86%, much higher than the historical disease-free survival of ~25% [29]. Subsequent Phase II trial of proton therapy in 68 patients with clinical Stage I used ten fractions of 6 Gy each. The 3-year local control was 74%, and disease specific survival was 72%. There was no significant toxicity, and the authors concluded that this approach was safe, with improved control compared to conventional radiation [30]. Two separate Japanese groups confirmed that this approach of focally delivered high-dose particle therapy is promising [31, 32].

Stereotactic Body Radiation Therapy

In the interim, technological advances associated with photon therapy allowed the development of SBRT, which uses immobilization techniques and stereotactic image-guided localization of the tumor prior to each radiation treatment to deliver very high fractional dose safely (Fig. 14.2). A dose-escalation Phase I trial from Indiana University showed that dose-limiting toxicity for smaller peripheral tumors (≤5 cm) was not reached even after delivering an essentially ablative dose of 20 Gy in three fractions [33]. Based on these results, the investigators enrolled 70 Stage I patients on a Phase II protocol, delivering 20 Gy × 3 fractions to T1 tumors and 22 Gy × 3 fractions to T2 tumors. With a median follow-up of 4.2 years, their 3-year local control rate was 88%, nodal failure occurred in 9%, and distant metastases developed in 13% of patients. Grade 3 or greater late toxicity occurred in 16% of patients. Of note, Grade 3 or greater toxicity occurred more frequently in central lesions (27%) rather than in peripheral lesions (10%), though the difference did not reach statistical significance. RTOG subsequently performed a multi-institutional Phase II trial (RTOG 0236) using the Indiana University scheme of 20 Gy in three fractions to treat 59 inoperable patients. Eligible patients had biopsy-proven peripheral tumors, cT1-T3 N0, >2 cm away from the bronchial tree, who were not surgical candidates. It is important to note that the 20 Gy prescribed dose was calculated without correcting for tissue heterogeneities such as lung and bone, which was the historical standard. As treatment planning software became more robust over time, heterogeneity corrections were used more widely, and the 20 Gy uncorrected dose was reported as 18 Gy corrected dose. The primary endpoint was local control and with a median follow-up

Fig. 14.2 Radiation dose delivered to a primary lung tumor by stereotactic technique (SBRT). The rapid dose fall-off limits dose to adjacent normal structures

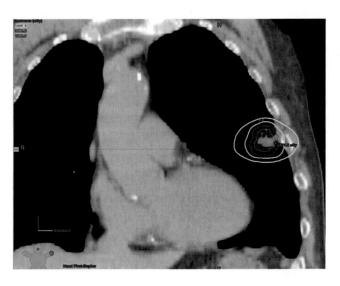

of 34 months, the estimated 3-year local control rate was 97.6%, lobar control rate was 90.6%, and locoregional control was 87.2%. The 3-year disease-free survival was 48.5%, and overall survival was 55.8%, which is dramatically superior to conventional radiation results. Approximately 15.3% of patients experienced a Grade 3 or Grade 4 toxicity. These results were encouraging for this compromised population [34].

It is not clear, however, which radiation dose schedule offers the best tumor control and the least toxicity. There are now multiple published reports available, most utilizing between one and five fractions. Single-fraction experience demonstrating that 26 Gy is feasible for both primary lung tumors and lung metastases was initially published by Wulf et al., showing no toxicity and no local failures, with a median follow-up of 11 months [35]. Several other groups have published studies demonstrating the safety and efficacy of a single-fraction approach, with highest dose reported by Hara et al. [36]. The authors treated 59 patients (both primary NSCLC and lung metastases) with single-fraction doses ranging from 26 to 34 Gy. The 2-year local control rate for patients treated with >30 Gy was 83%, and the overall survival was 41%. Conversely, multiple Japanese groups have reported on their experience with various multifraction schemas [37]; on a recent practice survey, the majority of institutions were using 12 Gy×4 fractions [38]. In an effort to optimize the SBRT dose schedule, RTOG is currently carrying out a randomized Phase II protocol (RTOG 0915) comparing 34 Gy × 1 fraction with 12 Gy × 4 fractions to select the most favorable in terms of toxicity and efficacy. This regimen will be compared against the current RTOG standard of 20 Gy (18 Gy heterogeneity corrected) × 3 fractions.

The majority of patients treated with stereotactic radiation thus far have been surgically inoperable. Comparison of outcomes between surgery and radiation therapy is complicated by issues of patient selection and by clinical vs. surgical staging. Patients who are not surgical candidates and are referred for radiation therapy typically have a severe pulmonary or cardiac compromise, with a limited life-expectancy. The University of Colorado experience in the management of patients with severe COPD (FEV1 < 50% or symptoms interfering with activities of daily living) in the 1960s showed their 5-year overall survival to be 41% compared with the age-matched survival of 86% ($p < 0.01$). This difference persisted at 10-years (17% vs. 69%) [39]. Furthermore, complicating the comparison with surgery, based on results from CALGB trial 96761, is that only 62% of clinically suspected Stage I NSCLC actually have pathologic Stage I disease; the remainder were benign diseases (9%), other histological malignancies (4%), or higher stages (24%) [40]. It is, therefore, difficult to directly compare outcomes of the relatively healthy, pathologically staged Stage I patients undergoing surgery with the relatively ill, clinically staged Stage I patients undergoing nonsurgical management such as radiation therapy. Japanese investigators reported on a subset of 87 patients who were healthy, but refused surgery, and were treated as part of a 245-patient SBRT cohort. With a median follow-up of 3.2 years, their 5-year overall survival was 71%, which compares favorably with surgical outcomes [37]. Demonstration of excellent local control in inoperable patients, the Japanese experience in operable patients and the fact that SBRT is an outpatient, well-tolerated procedure with relatively low toxicity has led to trials comparing SBRT to surgical alternatives. RTOG has completed accrual of a Phase II trial (RTOG 0618) to evaluate the 20 Gy × 3 fractions in operable patients in May 2010; the results are pending maturity. More recently, randomized Phase III trials have been opened in the USA, a collaboration of RTOG and ACOSOG (RTOG 1021), and in The Netherlands (NCT00687986).

Conclusion

In conclusion, lung cancer continues to be a disease with a significant epidemiological impact. Small-cell lung cancer is essentially a systemic disease, and chemotherapy serves as the primary treatment modality, with concurrent radiation for localized disease. Non-small cell lung cancer management is stage dependent. In Stage I disease, surgical resection with lobectomy is the standard of care, whereas stereotactic radiation therapy and other localized techniques are alternatives for the nonoperative patient; potential benefits for operative candidates are being prospectively evaluated. Multidisciplinary management, or at least evaluation, is recommended.

References

1. Dempke WC, Suto T, Reck M. Targeted therapies for non-small cell lung cancer. Lung Cancer. 2010;67(3):257–74. Epub 2009 Nov 14.
2. AJCC Cancer Staging Handbook. American Joint Committee On Cancer. 7th ed. New York: Springer; 2010.
3. Azzoli CG, Baker Jr S, Temin S, Pao W, Aliff T, Brahmer J, et al. American Society of Clinical Oncology Clinical Practice Guideline update on chemotherapy for stage IV non-small-cell lung cancer. J Clin Oncol. 2009;27(36):6251–66. Epub 2009 Nov 16.
4. Robinson LA, Ruckdeschel JC, Wagner H Jr, Stevens CW, American College of Chest Physicians. Treatment of non-small cell lung cancer-stage IIIA: ACCP evidence-based clinical practice guidelines (2nd ed.). Chest. 2007;132(3 Suppl):243 S–65 S.
5. National Comprehensive Cancer Network. NCCN clinical practice guidelines in oncology, non-small cell lung cancer, v2.2010. http://www.nccn.org/professionals/physician_gls/PDF/nscl.pdf. Accessed 1 Dec 2010.
6. Pisters KM, Evans WK, Azzoli CG, Kris MG, Smith CA, Desch CE, et al., Cancer Care Ontario, American Society of Clinical Oncology. Cancer Care Ontario and American Society of Clinical Oncology adjuvant chemotherapy and adjuvant radiation therapy for stages I-IIIA resectable non small-cell lung cancer guideline. J Clin Oncol. 2007;25(34):5506–18. Epub 2007 Oct 22.
7. Klotz L, Zhang L, Lam A, Nam R, Mamedov A, Loblaw A. Clinical results of long-term follow-up of a large, active surveillance cohort with localized prostate cancer. J Clin Oncol. 2010;28(1):126–31. Epub 2009 Nov 16.
8. Raz DJ, Zell JA, Ou SH, Gandara DR, Anton-Culver H, Jablons DM. Natural history of stage I non-small cell lung cancer: implications for early detection. Chest. 2007;132(1):193–9. Epub 2007 May 15.
9. Morrison R, Deeley TJ, Cleland WP. The treatment of carcinoma of the bronchus: a clinical trial to compare surgery and supervoltage radiotherapy. Lancet. 1963;281(7283):683–4.
10. National Institute for Clinical Excellence. The diagnosis and treatment of lung cancer: methods, evidence, and guidance. http://www.nice.org.uk/nicemedia/pdf/cg024fullguideline.pdf. Accessed 1 Dec 2010.
11. Jensik RJ, Faber LP, Millov FJ, et al. Segmental resection for lung cancer – a fifteen-year experience. J Thorac Cardiovasc Surg. 1973;66:563–72.
12. Ginsberg RJ, Rubinstein LV. Randomized trial of lobectomy versus limited resection for T1 N0 non-small cell lung cancer. Lung Cancer Study Group. Ann Thorac Surg. 1995;60(3):615–22. discussion 622–3.
13. Lederle FA. Lobectomy versus limited resection in T1 N0 lung cancer. Ann Thorac Surg. 1996;62(4):1249–50.
14. Okada M, Yoshikawa K, Hatta T, Tsubota N. Is segmentectomy with lymph node assessment an alternative to lobectomy for non-small cell lung cancer of 2 cm or smaller? Ann Thorac Surg. 2001;71(3):956–60. discussion 961.
15. Koike T, Yamato Y, Yoshiya K, Shimoyama T, Suzuki R. Intentional limited pulmonary resection for peripheral T1 N0 M0 small-sized lung cancer. J Thorac Cardiovasc Surg. 2003;125(4):924–8.
16. Nakamura H, Kawasaki N, Taguchi M, Kabasawa K. Survival following lobectomy vs limited resection for stage I lung cancer: a meta-analysis. Br J Cancer. 2005;92(6):1033–7.
17. Chamogeorgakis T, Ieromonachos C, Georgiannakis E, Mallios D. Does lobectomy achieve better survival and recurrence rates than limited pulmonary resection for T1N0M0 non-small cell lung cancer patients? Interact Cardiovasc Thorac Surg. 2009;8(3):364–72. Epub 2008 Jul 18.
18. Mery CM, Pappas AN, Bueno R, Colson YL, Linden P, Sugarbaker DJ, et al. Similar long-term survival of elderly patients with non-small cell lung cancer treated with lobectomy or wedge resection within the surveillance, epidemiology, and end results database. Chest. 2005;128(1):237–45.
19. Lyons G, Quadrelli S, Silva C, Vera K, Iotti A, et al. Analysis of survival in 400 surgically resected non-small cell lung carcinomas: towards a redefinition of the T factor. J Thorac Oncol. 2008;3(9):989–93.
20. British Thoracic Society, Society of Cardiothoracic Surgeons of Great Britain and Ireland Working Party. BTS guidelines: guidelines on the selection of patients with lung cancer for surgery. Thorax. 2001;56(2):89–108.
21. Colice GL, Shafazand S, Griffin JP, Keenan R, Bolliger CT, American College of Chest Physicians. Physiologic evaluation of the patient with lung cancer being considered for resectional surgery: ACCP evidenced-based clinical practice guidelines (2nd ed.). Chest. 2007;132(3 Suppl):161 S–77 S.
22. Lee W, Daly BD, DiPetrillo TA, Morelli DM, Neuschatz AC, Morr J, et al. Limited resection for non-small cell lung cancer: observed local control with implantation of I-125 brachytherapy seeds. Ann Thorac Surg. 2003;75(1):237–42. discussion 242–3.
23. Santos R, Colonias A, Parda D, Trombetta M, Maley RH, Macherey R, et al. Comparison between sublobar resection and 125Iodine brachytherapy after sublobar resection in high-risk patients with Stage I non-small-cell lung cancer. Surgery. 2003;134(4):691–7. discussion 697.
24. Qiao X, Tullgren O, Lax I, Sirzén F, Lewensohn R. The role of radiotherapy in treatment of stage I non-small cell lung cancer. Lung Cancer. 2003;41(1):1–11.

25. Wisnivesky JP, Bonomi M, Henschke C, Iannuzzi M, McGinn T. Radiation therapy for the treatment of unresected stage I-II non-small cell lung cancer. Chest. 2005;128(3):1461–7.
26. Mehta M, Scrimger R, Mackie R, Paliwal B, Chappell R, Fowler J. A new approach to dose escalation in non-small-cell lung cancer. Int J Radiat Oncol Biol Phys. 2001;49(1):23–33.
27. Bradley J, Graham MV, Winter K, Purdy JA, Komaki R, Roa WH, et al. Toxicity and outcome results of RTOG 9311: a phase I-II dose-escalation study using three-dimensional conformal radiotherapy in patients with inoperable non-small-cell lung carcinoma. Int J Radiat Oncol Biol Phys. 2005;61(2):318–28.
28. Slotman BJ, Antonisse IE, Njo KH. Limited field irradiation in early stage (T1-2 N0) non-small cell lung cancer. Radiother Oncol. 1996;41(1):41–4.
29. Bush DA, Slater JD, Bonnet R, Cheek GA, Dunbar RD, Moyers M, et al. Proton-beam radiotherapy for early-stage lung cancer. Chest. 1999;116(5):1313–9.
30. Bush DA, Slater JD, Shin BB, Cheek G, Miller DW, Slater JM. Hypofractionated proton beam radiotherapy for stage I lung cancer. Chest. 2004;126(4):1198–203.
31. Nihei K, Ogino T, Ishikura S, Nishimura H. High-dose proton beam therapy for Stage I non-small-cell lung cancer. Int J Radiat Oncol Biol Phys. 2006;65(1):107–11.
32. Hata M, Tokuuye K, Kagei K, Sugahara S, Nakayama H, Fukumitsu N, et al. Hypofractionated high-dose proton beam therapy for stage I non-small-cell lung cancer: preliminary results of a phase I/II clinical study. Int J Radiat Oncol Biol Phys. 2007;68(3):786–93. Epub 2007 Mar 26.
33. McGarry RC, Papiez L, Williams M, Whitford T, Timmerman RD. Stereotactic body radiation therapy of early-stage non-small-cell lung carcinoma: phase I study. Int J Radiat Oncol Biol Phys. 2005;63(4):1010–5. Epub 2005 Aug 22.
34. Timmerman R et al. Stereotactic body radiation therapy for inoperable early stage lung cancer. JAMA. 2010;303(110):1070–6.
35. Wulf J, Baier K, Mueller G, Flentje MP. Dose–response in stereotactic irradiation of lung tumors. Radiother Oncol. 2005;77(1):83–7. Epub 2005 Oct 4.
36. Hara R, Itami J, Kondo T, Aruga T, Uno T, Sasano N, et al. Clinical outcomes of single-fraction stereotactic radiation therapy of lung tumors. Cancer. 2006;106(6):1347–52.
37. Onishi H, Shirato H, Nagata Y, Hiraoka M, Fujino M, Gomi K, et al. Hypofractionated stereotactic radiotherapy (HypoFXSRT) for stage I non-small cell lung cancer: updated results of 257 patients in a Japanese multi-institutional study. J Thorac Oncol. 2007;2(7 Suppl 3):S94–100.
38. Nagata Y, Hiraoka M, Mizowaki T, Narita Y, Matsuo Y, Norihisa Y, et al. Survey of stereotactic body radiation therapy in Japan by the Japan 3-D Conformal External Beam Radiotherapy Group. Int J Radiat Oncol Biol Phys. 2009;75(2):343–7.
39. Sahn SA, Nett LM, Petty TL. Ten year follow-up of a comprehensive rehabilitation program for severe COPD. Chest. 1980;77(2 Suppl):311–4.
40. D'Cunha J, Herndon JE 2nd, Herzan DL, Patterson GA, Kohman LJ, Harpole DH et al., Cancer and Leukemia Group B. Poor correspondence between clinical and pathologic staging in stage 1 non-small cell lung cancer: results from CALGB 9761, a prospective trial. Lung Cancer. 2005;48(2):241–6. Epub 2005 Jan 4.

Chapter 15
Radiofrequency Ablation, Microwave Ablation, and Cryoablation for Lung Tumors

Tracey G. Simon and Damian E. Dupuy

Introduction

The current standard of care for patients with early stage pulmonary neoplasms is surgical resection. However, only approximately 15% of patients are surgical candidates, due to advanced disease stage and/or severe medical comorbidities [1, 2]. For such patients, the treatment options are limited, and the 5-year survival is poor ranging from 5% to 12% [3].

The development of noninvasive strategies – such as radiofrequency ablation (RFA), microwave ablation (MWA), or cryoablation – have provided new therapeutic options for medically inoperable lung cancer patients. Both RFA and MWA are heat-based ablation methods that cause cell death by thermocoagulation. Cryoablation, however, causes the formation of intra- and extracellular ice crystals in the target tissue and causes tumor cell death by freezing. Owing to the development of small-diameter applicators, all three ablation techniques can be performed percutaneously under image guidance, as well as laparoscopically or intraoperatively [4]. The advantages of these therapies over invasive surgery include reduced morbidity and mortality, decreased cost, and the ability to be performed on an outpatient basis [5].

This section seeks to describe the role of image-guided thermal ablation (RFA, MWA, and cryoablation) in the treatment of lung neoplasms.

Patient Selection

Image-guided ablation is useful as a definitive therapy in patients who are not surgical candidates – be that due to age, comorbid conditions, or poor cardiopulmonary reserve. It is an effective treatment option for patients with primary non-small cell lung cancer, as well as for those who present with a finite number (less than five or six) of biologically favorable metastases, such as sarcomas, renal cell carcinoma, colorectal carcinoma, and breast carcinoma, in addition to treatment of primary non-small cell lung cancer.

Further, image-guided thermal ablation is an effective palliative therapy and has been used successfully to control tumor recurrence in patients who are ineligible for repeat radiation, as well as to limit chest wall pain and brachial plexus involvement [6]. There is no lower limit to a patient's pulmonary function that would preclude them from thermal ablation; many successfully treated patients have presented with low forced expiratory volume (FEV1) or low diffusion capacity (DLCO). However, if the comorbid conditions and performance status indicate that a patient may have survival of less than a year, treatment with thermal ablation may not be indicated.

T.G. Simon (✉) • D.E. Dupuy
Department of Diagnostic Imaging, Warren Alpert Medical School of Brown University,
Rhode Island Hospital, Providence, RI, USA
e-mail: tracey_simon@brown.edu

P.R. Mueller and A. Adam (eds.), *Interventional Oncology: A Practical Guide for the Interventional Radiologist*,
DOI 10.1007/978-1-4419-1469-9_15, © Springer Science+Business Media, LLC 2012

Radiofrequency Ablation

Radiofrequency ablation (RFA) is a minimally invasive technique used in the management of inoperable non-small cell lung cancer, as well as in palliative treatment for patients with pulmonary metastases. First reported in human lungs in 2000, it has been shown to be an effective treatment for both primary and metastatic tumors, with negligible mortality, low morbidity, and dramatic improvements in quality of life [7].

Lung cancer patients selected for RFA generally fall into two groups: a local control group and a palliative group. The local control group is comprised of patients with primary or metastatic pulmonary neoplasms, who are ineligible for surgery due to advanced disease stage and/or comorbid conditions. Among these patients, RFA has been shown to be highly successful, with survival rates of 70% at 1 year and 48% at 2 years [8, 9]. Table 15.1 summarizes clinical outcomes in lung ablation. These survival rates compare favorably to surgical cohorts. RFA is most successful in the treatment of lung lesions less than 3 cm; such patients demonstrate high rates of complete tumor necrosis (69–91%), longer median time to disease recurrence (45 months), and less impaired survival, than do patients with larger (>3 cm) tumors [10–12] (Fig. 15.1). The large, multicenter Radiofrequency Ablation of Pulmonary Tumors Response Evaluation (RAPTURE) trial showed that post-RFA, 2-year survival rates were 48%, and cancer-specific survival rates were 92% [9].

On the other hand, RFA can also be implemented for the palliative treatment of larger neoplasms, as well. It has been shown to successfully debulk large lung tumors – especially those involving the chest wall or pleura. Further, in such patients, RFA has well-documented ability to alleviate pain, cough, hemoptysis, and dyspnea, as well as to lessen pain from bony metastases [13, 14].

In the lung, the aerated tissue acts as an insulator, concentrating the thermal energy at the site of the lesion; at the same time, the vascular flow and air exchange serve to distribute heat away from normal parenchyma [15]. While this "heat-sink" effect serves to protect the proximal normal parenchyma and vasculature, it also limits the therapeutic effects of the RF treatment, by limiting the ablation margins, which are critical in the prevention of local disease recurrence. This can be overcome by the infusion of saline or via the use of multiple needle electrodes, both of which serve to promote electrical conduction and reduce the high impedance created by aerated lung tissue [16].

Benefits

Unlike surgery or external-beam radiation therapy (XRT), repeated RF ablations can easily be performed on a patient without additional morbidity or mortality. For tumors smaller than 3 cm, excellent short-term local control has been documented, and tumors can be covered by a complete ablation zone by one electrode, in a single-treatment session [4]. Further, RFA can be used synergistically with other treatments, such as XRT or brachytherapy [17].

Risks and Complications

In the treatment of lung tumors larger than 3 cm, RFA shows less local control, and both disease recurrence and the need for repeated ablations markedly increases [18]. To date, no report has examined the possibility of utilizing multiple RFA probes in the treatment of large pulmonary malignancies.

Contraindications for RFA are few, including only recent use of anticoagulants and uncontrollable bleeding diathesis. Complications include pneumothorax (30–35%) (Fig. 15.2), pleural effusion (4–30%), pulmonary abscess (1–6%), and pneumonia (1.2%); exacerbation of chronic obstructive pulmonary disease (COPD) or acute respiratory distress syndrome (ARDS), hemoptysis, hemothorax, bronchopleural fistula, parenchymal hemorrhage, acute renal failure, vocal cord paralysis, phrenic nerve injury, atrial fibrillation, pulmonary embolus, skin burns (secondary to inappropriate placement of grounding pads), tumor tract seeding, and pneumopathy are rare [19, 20]. Inflammation-related complications – specifically interstitial pneumonia and aseptic pleuritis – have been reported at a rate of 1.2%; the risk factors for these events have been shown to be: previous XRT therapy and tumor size larger than 4 cm [21]. Fortunately, for the most common complication, namely pneumothorax, this is easily treated or self-limited and resolves without intervention. In patients with persistent air leaks despite pleural drainage, pleurodesis, blood patches, and bronchoscopic fibrin injections may need to be performed because often times patients with emphysema and persistent air leaks develop multiple small pleural tears from architectural distortion and pleural adhesions in addition to the electrode puncture site.

Table 15.1 Summary table of lung thermal ablation literature (Adapted from a table to be published in "Image Guided Thermal Ablation of Lung Malignancies," *Radiology*)

Author	Title	Journal	Number of patients	Indications	Local control rate	Survival
RFA						
Lee JM, Jin GY, Goldberg SN, Lee YC, Chung GH, Han YM, Lee SY, Kim CS	Percutaneous radiofrequency ablation for inoperable non-small cell lung cancer and metastases: preliminary report	Radiology 2004; 230:125–134	30 Patients; 27 NSCLC, 5 lung metastases	Local control	Complete necrosis in all six patients with tumors <3 cm; 23% complete ablation lesions >3 cm; 50% tumor necrosis among 20 lesions with incomplete necrosis; 5 mm well-demarcated nonenhancing zone of ground glass opacity surrounding ablated lesion in 8/12 cases of complete necrosis	No local tumor recurrence at 22.2 months
Akeboshi M, Yamakado K, Nakatsuka A, et al.	Percutaneous radiofrequency ablation of lung neoplasms: initial therapeutic response	J Vasc Interv Radiol 2004; 15:463–470	31 Patients; 54 tumors (primary lung, $n=13$; metastases, $n=41$)	Local control	69% Complete tumor necrosis in 36 lesions <3 cm; 39% complete necrosis in 18 tumors >3 cm	Not reported
Yasui K, Kanazawa S, Sano Y, et al.	Thoracic tumors treated with CT-guided radiofrequency ablation: initial experience	Radiology 2004; 231:850–857	35 Patients; 99 tumors (primary lung, $n=3$; metastases, $n=96$)	Local control	91% Complete tumor necrosis among 99 neoplasms mean diameter of 1.9 cm	Not reported
Herrera LJ, Fernando HC, Perry Y, et al.	Radiofrequency ablation of pulmonary malignant tumors in nonsurgical candidates	J Thorac Cardiovasc Surg 2003; 125:929–937	18 Patients; 33 tumors	Local control	Response: complete, 6%; partial, 44%; stable, 33%; progressed, 17%	Not reported
Fernando HC, De Hoyos A, Landreneau RJ, et al.	Radiofrequency ablation for the treatment of non-small cell lung cancer in marginal surgical candidates	J Thorac Cardiovasc Surg 2005; 129:639–644	18 Patients (13 from a percutaneous approach); metastases, $n=13$; primary lung, $n=5$; 33 tumors	Local control	Disease progression was seen in eight nodules (38%) in six patients (33%)	Overall mean survival was 20.97 months; median survival not reached. Mean progression free interval for stage I vs. other stages was 17.6 months vs. 14.98 months (NS)
Pennathur A, Luketich JD, Abbas G, et al.	Radiofrequency ablation for the treatment of stage I non-small cell lung cancer in high-risk patients	J Thorac Cadiovasc Surg 2007; 134:857–864	19 Patients	Local control	Local control was 58%	Overall survival at 1 year was 95%

(continued)

Table 15.1 (continued)

Author	Title	Journal	Number of patients	Indications	Local control rate	Survival
Lencioni RR, Crocetti L, Cioni R, et al.	Response to radiofrequency ablation of pulmonary tumours: a prospective, intention-to-treat, multicentre clinical trial (the RAPTURE study)	Lancet Oncol 2008; 9:621–628	106 Patients; 183 tumors (primary, 33; metastatic, 150)	Local control	88% Local control at 1 year	Overall survival primary lung cancer patients 70% at 1 year and 48% at 2 years. Overall survival colorectal metastatic patients 89% at 1 year and 60% at 2 years
Simon CJ, Dupuy DE, DiPetrillo TA, et al.	Pulmonary radiofrequency ablation: long-term safety and efficacy in 153 patients	Radiology 2007; 243:268–275	153 Patients; 189 tumors (primary, 116; metastases, 73)	Local control and palliation	The 1, 2, 3, 4 and 5-year local tumor progression-free rates, respectively, were 83%, 64%, 57%, 47%, and 47% for tumors ≤ 3 cm, and 45%, 25%, 25%, 25%, and 25% for tumors >3 cm	The overall 1-, 2-, 3-, 4-, and 5-year survival rates, respectively, for stage I non-small cell lung cancer were 78%, 57%, 36%, 27%, and 27%; survival rates for colorectal pulmonary metastasis were 87%, 78%, 57%, 57%, and 57%
Kang S, Luo R, Liao W, et al.	Single group study to evaluate the feasibility and complications of radiofrequency ablation and usefulness of posttreatment positron emission tomography in lung tumours	World J Surg Oncol 2004; 2:30:1–6	50 Patients (primary lung $n=23$; metastases $n=27$); 120 tumors; 17 patients had single lesions	Local control	Tumors ≤ 3.5 cm were completely killed after RFA. In tumors >3.5 cm, the part within 3.5 cm was killed. While CT showed that tumors became larger 1–2 weeks after RFA procedure. PET demonstrated tumor destruction in 70% cases, compared with 38% in CT	Not reported
Yan T, King J, Sjarif A, Glenn D, Steinke K, Morris D	Percutaneous radiofrequency ablation of pulmonary metastases from colorectal carcinoma: prognostic determinants for survival	Ann Surg Oncol 2006; 13:1529–1537	55 Patients with colorectal metastases	Local control	Not reported	Even though 30/55 patients had previously resected liver metastases, overall median survival was 33 months. The 1-, 2-, and 3-year actuarial survival was 85%, 64%, and 46%, respectively. In univariate analysis lesion size, location, and need for repeat RFA were predictive of survival. In a multivariate model only lesion size remained predictive

de Baere T, Palussiere J, Auperin A, et al.	Midterm local efficacy and survival after radiofrequency ablation of lung tumors with minimum follow-up of 1 year: prospective evaluation	Radiology 2006; 240:587–596	60 Patients; 100 tumors	Local control	93% Local control at 18 months	Overall survival and lung disease-free survival rates at 18 months were 71% and 34%, respectively
Dupuy DE, DePetrillo T, Gandhi S, et al.	Radiofrequency ablation followed by conventional radiotherapy for medically inoperable stage I non-small cell lung cancer	Chest 2006; 129:738–745	24 Patients	Local control	92% Local control	The cumulative survival rates for patients with stage IA at the end of 12, 24, and 56 months were 92%, 62%, and 46%, respectively. For stage IB, the cumulative survival rates at 12, 24, and 60 months were 73%, 42%, and 31%, respectively
Thanos L, Mylona S, Pomoni M, et al.	Percutaneous radiofrequency thermal ablation of primary and metastatic lung tumors	Eur J Cardiothorac Surg 2006; 30:797–800	22 Patients (14 primary lung cancer; 8 metastatic lung neoplasms)	Local control	Not reported	The 3-year overall survival 42% for metastatic patients and 14% for primary lung cancer patients
Microwave ablation						
Feng W, Liu W, Li C, et al.	Percutaneous microwave coagulation therapy for lung cancer	Chin J Oncol (ChungHua Chung Liu Tsa Chih) 2002; 24:388–390	20 Patients; 28 lesions (8 primary, 12 metastatic)	Local control	57% Local response rate	Not reported
Wolf F, DiPetrillo T, Machan J, DiPetrillo TA, Mayo-Smith WW, Dupuy DE	Microwave ablation of lung malignancies: effectiveness, CT findings and safety in 50 patients	Radiology 2008; 247:871–879	50 Patients (primary lung $n=30$; metastases $n=20$)	Local control	Primary local control 74% at median follow-up of 10 months, with 6% additional secondary local control for a total of 80% local control rate	The 1-, 2-, and 3-year actuarial survival rates were 65%, 55%, and 45%, respectively
Cryoablation						
Wang H, Littrup PJ, Duan Y, Zhang Y, Feng H, Nie Z	Thoracic masses treated with percutaneous cryotherapy: initial experience with more than 200 procedures	Radiology 2005; 235:289–298	187 Patients; 234 tumors (primary lung, 196; metastases, 38); (stage I $n=5$, stage II $n=17$, stage IIIA $n=20$, stage IIIB $n=60$, stage IV $n=63$)	Local control and palliation	Not reported	The mean Karnofsky performance score increased from 75.2 ± 1.3 before to 82.6 ± 1.4 1-week after cryoablation (Student's $t=3.87$, $P<0.01$); survival not reported

(continued)

Table 15.1 (continued)

Author	Title	Journal	Number of patients	Indications	Local control rate	Survival
Kawamura M, Izumi Y, Tsukada N, et al.	Percutaneous cryoablation of small pulmonary malignant tumors under computed tomographic guidance with local anesthesia for nonsurgical candidates	J Thorac Cardiovasc Surg 2006; 131:1007–1113	20 Patients; 35 tumors; all had metastatic tumors	Local control	80% Local control rate	The 1-year survival of 90%
Zemylak A, Moore WH, Bilfinger TV	Comparison of survival after sublobar resections and ablative therapies for stage I non-small cell lung cancer	J Am Coll Surg 2010; 211:68–72	64 Patients (25 sublobar resection, 12 RFA, 27 cryoablation)	Local control	Not reported	The 3-year cancer-specific and cancer-free survival for SLR 90.6/60.6%, for RFA 87.5/50%, and cryoablation 90.2/45.6%
Laser ablation						
Rosenberg C, Puls R, Hegenscheid K, et al.	Laser ablation of metastatic lesions of the lung: long-term outcome	Am J Roentgenol 2009; 92:785–792	64 Patients; 108 metastatic tumors	Local control	The primary local control rate was 78% (85 of 108 tumors). In the cases of 10 of 13 tumors on which ablation was repeated because of the finding of local tumor progression at follow-up despite an initial record of complete ablation, the repeated treatment was successful, resulting in a secondary local control rate of 72% (78 of 108 tumors)	The 1-, 2-, 3-, 4-, and 5-year survival rates after ablative therapy were 81%, 59%, 44%, 44%, and 27%, respectively

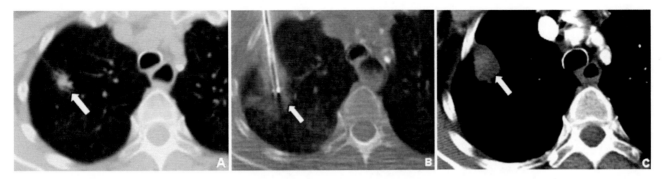

Fig. 15.1 A 78-year-old woman with biopsy-proven right upper lobe bronchoalveolar carcinoma was referred for radiofrequency ablation (RFA). (**a**) Axial noncontrast computed tomography (CT) shows the 1.5 cm mass in the patient's right lower lobe (*arrow*). (**b**) Axial fluoroscopic CT taken during the RFA procedure shows the RFA applicator placed appropriately within the mass (*arrow*) and the ensuing surrounding ground glass halo after treatment. (**c**) Axial CT image from 30-month follow-up, after the RFA procedure, shows a nonenhancing residual scar (*arrow*)

Additionally, the heat energy generated by the RFA treatment can cause thermal damage to proximal structures, such as central bronchi, trachea, heart, nerves, and esophagus. Consequently, central, mediastinal, or hilar lesions carry greater risk of damage and treatment-related complications; and it is commonly accepted that lesions within 1 cm of a major vessel or bronchus are less optimal candidates for RFA therapy, and in these instances combination therapy with radiation is likely to be more efficacious [22].

Technical Considerations

RFA techniques vary depending on the electrode system used, so that the application of energy from the electrode creates a maximal zone of tissue necrosis, encompassing both the tumor and a margin of normal surrounding tissue. Studies have shown that a margin of 8 mm for adenocarcinoma and a margin of 6 mm for squamous cell carcinoma will successfully encompass 95% of a primary non-small cell lung cancer neoplasm [23].

Two of the RF systems make deployable-array RF electrodes: Radiotherapeutics (Boston Scientific, Natick, Massachusetts) and RITA Medical Systems Inc. (AngioDynamics, Latham, New York). The Boston Scientific electrode has tines that curve backward at the handle and, therefore, is most effective when deployed into the deep portion of a tumor. The RITA electrode has tines that curve forward and laterally and, therefore, is best inserted on the near surface of the tumor. Because the Boston Scientific electrode only measures impedance, treatment time is determined by the rise in impedance during active tumor heating. The RITA system, on the other hand, measures temperature throughout the ablation via multiple peripheral thermocouples and infuses saline into the tissue via multiple perfusion electrodes. This serves to enhance the distribution of tissue heating during the procedure.

The third system (Cool-tip™, Covidien, Boulder, Colorado) exists as a single or triple "cluster" electrode (composed of three single electrodes spaced 5 mm apart); this tip is positioned at the deepest aspect of the tumor.

Microwave Ablation

Microwave ablation (MWA) has been most commonly used in the treatment of hepatic, pulmonary, and renal neoplasms. As a percutaneous treatment of lung neoplasms, the localized nature of this energy is ideally suited, since neoplastic tissue is destroyed and the remaining functional parenchyma is preserved [24]. However, to date, there are few reports of MWA for lung neoplasms. The largest study, by Wolf et al., examined 50 patients who underwent 66 percutaneous MWA treatments for intraparenchymal pulmonary lesions: 1-year local control was shown to be $67 \pm 10\%$ with a mean distant-recurrence rate of 16.2 ± 1.3 months [25].

Percutaneous MWA is the treatment of choice for lesions that are larger than 4 cm in diameter and those which are located close to a vessel that is larger than 3 mm in diameter, as it is less affected from the heat-sink effect observed with

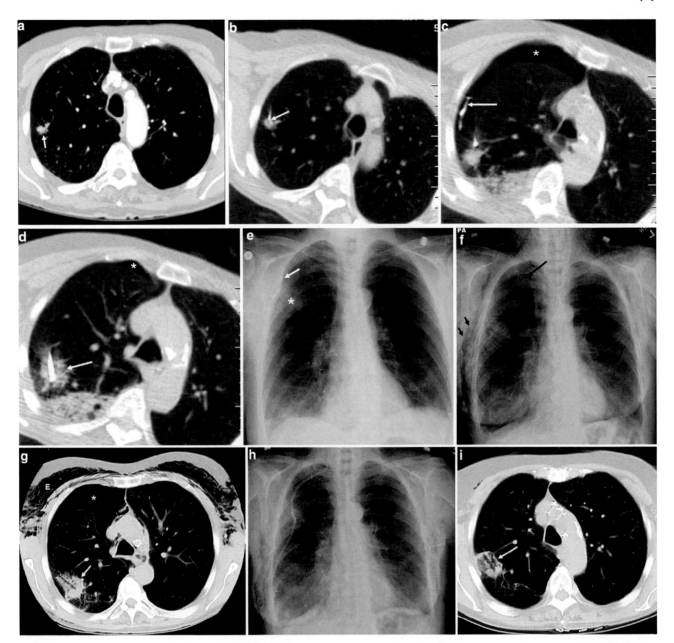

Fig. 15.2 A 72-year-old woman with severe chronic obstructive pulmonary disease (COPD) with right upper mass detected on CT pulmonary angiogram due to shortness of breath. (**a**) Axial image from CT shows irregular right upper lobe mass (*arrow*) suspicious for bronchogenic carcinoma. (**b**) CT fluoroscopic image from needle biopsy (*arrow*) yielded non-small cell lung cancer with onsite cytopathology. (**c**) Axial CT-fluoroscopic image shows a pneumothorax (*asterisk*) that required a chest tube (*arrow*) as the patient was undergoing placement of radiofrequency (RF) electrode into the mass. (**d**) Axial CT-fluoroscopic image after pneumothorax reduction (*asterisk*) shows RF electrode within the mass and the immediate posttreatment halo related to interstitial edema (*arrow*). (**e**) Chest X-ray 2 h after the procedure shows satisfactory chest tube placement and the typical hazy opacity from the RFA (*asterisk*). The pneumothorax had resolved. (**f**) The air leak resolved, and the chest tube was removed 2 days later. However, 2 h after chest tube removal the patient complained of chest swelling. Chest X-ray shows pneumothorax (*arrow*) and extensive subcutaneous emphysema (*arrows*). (**g**) Repeat CT scan 1 day shows the recurrent pneumothorax (*asterisk*) and extensive subcutaneous emphysema (*E*). Note the RF treatment halo (*arrow*). (**h**) After apical chest tube was placed that same day, a repeat chest X-ray shows improvement in subcutaneous emphysema and pneumothorax. (**i**) Follow-up baseline Chest CT 3 weeks later shows typical cavitary changes with bubble lucencies of the treated mass (*arrow*) and near complete resolution of the subcutaneous emphysema

RFA [26] (Fig. 15.3). MWA is usually performed with the patient under conscious sedation; however, general anesthesia may also be used in cases where pain control may be more difficult, as in cases of painful chest wall tumors.

The tumor is localized by computed tomography (CT), and the approach is determined based on its size and location. A microwave antenna is inserted directly into the target tumor, so that the feedpoint (focus of microwave energy emission) portion is surrounded by target tumor tissue. The antenna is then connected to the microwave generator by a coaxial cable.

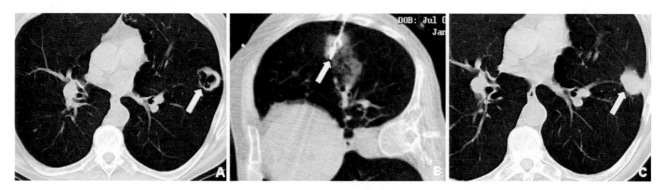

Fig. 15.3 An 82-year-old man with biopsy-proven squamous cell carcinoma in the left upper lobe was referred for microwave ablation (MWA). (**a**) Axial noncontrast CT shows a 2.5 cm cavitary mass in the left lobe (*arrow*). (**b**) Axial fluoroscopic CT showing one of three MW applicators positioned within the mass (*arrow*). (**c**) Axial CT image taken 8 months post-MWA procedure, showing residual thermal scar (*arrow*)

During treatment, an electromagnetic wave of high intensity is emitted from the noninsulated portion of the microwave antenna directly into the proximal tumor cells, causing oscillation of water molecules and tissue heating. Conductive heating of the shaft can lead to proximal tissue injury so the shaft is cooled by perfusing room temperature saline through a thin plastic sheath that surrounds the nonactive portion of the applicator shaft.

Benefits

In multiple organs, microwave ablation has been shown to have higher intratumor temperatures, larger ablation zones, faster ablation times, reduced heat-sink effect, and an improved convection profile, when compared with RFA [27]. Brace et al. recently conducted the first direct comparison of RFA and microwave ablation of pulmonary neoplasms, in a porcine model; they demonstrated that microwave ablation results in a larger, more spherical and faster-growing zone of ablation than is observed with RFA [28]. Consequently, MWA is the modality of choice for large (>4 cm) pulmonary malignancies.

Although previous reports have documented the ability of multiple RFA probes to be used simultaneously, to date, no work has documented the use of these devices in pulmonary neoplasms. MWA, in contrast, has been shown in several studies to effectively and safely treat lung tumors, when multiple microwave applicators are simultaneously employed [25].

Risks and Complications

Recent studies have shown that complications include cavitation (43%), pneumothorax (39%), hemoptysis (0.06%), and skin burns (0.01%) [28]. Skin burns are less of a risk with microwave ablation than with RFA, because no electrical current is generated, and therefore, the system does not need to be grounded. However, thermal injury can nonetheless occur, when applicators are placed too close to the skin. Cavitary changes have been shown to have a statistically significant inverse relationship to cancer-specific mortality ($P=0.02$) [25]. This may be explained by the fact that cavitation results from more-complete tumor kill and tissue thermocoagulation.

Technical Considerations

The microwave system available in the USA (Evident™, Covidien, Boulder, Colorado; Avecure™, Medwaves, San Diego, California; Microtherm X™, BSD Medical, Salt Lake City, Utah; Certus 140™, Neuwave, Madison, Wisconsin; Amica™, Hospital Service, Rome, Italy; Acculis MTA™, Microsulis Medical Limited, Hampshire, UK) makes use of a 915- or 2,450-MHz generator and straight antennas. Cooling of the antenna's shaft with room temperature fluid of carbon dioxide gas for most of the systems reduces conductive heating of the nonactive portion of the applicator, and spares damage to adjacent skin and tissues.

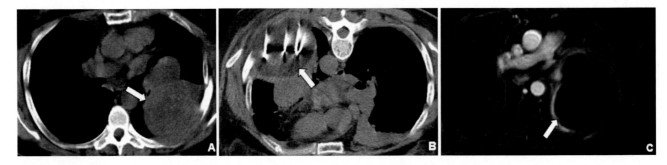

Fig. 15.4 A 66-year-old woman with recurrent chest wall primitive neuroendocrine tumor was referred for cryoablation for pain palliation. (**a**) Axial noncontrast CT shows a 10-cm mass in the left lower lobe (*arrow*), abutting the patient's ribs. (**b**) Axial noncontrast CT shows three of seven percutaneous cryoprobes positioned within the mass (*arrow*), and the surrounding low-density ice ball after the second freeze cycle. (**c**) Gadolinium-enhanced subtraction T1-weighted axial MR image taken 2 days postcryoablation, at the same level as (**b**), shows the large area of nonenhancement consistent with tumor necrosis (*arrow*)

Cryoablation

Unlike RFA and MWA, which exert their tumoricidal effects from the generation of heat, cryoablation results in the generation of intra- and extracellular ice crystals, which in turn cause protein denaturation, intracellular dehydration and pH changes, ischemic necrosis via vascular injury, cellular edema, and activation of antitumor immune responses.

Historically, cryotherapy has been considered to be mainly an intraoperative procedure for the treatment of prostate or liver lesions, although extensive research has documented the value of endobronchial cryotherapy for the treatment of early bronchial carcinomas [25]. Until the recent development of smaller-diameter cryoprobes (1.5–2.4 mm), cryoablation carried a greater risk of inflammatory responses, blood loss, and complications than RFA or MWA, and was more difficult to perform percutaneously [29]. With the advent of smaller-diameter cryoprobes, this is no longer the case, and interest has grown in this percutaneous technique. More recently, the development of cryoprobes with smaller diameters has enabled researchers to evaluate the role of percutaneous cryotherapy for lung neoplasms (Fig. 15.4). In a large cohort study, Wang et al. demonstrated efficacy and palliative benefits, in terms of Karnofsky Performance Status scale and general health status ratings [30]. More recently, Kawamura et al. examined cryoablation outcomes in 35 patients with metastatic lung lesions and showed overall local control of 80%, and 1-year Kaplan–Meier survival of 89% [31].

Risks and Complications

Two studies (Wang et al. and Kawamura et al.) have examined the efficacy and complications associated with this treatment. Wang et al. demonstrate the efficacy and palliative benefits of cryoablation for lung neoplasms in terms of Karnofsky Performance Status scale and general health status ratings [30]. In addition, their study shows a low rate of cryoablation-related complications (pneumothorax, 12%; self-limited hypertension, 33%; pleural effusion 14%) for cryoablation as a treatment of pulmonary or thoracic primary and metastatic neoplasms [31]. Kawamura et al. reported similarly encouraging efficacy data: among 35 patients with metastatic lung lesions treated with cryoablation, overall local control was 80%, and 1-year Kaplan–Meier survival was 89% [31]. These results show that cryoablation has an acceptable safety profile and can result in sufficient local control of both primary and metastatic tumors.

Conclusions

Image-guided ablation techniques provide a safe and effective alternative to traditional cancer therapies. They demonstrate low morbidity and mortality, lower procedural cost, synergy with other cancer treatments, and the ability to be performed on an outpatient basis. Continued development of these technologies, as well as further examinations of local control and survival, will enable clinicians to continue improving the quality of care for patients with lung cancer.

References

1. D'Amico T. Local control without resection. J Thorac Cardiovasc Surg. 2003;125:787–8.
2. Ginsberg RJ, Vokes EE, Raben A. Cancer of lung: non-small cell lung cancer. In: Mitchell JB, Johnson DH, Turrisi AT, editors. Lung cancer: principles and practice of oncology. 5th ed. Philadelphia, PA: Lippincott-Raven; 1996. p. 849–57.
3. Ihde DC, Minna JD. Non-small cell lung cancer. II. Treatment. Curr Probl Cancer. 1991;15:105–54.
4. Simon C, Dupuy DE. Current role of image-guided ablative therapies in lung cancer. Expert Rev Anticancer Ther. 2005;5(4):657–66.
5. Bojarski J, Dupuy D, Mayo-Smith W. CT imaging findings of pulmonary neoplasms after treatment with radiofrequency ablation: results in 32 tumors. AJR Am J Roentgenol. 2005;185:466–71.
6. Grieco CA, Simon CJ, Mayo-Smith WW, DiPetrillo TA, Ready NE, Dupuy DE. Image-guided percutaneous thermal ablation for the palliative treatment of chest wall masses. Am J Clin Oncol. 2007;30:361–7.
7. Steinke K, Sewell PE, Dupuy D, et al. Pulmonary radiofrequency ablation – an international study survey. Anticancer Res. 2004;24:339–43.
8. Dupuy DE, DiPetrillo T, Gandhi S, et al. Radiofrequency ablation followed by conventional radiotherapy for medically inoperable stage 1 non-small cell lung cancer. Chest. 2006;3:738–40.
9. Lencioni R, Crocetti L, Cioni R. Response to radiofrequency ablation of pulmonary tumours: a prospective, intention-to-treat, multicentre clinical trial (the RAPTURE study). Lancet Oncol. 2008;9(7):621–8.
10. Akeboshi M, Yamakado K, Nakasuka A, et al. Percutaneous radiofrequency ablation of lung neoplasms: initial therapeutic response. J Vasc Interv Radiol. 2004;15:463–70.
11. Yasui K, Kanazawa A, Sano Y, et al. Thoracic tumors treated with CT-guided radiofrequency ablation: initial experience. Radiology. 2004;231:850–7.
12. Simon CJ, Dupuy DE, DiPetrillo TA, et al. Pulmonary radiofrequency ablation: long-term safety and efficacy in 153 patients. Radiology. 2007;243:268–75.
13. Lee JM, Jin GY, Goldberg SN, et al. Percutaneous radiofrequency ablation for inoperable non-small cell lung cancer and metastases: preliminary report. Radiology. 2004;230(1):125–34.
14. Callstrom MR, Charboneau JW, Goetz MP, et al. Painful metastases involving bone: feasibility of percutaneous CT and US-guided radiofrequency ablation. Radiology. 2002;224(1):87–97.
15. Ahmed M, Liu Z, Afzal KS, et al. Radiofrequency ablation: effect of surrounding tissue composition on coagulation necrosis in a canine tumor model. Radiology. 2004;230:761–7.
16. Gananadha S, Morris DL. Saline infusion markedly reduces impedance and improves efficacy of pulmonary radiofrequency ablation. Cardiovasc Intervent Radiol. 2004;27:361–5.
17. Jain SK, Dupuy DE, Cardarelli GA, et al. Percutaneous radiofrequency ablation of pulmonary malignancies: combined treatment with brachytherapy. AJR Am J Roentgenol. 2003;181(3):711–5.
18. Abbas G, Schuchert MJ, Pennathur A, et al. Ablative treatments for lung tumors: radiofrequency ablation, stereotactic radiosurgery, and microwave ablation. Thorac Surg Clin. 2007;17(2):261–71.
19. Herrera LJ, Fernando HC, Perry Y, et al. Radiofrequency ablation of pulmonary malignant tumors in nonsurgical candidates. J Thorac Cardiovasc Surg. 2003;125(4):929–37.
20. Pennathur A, Luketich JD, Abbas G, et al. Radiofrequency ablation for the Treatment of Stage I non-small cell lung cancer in high-risk patients. J Thorac Cardiovasc Surg. 2007;134(4):857–64.
21. Nomura M, Yamakado K, Nomoto Y. Complications after lung radiofrequency ablation: risk factors for lung inflammation. Br J Radiol. 2008;81:244–9.
22. Ambrogi MC, Lucchi M, Dini P, et al. Percutaneous radiofrequency ablation of lung tumors: results in the midterm. Eur J Cardiothorac Surg. 2006;30:177–83.
23. Giraud P, Antoine M, Larrouy A, et al. Evaluation of microscopic tumor extension in non-small cell lung cancer for three-dimensional conformal radiotherapy planning. Int J Radiat Oncol Biol Phys. 2000;48:1015–24.
24. McGovern FJ, Wood BJ, Goldberg SN, Mueller PR. Radiofrequency ablation of renal cell carcinoma via image-guided needle electrodes. J Urol. 1999;161:599–600.
25. Wolf FJ, Grand DJ, Machan JT, et al. Microwave ablation of lung malignancies: effectiveness, CT findings, and safety in 50 patients. Radiology. 2008;247(3):871–9.
26. Carrafiello G, Lagana D, Mangini M, et al. Microwave tumor ablation: principles, clinical applications and review of preliminary experiences. Int J Surg. 2008;6 Suppl 1:S65–9.
27. Simon CJ, Dupuy DE, Mayo-Smith WW. Microwave ablation: principles and applications. Radiographics. 2005;25:S69–83.
28. Brace CL, Hinshaw JL, Laeseke PF, et al. Pulmonary thermal ablation: comparison of radiofrequency and microwave devices by using gross pathologic and CT findings in a swine model. Radiology. 2009;251(3):701–11.
29. Deygas N, Froudarakis M, Ozenne G, et al. Cryotherapy in early superficial bronchogenic carcinoma. Chest. 2001;120:26–31.
30. Wang H, Littrup P, Duan Y, et al. Thoracic masses treated with percutaneous cryotherapy: initial experience with more than 200 procedures. Radiology. 2005;235:289–98.
31. Kawamura M, Izumi Y, Tsukada N, et al. Percutaneous cryoablation of small pulmonary malignant tumors under computed tomographic guidance with local anesthesia for nonsurgical candidates. J Thorac Cardiovasc Surg. 2006;131:1007–13.

Part V
Bone

Chapter 16
Radiation Therapy of Bone Metastasis

Georges Noel, Pierre Truntzer, and Sébastien Guihard

Introduction

Bone metastases often present as the first evidence of disseminated disease in cancer patients, and the most common primary sites are breast, prostate, and lung. Treatment of bone metastases with radiation has proven successful. Radiation therapy is an efficient treatment of tumor cells, even with a relatively low dose. In addition, even in low doses, radiation is well-known as an anti-inflammatory treatment for benign lesions. Some authors have described advantages in the use of radiation in terms of bone reconstruction, recognizing, however, that this radiation effect is not major and probably occurs late after the end of treatment. Lastly, in addition to relieving pain, radiotherapy may prevent pathological fractures, maintain activity and mobility, and, rarely, prolong survival. Although almost all the patients eventually die of their disease, some survive for several years. Finding the optimal palliative treatment with both a short- and long-term perspective is, therefore, crucial. It is difficult to determine the best irradiation schedule to lead to these goals. There is no established relationship between tumor histology and the radiation dose necessary for pain relief [1].

The biological effectiveness of radiotherapy depends on the total dose and the dose per fraction. Different radiation schedules can be compared using the equivalent dose in 2-Gy fractions (EQD2), which takes into account the total dose and the dose per fraction. The EQD2 is calculated with the equation, as derived from the linear-quadratic model:

$$EQD2 = D[(d + \alpha / \beta) / 2Gy + \alpha / \beta],$$

where D is the total dose, d is the dose per fraction, a is the linear (first-order dose-dependent) component of cell killing, and the α/β is the dose at which both components of cell killing are equal. Assuming an α/β ratio of 10 Gy for tumor kill, the EQD2 of the radiation schedules are (12 Gy for 1×8 Gy), (32.5 Gy for 10×3 Gy), (39.1 Gy for 15×2.5 Gy), and (40 Gy for 20×2 Gy); however, this model is discussed for the high single-dose.

Arguably the most commonly used modality (Ben-Josef) [2], external beam radiotherapy has been investigated in multiple randomized controlled trials [3–21]. These dose-finding trials have almost universally demonstrated the equivalence of multiple- and single-fraction (SF) radiotherapy schedules for the palliation of pain owing to uncomplicated bone metastases, despite different inclusion criteria, primary endpoints, and randomization arms. The limited survival of most patients with bone metastasis argues for the use of the shortest, most effective schedule to decrease the time invested in medical appointments near the end of a patient's life [22]. Schedules prescribed as a multifraction course when single fraction is appropriate places all patients at a disadvantage and overextends many centers' already-strained resources [23]. Furthermore, single-fraction treatment complies with MacKillop's rules for palliative radiotherapy: courses should be no longer than necessary to achieve their therapeutic goal and should consume no more resources than required [24]. One of the criticisms of these studies was the low number of patients who returned mailed questionnaires at variable times after the end of the studies [21]. The previously suggested drawbacks of single fraction have been already refuted [25–28]. Authors have indicated the superiority of multiple-fraction treatment, especially for patients with a more favorable prognosis and a longer survival time. However, in long surviving patients (≥12 months), the response rate in terms of dose palliation was not significantly different [after 8 Gy in one fraction (87%) and 24 Gy in six fractions (85%)]. The

G. Noel (✉) • P. Truntzer • S. Guihard
Department of Radiotherapy, Centre de lutte contre le Cancer Paul Strauss, Strasbourg, France
e-mail: gnoel@strasbourg.fnclcc.fr

P.R. Mueller and A. Adam (eds.), *Interventional Oncology: A Practical Guide for the Interventional Radiologist,*
DOI 10.1007/978-1-4419-1469-9_16, © Springer Science+Business Media, LLC 2012

duration of response and progression rates were similar [28], indicating that patients with relatively favorable prognosis do not necessarily outlive the effects of single-dose irradiation. The same conclusion of noninferiority of single dose was demonstrated for neuropathic pain [27]. In terms of reirradiation, patients treated with a single dose were retreated more frequently, at an earlier time during follow-up and at a lower pain score [20]. This assumes practitioner bias as opposed to the real necessity of reirradiation. In a long-term follow-up study, Sande et al. showed that patients in the single-fraction arm received significantly more reirradiations as compared to the multiple-fraction arm (27% vs. 9%, $p=0.002$). This study indicated no difference between radiotherapy with 8 Gy × 1 and 3 Gy × 10 for the majority of patients with painful bone metastases, also in the long-term perspective. Most importantly, patient follow-up in this study occurred until death, and the trial showed no disadvantages for 8 Gy × 1 compared to 3 Gy × 10. Despite the fact that single-fraction treatment will imply an approximately 2.5-fold greater need for reirradiation, single-fraction treatment is considered more convenient for the patient [29].

A temporary worsening of pain shortly after palliative radiotherapy is clinically common and can be problematic, particularly for those receiving single fraction. Loblaw et al. reported that one-third of the patients complained of the pain flare that lasted a median of 3 days [30].

Some patients with bone metastases develop spinal cord compression. It has been estimated that this occurs in about 5–10% of cancer patients during the course of their disease. Patchell et al. showed that surgery for decompression before radiation increases the life of patients with relatively good mobility compared to radiation alone [31]. Radiotherapy was delivered at a total dose of 30 Gy in ten fractions. However, Rades et al. showed that, in a retrospective study of 922 patients, escalation of radiation dose to >30 Gy in ten fractions did not improve the outcome in terms of motor function, local control, or survival, but did increase the treatment time for these frequently debilitated patients. Therefore, doses >30 Gy in ten fractions are not recommended [32]. Furthermore, in a series of 308 patients older than 74 years, 20 Gy in five fractions of 4 Gy is probably enough to obtain a maximal efficiency/side-effect ratio [33]. To prevent compression, it is not possible to recommend single-fraction irradiation.

Reirradiation may be considered in three scenarios: (1) no pain relief or pain progression after initial radiotherapy, (2) partial response with initial radiotherapy and the hope of achieving further pain reduction with more radiotherapy, and (3) partial or complete response with initial radiotherapy but subsequent recurrence of pain. Classically, it has been reported that pain relief can be noted up to 1 month after the end of irradiation. At this time, if the pain relief is insufficient or if pain progresses, it is possible to prepare for new irradiation. A specific schedule is difficult to recommend, but often a single-fraction treatment is performed after an inefficient multiple-fraction treatment and vice versa.

Interpretation of results of these different randomized studies has been made more difficult by methodological deficiencies, such as short duration of follow-up; small number of patients, which limits the study's statistical power; differences in pain evaluation in terms of scale; and time of evaluation. End points differ as well: pain relief, analgesic decrease, spinal cord compression, fracture, or reirradiation. Thus meta-analyses are definitively needed to show the results of single dose.

Meta-analyses have reported an overall response rate of approximately 60% (intent-to-treat) with a complete response rate of 33% at 4 weeks [34–36]. In the meta-analysis by Chow et al., a total of 16 randomized trials from 1986 onward were identified. This represents seven new trials compared to the two previously published meta-analyses. For intention-to-treat patients, the overall response (OR) rates for pain were similar for single-fraction schedule at 1,468 (58%) of 2,513 patients and multiple-fraction radiotherapy at 1,466 (59%) of 2,487 patients. The complete response (CR) rates for pain were 23% (545 of 2,375 patients) for single-fraction schedule and 24% (558 of 2,351 patients) for multiple-fraction radiotherapy. No significant differences were found in response rates. Trends showing an increased risk for single-fraction radiotherapy arm patients in terms of pathological fractures and spinal cord compressions were observed, but neither were statistically significant ($p=0.75$ and $p=0.13$, respectively). The likelihood of retreatment was 2.5-fold higher (95% CI, 1.76–3.56) in single-fraction treatment compared to multiple-fraction treatment arm patients ($p=0.00001$). Repeated analysis of these end points, excluding dropout patients, did not alter the conclusions. Generally, no significant differences with respect to acute toxicities were observed between the groups [36].

Because of the development of stereotactic radiotherapy with a low number of high-dose fractions, the interest in short treatments has increased. In stereotactic radiotherapy, as it is classically defined, the growth of malignant tumors is arrested with a single, high dose of focused ionizing radiation. Until just a few years ago, stereotactic radiotherapy could only be used to treat pathological lesions in the brain and skull. Persuasive scientific evidence (level 2 evidence) has now accumulated to demonstrate the benefit of stereotactic radiotherapy for brain metastases [37, 38]. The resulting clinical attractiveness of the method has led to the application of the stereotactic radiotherapy concept extracranially as well, particularly in the spine. Generalized metastatic involvement of the axial skeleton is certainly not an indication for stereotactic radiotherapy, but radiosurgical treatment may well be reasonable for one or two metastatic tumors in the spine. In such situations, a single dose or a low-numbered fraction of radiation with a steep dose fall-off outside the tumor is more effective and less fraught with complications than fractionated radiotherapy [39]. Furthermore, stereotactic radiotherapy requires only a few hours, much less time than fractionated radiotherapy, and can, in principle, always be performed on an outpatient basis. This may be an advantage for patients with advanced malignant disease who often require multimodal treatment. For these types of malignant tumors in the spine, the results of such radiotherapy are relatively uniform, varying only to a small degree from one type of primary tumor to another. Tumor growth can be effectively arrested by stereotactic radiotherapy in up to 96% of cases (81–96%) [39–47]. Stereotactic radiotherapy can also be used to treat tumors that have recurred after fractionated radiotherapy [39] and surgery [39, 45, 48]. Pain is suppressed in 80–90% in few days, less than 1 week.

In a systematic review [49], there is a lack of firm evidence relating the fractionation schedule to the prevention of pathologic fracture, because no study has evaluated the risk of pathologic fracture prior to treatment. Although the pathologic fracture rate was significantly higher after single-fraction radiotherapy than after multifraction in the Dutch study [18], the absolute difference was only 2%. The Radiation Therapy Oncology Group (RTOG) study, on the other hand, showed a higher fracture rate following high-dose fractionation (40 Gy) than low-dose treatment (20 Gy) in patients with a solitary metastasis [19].

In the literature, the reporting of adverse effects has been generally poor, and there are no obvious differences between the fractionation schedules studied, at least in the incidence of nausea, vomiting, diarrhea, and pathological fractures; however, the analysis can be biased due to short follow-up time and no systematic appointments with the radiation oncologist after irradiation. The multiplication of fields for the irradiation of the spinal bone is probably important to reduce side effects, mainly vomiting when the epigastric area (D12-L2) is irradiated, and a technique with three fields (anterior and two postero-oblique fields) limits the risk of diarrhea compared to a anteroposterior field technique. For lesions near the kidneys, the dose delivered to these organs is superior with the three-fields' technique but rarely leads to renal insufficiency. Pain flare can be avoided by prescribing steroids during treatment days. Chow et al. showed that dexamethasone might be effective in the prophylaxis of radiation-induced pain flare after palliative radiotherapy for bone metastases [50]. More importantly, analgesic treatment needs to be regularly evaluated after irradiation. If pain decreases after irradiation and the dosage is not adapted, morphine-related complications may be observed.

There is no limit to the use of single-fraction treatment; however, no study has specifically addressed large-volume treatment (i.e., wide-field, hemibody irradiation). Although average treatment volumes were not reported in any of the single-fraction trials, a significant proportion of patients did receive treatments to the lumbar spine and pelvis, but some trials excluded patients with large volume, 400 cm^2 [10], 200 cm^2 or 150 cm^2 if digestive tract was included in the field [4]. Some other exclusion criterion has been regularly imposed in trials (bone fracture, spinal cord compression, or bone metastases localized in cervical spine). This criterion could be factors of choice in advantages of multiple-fractionated irradiation.

Owing to the resource advantages [35, 51], patient convenience [35], and cost-effectiveness [34, 35, 51], SF regimens should be in widespread use. Additional benefits include the potential for increased accessibility, fewer medical appointments, and shorter hospital admissions [35, 51]. Clinical practice guidelines [49] and consensus documents [52] published since 1999 have recommended single-fraction treatment as the new standard of care.

However, according to previous patterns of practice surveys, single-fraction schedules have remained underused globally [2, 53–64]. Overall, 11–42% of radiation oncologists would use single-fraction radiotherapy. The reasons proposed for this reticence have included regional variation in participation in related randomized controlled trials, a lack of experience with large single-fraction sizes, and the influence of reimbursement [59, 60]. Other factors not included in the published data have been reported to strongly influence prescription patterns include patient, tumor, and institutional factors, as well as physician attitudes [23]. Recently, Fairchild et al. analyzed practices of members of scientific societies [American Society for Radiology Oncology (ASTRO), Canadian Association of Radiation Oncology (CARO), Royal Australian and New Zealand College of Radiologists], where members had completed an Internet-based survey. Authors showed that from a total of 962 respondents, three-quarters ASTRO members, described 101 different dose schedules in common use (range, 3 Gy/1 fraction to 60 Gy/20 fractions). The overall median dose was 30 Gy/10 fractions. SF schedules were used the least often by ASTRO members practicing in the USA and most often by CARO members. Case, membership affiliation, country of training, location of practice, and practice type were independently predictive of the use of SF. The principal factors considered when prescribing were prognosis, risk of spinal cord compression, and performance status. The authors concluded that, despite abundant evidence, most radiation oncologists continue to prescribe multifraction schedules for patients who fit the eligibility criteria of previous randomized controlled trials [64].

External beam radiotherapy is not the only way of palliating the pain of bone metastases using ionizing radiation. Patients with osteoblastic metastases from prostate cancer may get excellent pain control from targeted radiotherapy with strontium. The response rates with external irradiation and strontium (^{89}Sr) are similar. In a randomized trial, patients with localized disease achieved pain relief in 65.9% following ^{89}Sr treatment, compared with 61% following conventional radiotherapy [65]. Strontium therapy is also of value in patients with widespread disease, which cannot be encompassed with localized radiotherapy fields, but hemibody radiotherapy offers a useful alternative [7].

In an editorial, Kachnic and Berk [66] questioned how much more evidence is needed for palliative single-fraction radiation therapy to become a standard practice. Radiation treatment is effective in palliating painful bone metastases, but multiple fraction remains the most common referral from medical-oncology and palliative-care colleagues. Updated systematic reviews provide further evidence of equivalency between single- and multiple-fraction treatments in terms of pain relief. The challenge is to identify which group of patients would benefit from multiple-faction treatment. Radiation departments should critically examine their current practice based on the evidence and standard guidelines proposed by Wu et al. to maximize the efficient use of limited radiation resources [49].

According to Wu et al.'s recommendations [49], for patients to whom the treatment objective is pain relief, a single 8-Gy treatment prescribed to the appropriate target volume is recommended as the standard dose-fractionation schedule for the treatment of symptomatic and uncomplicated bone metastases. This recommendation applies to adult patients with single or multiple radiographically confirmed bone metastases of any histology corresponding to painful areas in previously nonirradiated areas without pathologic fractures or spinal cord/cauda equina compression. It does not apply to the management of malignant primary bone tumor.

Patients and referring physicians should be advised that repeat irradiation to the treated area may be possible. There is insufficient evidence at this time to make a dose-fractionation recommendation for other treatment indications, such as long-term disease control for patients with solitary bone metastasis, prevention/treatment of cord compression, prevention/treatment of pathologic fractures, and treatment of soft-tissue masses associated with bony disease.

References

1. Poulsen HS, Nielsen OS, Klee M, Rorth M. Palliative irradiation of bone metastases. Cancer Treat Rev. 1989;16:41–8.
2. Ben-Josef E, Shamsa F, Williams AO, Porter AT. Radiotherapeutic management of osseous metastases: a survey of current patterns of care. Int J Radiat Oncol Biol Phys. 1998;40:915–21.
3. Cole DJ. A randomized trial of a single treatment versus conventional fractionation in the palliative radiotherapy of painful bone metastases. Clin Oncol (R Coll Radiol). 1989;1:59–62.
4. Gaze MN, Kelly CG, Kerr GR, et al. Pain relief and quality of life following radiotherapy for bone metastases: a randomised trial of two fractionation schedules. Radiother Oncol. 1997;45:109–16.
5. Hartsell WF, Scott CB, Bruner DW, et al. Randomized trial of short- versus long-course radiotherapy for palliation of painful bone metastases. J Natl Cancer Inst. 2005;97:798–804.
6. Hirokawa Y, Wadasaki K, Kashiwado K, et al. A multi-institutional prospective randomized study of radiation therapy of bone metastases. Nippon Igaku Hoshasen Gakkai Zasshi. 1988;48:1425–31.
7. Hoskin PJ, Ford HT, Harmer CL. Hemibody irradiation (HBI) for metastatic bone pain in two histologically distinct groups of patients. Clin Oncol (R Coll Radiol). 1989;1:67–9.
8. Hoskin PJ, Price P, Easton D, et al. A prospective randomised trial of 4 Gy or 8 Gy single doses in the treatment of metastatic bone pain. Radiother Oncol. 1992;23:74–8.
9. Jeremic B, Shibamoto Y, Acimovic L, et al. A randomized trial of three single-dose radiation therapy regimens in the treatment of metastatic bone pain. Int J Radiat Oncol Biol Phys. 1998;42:161–7.
10. Kaasa S, Brenne E, Lund JA, et al. Prospective randomised multicenter trial on single fraction radiotherapy (8 Gy×1) versus multiple fractions (3 Gy×10) in the treatment of painful bone metastases. Radiother Oncol. 2006;79:278–84.
11. Kagei K, Suzuki K, Shirato H, Nambu T, Yoshikawa H, Irie G. A randomized trial of single and multifraction radiation therapy for bone metastasis: a preliminary report. Gan No Rinsho. 1990;36:2553–8.
12. Koswig S. Budach V [Remineralization and pain relief in bone metastases after different radiotherapy fractions (10 times 3 Gy vs. 1 time 8 Gy). A prospective study]. Strahlenther Onkol. 1999;175:500–8.
13. Madsen EL. Painful bone metastasis: efficacy of radiotherapy assessed by the patients: a randomized trial comparing 4 Gy×6 versus 10 Gy×2. Int J Radiat Oncol Biol Phys. 1983;9:1775–9.
14. Nielsen OS, Bentzen SM, Sandberg E, Gadeberg CC, Timothy AR. Randomized trial of single dose versus fractionated palliative radiotherapy of bone metastases. Radiother Oncol. 1998;47:233–40.
15. Niewald M, Tkocz HJ, Abel U, et al. Rapid course radiation therapy vs. more standard treatment: a randomized trial for bone metastases. Int J Radiat Oncol Biol Phys. 1996;36:1085–9.
16. Okawa T, Kita M, Goto M, Nishijima H, Miyaji N. Randomized prospective clinical study of small, large and twice-a-day fraction radiotherapy for painful bone metastases. Radiother Oncol. 1988;13:99–104.
17. Price P, Hoskin PJ, Easton D, Austin D, Palmer SG, Yarnold JR. Prospective randomised trial of single and multifraction radiotherapy schedules in the treatment of painful bony metastases. Radiother Oncol. 1986;6:247–55.
18. Steenland E, Leer JW, van Houwelingen H, et al. The effect of a single fraction compared to multiple fractions on painful bone metastases: a global analysis of the Dutch Bone Metastasis Study. Radiother Oncol. 1999;52:101–9.
19. Tong D, Gillick L, Hendrickson FR. The palliation of symptomatic osseous metastases: final results of the Study by the Radiation Therapy Oncology Group. Cancer. 1982;50:893–9.
20. van der Linden YM, Lok JJ, Steenland E, et al. Single fraction radiotherapy is efficacious: a further analysis of the Dutch Bone Metastasis Study controlling for the influence of retreatment. Int J Radiat Oncol Biol Phys. 2004;59:528–37.
21. Anonymous. 8 Gy single fraction radiotherapy for the treatment of metastatic skeletal pain: randomised comparison with a multifraction schedule over 12 months of patient follow-up. Bone Pain Trial Working Party. Radiother Oncol. 1999;52:111–21.
22. Kirkbride B, Barton P. Palliative radiation therapy. J Palliat Med. 1999;2:87–97.

23. Bradley NM, Husted J, Sey MS, et al. Review of patterns of practice and patients' preferences in the treatment of bone metastases with palliative radiotherapy. Support Care Cancer. 2007;15:373–85.

24. Mackillop WJ. The principles of palliative radiotherapy: a radiation oncologist's perspective. Can J Oncol. 1996;6 Suppl 1:5–11.

25. Rose CM, Kagan AR. The final report of the expert panel for the radiation oncology bone metastasis work group of the American College of Radiology. Int J Radiat Oncol Biol Phys. 1998;40:1117–24.

26. van den Hout WB, van der Linden YM, Steenland E, et al. Single- versus multiple-fraction radiotherapy in patients with painful bone metastases: cost-utility analysis based on a randomized trial. J Natl Cancer Inst. 2003;95:222–9.

27. Roos DE, Turner SL, O'Brien PC, et al. Randomized trial of 8 Gy in 1 versus 20 Gy in 5 fractions of radiotherapy for neuropathic pain due to bone metastases (Trans-Tasman Radiation Oncology Group, TROG 96.05). Radiother Oncol. 2005;75:54–63.

28. van der Linden YM, Steenland E, van Houwelingen HC, et al. Patients with a favourable prognosis are equally palliated with single and multiple fraction radiotherapy: results on survival in the Dutch Bone Metastasis Study. Radiother Oncol. 2006;78:245–53.

29. Sande TA, Ruenes R, Lund JA, et al. Long-term follow-up of cancer patients receiving radiotherapy for bone metastases: results from a randomised multicentre trial. Radiother Oncol. 2009;91:261–6.

30. Loblaw DA, Wu JS, Kirkbride P, et al. Pain flare in patients with bone metastases after palliative radiotherapy – a nested randomized control trial. Support Care Cancer. 2007;15:451–5.

31. Patchell RA, Tibbs PA, Regine WF, et al. Direct decompressive surgical resection in the treatment of spinal cord compression caused by metastatic cancer: a randomised trial. Lancet. 2005;366:643–8.

32. Rades D, Karstens JH, Hoskin PJ, et al. Escalation of radiation dose beyond 30 Gy in 10 fractions for metastatic spinal cord compression. Int J Radiat Oncol Biol Phys. 2007;67:525–31.

33. Rades D, Hoskin PJ, Karstens JH, et al. Radiotherapy of metastatic spinal cord compression in very elderly patients. Int J Radiat Oncol Biol Phys. 2007;67:256–63.

34. Sze WM, Shelley MD, Held I, Wilt TJ, Mason MD. Palliation of metastatic bone pain: single fraction versus multifraction radiotherapy – a systematic review of randomised trials. Clin Oncol (R Coll Radiol). 2003;15:345–52.

35. Wu JS, Wong R, Johnston M, Bezjak A, Whelan T. Meta-analysis of dose-fractionation radiotherapy trials for the palliation of painful bone metastases. Int J Radiat Oncol Biol Phys. 2003;55:594–605.

36. Chow E, Loblaw A, Harris K, et al. Dexamethasone for the prophylaxis of radiation-induced pain flare after palliative radiotherapy for bone metastases: a pilot study. Support Care Cancer. 2007;15:643–7.

37. Muacevic A, Wowra B, Siefert A, et al. Microsurgery plus whole brain irradiation versus Gamma Knife surgery alone for treatment of single metastases to the brain: a randomized controlled multicentre phase III trial. J Neurooncol. 2008;87:299–307.

38. Smith ML, Lee JY. Stereotactic radiosurgery in the management of brain metastasis. Neurosurg Focus. 2007;22(E5):1–8.

39. Sahgal A, Larson DA, Chang EL. Stereotactic body radiosurgery for spinal metastases: a critical review. Int J Radiat Oncol Biol Phys. 2008;71:652–65.

40. Chang EL, Shiu AS, Mendel E. Phase I/II study of stereotactic body radiotherapy for spinal metastasis and its pattern of failure. J Neurosurg Spine. 2007;7(2):151–60.

41. Degen JW, Gagnon GJ, Voyadzis JM. CyberKnife stereotactic radiosurgical treatment of spinal tumors for pain control and quality of life. J Neurosurg Spine. 2005;2:540–9.

42. Gerszten PC, Burton SA, Ozhasoglu C, et al. Radiosurgery for spinal metastases: clinical experience in 500 cases from a single institution. Spine. 2007;32:193–9.

43. Gibbs IC, Kamnerdsupaphon P, Ryu MR. Image-guided robotic radiosurgery for spinal metastases. Radiother Oncol. 2007;82:185–90.

44. Jin JY, Ryu S, Rock J. Evaluation of residual patient position variation for spinal radiosurgery using the Novalis image guided system. Med Phys. 2008;35:1087–93.

45. Rock JP, Ryu S, Shukairy MS. Postoperative radiosurgery for malignant spinal tumors. Neurosurgery. 2006;58:891–8.

46. Ryu S, Fang Yin F, Rock J. Image-guided and intensity-modulated radiosurgery for patients with spinal metastasis. Cancer. 2003;97:2013–8.

47. Yamada Y, Lovelock DM, Yenice KM. Multifractionated imageguided and stereotactic intensity-modulated radiotherapy of paraspinal tumors: a preliminary report. Int J Radiat Oncol Biol Phys. 2005;62:53–61.

48. Gerszten PC, Germanwala A, Burton SA, et al. Combination kyphoplasty and spinal radiosurgery: a new treatment paradigm for pathological fractures. Neurosurg Focus. 2005;18:e8.

49. Wu JS, Wong RK, Lloyd NS, Johnston M, Bezjak A, Whelan T. Radiotherapy fractionation for the palliation of uncomplicated painful bone metastases – an evidence-based practice guideline. BMC Cancer. 2004;4:71.

50. Chow E, Harris K, Fan G, Tsao M, Sze WM. Palliative radiotherapy trials for bone metastases: a systematic review. J Clin Oncol. 2007;25:1423–36.

51. Booth M, Summers J, Williams MV. Audit reduces the reluctance to use single fractions for painful bone metastases. Clin Oncol (R Coll Radiol). 1993;5:15–8.

52. Chow E, Wu JS, Hoskin P, Coia LR, Bentzen SM, Blitzer PH. International consensus on palliative radiotherapy endpoints for future clinical trials in bone metastases. Radiother Oncol. 2002;64:275–80.

53. Crellin AM, Marks A, Maher EJ. Why don't British radiotherapists give single fractions of radiotherapy for bone metastases? Clin Oncol (R Coll Radiol). 1989;1:63–6.

54. Priestman TJ, Bullimore JA, Godden TP, Deutsch GP. The Royal College of Radiologists' Fractionation Survey. Clin Oncol (R Coll Radiol). 1989;1:39–46.

55. Lawton PA, Maher EJ. Treatment strategies for advanced and metastatic cancer in Europe. Radiother Oncol. 1991;22:1–6.

56. Maher EJ, Coia L, Duncan G, Lawton PA. Treatment strategies in advanced and metastatic cancer: differences in attitude between the USA, Canada and Europe. Int J Radiat Oncol Biol Phys. 1992;23:239–44.

57. Chow E, Danjoux C, Wong R, et al. Palliation of bone metastases: a survey of patterns of practice among Canadian radiation oncologists. Radiother Oncol. 2000;56:305–14.

58. Lievens Y, Kesteloot K, Rijnders A, Kutcher G, Van den Bogaert W. Differences in palliative radiotherapy for bone metastases within Western European countries. Radiother Oncol. 2000;56:297–303.

59. Lievens Y, Van den Bogaert W, Rijnders A, Kutcher G, Kesteloot K. Palliative radiotherapy practice within Western European countries: impact of the radiotherapy financing system? Radiother Oncol. 2000;56:289–95.

60. Roos DE. Continuing reluctance to use single fractions of radiotherapy for metastatic bone pain: an Australian and New Zealand practice survey and literature review. Radiother Oncol. 2000;56:315–22.

61. Adamietz IA, Schneider O, Muller RP. Results of a nationwide survey on radiotherapy of bone metastases in Germany. Strahlenther Onkol. 2002;178:531–6.

62. Barton R, Robinson G, Gutierrez E, Kirkbride P, McLean M. Palliative radiation for vertebral metastases: the effect of variation in prescription parameters on the dose received at depth. Int J Radiat Oncol Biol Phys. 2002;52:1083–91.

63. Gupta T, Sarin R. Palliative radiation therapy for painful vertebral metastases: a practice survey. Cancer. 2004;101:2892–6.

64. Fairchild A, Barnes E, Ghosh S, et al. International patterns of practice in palliative radiotherapy for painful bone metastases: evidence-based practice? Int J Radiat Oncol Biol Phys. 2009;75:1501–10.

65. Quilty PM, Kirk D, Bolger JJ, et al. A comparison of the palliative effects of strontium-89 and external beam radiotherapy in metastatic prostate cancer. Radiother Oncol. 1994;31:33–40.

66. Kachnic L, Berk L. Palliative single-fraction radiation therapy: how much more evidence is needed? J Natl Cancer Inst. 2005;97:786–8.

Chapter 17
Percutaneous Bone Tumor Management

Afshin Gangi, Georgia Tsoumakidou, Xavier Buy, Julien Garnon, Tarun Sabharwal, and Ricardo Douarte

Introduction

Skeletal tumor morbidity includes pain, hypercalcemia, pathological fracture, and spinal cord or nerve-root compression. Occasionally, bone metastatic disease may remain confined to the skeleton with the decline in quality-of-life and eventual death, primarily due to skeletal complications. The opportunities for improving the management of metastatic bone disease and bone tumors have never been greater. Recent developments have been accomplished in all aspects of cancer management. The improvements achieved on skeletal imaging, the use of reconstructive orthopedic surgery, and radiotherapy, and particularly the development of interventional radiology, bone-seeking radiopharmaceuticals, new endocrine and cytotoxic treatments, and the increasing use of bisphosphonates help prevent and/or treat skeletal complications [1].

During the past few decades, the role of interventional radiology has rapidly increased thanks to the development of a variety of techniques. Different image-guided percutaneous procedures can be used for treatment or pain palliation in patients with primary or secondary bone tumors. Curative ablation can be applied for the treatment of specific benign or in selected cases of localized malignant bone tumors. Pain palliation therapy of primary and secondary bone tumors can be achieved with safe, fast, effective, and tolerable percutaneous methods. The different ablation (chemical, thermal, and mechanical), cavitation (radiofrequency ionization), and consolidation (cementoplasty) techniques can be used separately or in combination. Each technique has its indications, with advantages and drawbacks.

- *Curative treatment*: The therapeutic goal is to completely and definitively ablate the tumor.
- *Palliative treatment*: The therapeutic goal is not complete ablation of the tumor, but pain palliation.

Consolidation Techniques:

- *Cementoplasty*: Percutaneous injection of methylmethacrylate that provides bone strengthening and pain relief. Cementoplasty is a symptomatic and not a curative treatment.

Ablation Techniques:

- *Chemical ablation*: Injection of ethanol is used to ablate osteolytic bone tumors, as well as to achieve pain management (neurolysis).
- *Thermal ablation procedures*:

    1. *Laser photocoagulation*: Thermoablation is produced with near-infrared wavelength lasers (neodymium:yttrium–aluminum–garnet [Nd:YAG], diode laser 800–1,000 nm).

A. Gangi (✉) • G. Tsoumakidou • X. Buy • J. Garnon • R. Douarte
Department of Radiology, University Hospital of Strasbourg, Strasbourg, France
e-mail: gangi@unistra.fr

T. Sabharwal
Department of Radiology, Guy's and St. Thomas' Hospital, London, UK

P.R. Mueller and A. Adam (eds.), *Interventional Oncology: A Practical Guide for the Interventional Radiologist*,
DOI 10.1007/978-1-4419-1469-9_17, © Springer Science+Business Media, LLC 2012

2. *Radiofrequency ablation*: Thermoablation is produced by altering the electric current at the tip of the electrode, causing local ionic agitation and subsequent frictional heat.

3. *Microwave ablation*: Electromagnetic waves cause agitation of ionic molecules and frictional heat, which results in tissue coagulative necrosis.

4. *Cryoablation*: The application of extreme cold aiming to destroy cells, by causing both direct cellular and vascular injury.

- *Radiofrequency ionization (decompression technique)*: A low-temperature bipolar technique that produces a plasma field at the tip of the electrode that breaks the intermolecular bonds, creating a cavity inside the tissue and leading to decompression.

- *High-intensity focused ultrasound*: A noninvasive technique that facilitates coagulative necrosis at a precise focal point in the body. The ability to focus and accurately target a lesion with high-intensity focused ultrasound (HIFU) by using real-time ultrasonography (US) or magnetic resonance imaging (MRI) guidance allows precise ablation of lesions of any shape without damage to surrounding structures.

In this chapter, each technique is presented in detail with reference to the mechanisms, the indications, and the results.

Cementoplasty

Principle

Percutaneous injection of polymethylmethacrylate cement (PMMA) provides pain relief and bone strengthening in patients with malignant bone tumors [2]. PMMA is highly resistant to compression forces, but susceptible to torsion forces. Due to its mechanical properties, the cement is suitable for treatment of fractures involving weight-bearing bones such as vertebral body, acetabulum, and in any bones subject to compression forces only. In opposition, injection in long diaphyses does not achieve sufficient bone strengthening, with possible fracture of the cement rod.

Indications

Patients with painful osteolytic tumors (metastasis, multiple myeloma, and lymphoma) located to the vertebral body, acetabulum and condyles and causing local pain, disability and with a risk of compression fracture are excellent indications for the technique. Cement can only prevent compression fractures. For lesions concerning long bones, such as the femoral diaphysis, surgical consolidation should be considered to avoid a pathological fracture [3]. Due to the multifocal nature of these lesions, surgical treatment is rarely undertaken [4]. Radiation therapy does not provide consolidation nor relieve pain, and the therapeutic response is generally delayed. In opposition, cement injection allows fast consolidation resulting in effective pain relief. The cementoplasty should be performed with a palliative intent. It does not stop tumor progression and thus, it should be considered as a complement, not a replacement to other treatments for cancer. When the bone tumor is associated with painful paraosseous soft-tissue invasion, cementoplasty can be combined with thermal ablation techniques, such as radiofrequency ablation or cryoablation [4, 5].

For spinal metastases, cement injection (vertebroplasty) can be performed at multiple levels according to the multifocal nature of the disease process (Fig. 17.1). However, vertebroplasty is specifically indicated for the management of local pain from metastatic disease and not for diffuse back pain with the involvement of entire spine. Cementoplasty has also been successfully used in extra-spinal tumor locations, such as the acetabulum, femoral condyles, tibial ends, talus, scapula, and calcaneus (Figs. 17.2 and 17.3). A detailed clinical examination with specific emphasis on neurological assessment must be carried out in conjunction with the imaging findings to rule out other causes of pain.

Contraindications of cementoplasty include irreversible coagulation disorders and acute infection. Spinal tumors with large rupture of the posterior wall should be considered with caution as the risk of epidural cement leakage is increased. Vertebral metastases causing neurological symptoms or instability are generally contraindicated for percutaneous treatment; however, in some cases, vertebroplasty can be combined with laminectomy and surgical fixation to avoid a complex surgical anterior approach. In cases of osteoblastic metastases, the cement injection can prove difficult or even impossible.

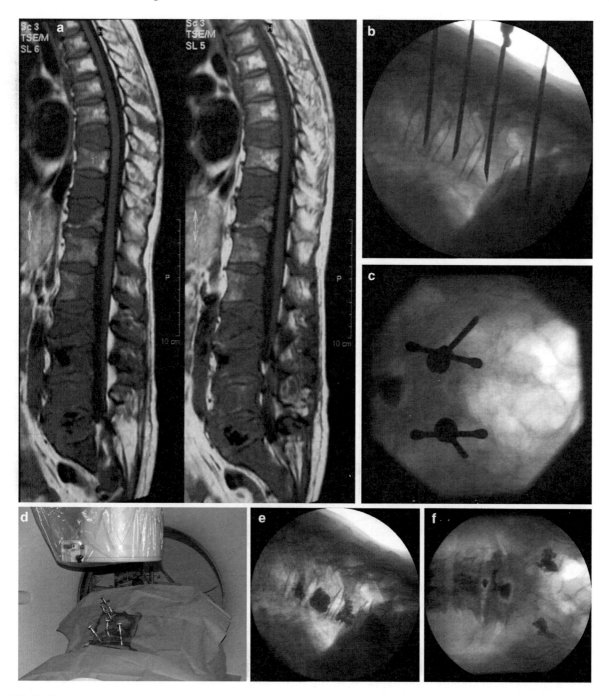

Fig. 17.1 Multiple painful vertebral metastases in a patient with breast carcinoma. (**a**) T1W magnetic resonance imaging (MRI) of a patient with multiple spinal metastases. A previous vertebroplasty has been performed at two levels (L3, L5). (**b–e** and **f**) Six levels vertebroplasty and sacroplasty were performed under general anesthesia

Technique

Cementoplasty can be performed under general anesthesia or conscious sedation, depending on the general status of the patient, his positioning, and the estimated procedural time [4, 6]. Strict asepsis is mandatory. Intraprocedural intravenous antibiotic prophylaxis (Cephazolin 1 mg) is recommended in immunocompromized patients, but there is no clear consensus on other patients. Local anesthesia of the whole pathway is performed with lidocaine 1% through a 22-gauge spinal needle. Under fluoroscopic guidance, a cementoplasty trocar (10–13 gauge) is advanced tandem to the spinal needle and introduced into the bone. For complex cases or if a thermal ablation is combined, the dual guidance [computed tomography (CT) and

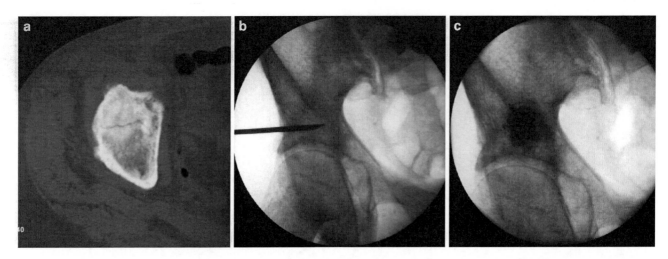

Fig. 17.2 Pathological fracture of the right acetabulum. (**a**) Axial computed tomography (CT) image confirming the pathological fracture of the acetabulum. (**b**) Anteroposterior fluoroscopic showing a 10-gauge vertebroplasty needle positioned in the acetabulum. (**c**) Cement delivery was performed under continuous fluoroscopic control

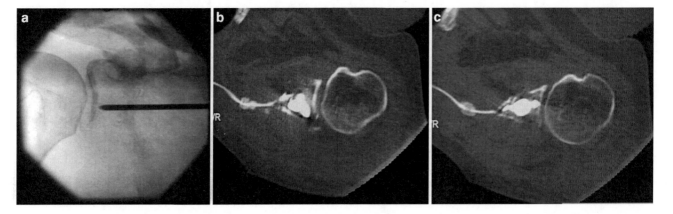

Fig. 17.3 (**a**–**c**) Osteolytic metastasis of the neck of scapula. Cementoplasty performed under combined CT and C-arm fluoroscopic guidance with excellent clinical result

fluoroscopy] allows precise needle placement, increases the operator comfort, and reduces the rate of complications. Because of the high radiation dose, CT–fluoroscopy should not be used in routine practice.

Lumbar vertebroplasty is generally performed via a unilateral transpedicular oblique approach. At the thoracic level, the unilateral intercostopedicular route is preferred to avoid both the spinal canal and the pleura. At the cervical level, the approach is anterolateral with a trajectory between the carotid artery laterally, and the thyroid gland and esophagus medially. For C1 and C2 levels, a direct transoral approach is described, which is the most direct route to avoid the neural and vascular structures. When cementoplasty of the sacral wings is needed, the sacral puncture is commonly performed via a posterior approach; an oblique posterolateral approach through the iliac wing is sometimes necessary for cementoplasty of the S1–S2 vertebral bodies.

For acetabular cementoplasty, the approach can be anterolateral through the iliac wing (avoiding the femoral nerve) or posterolateral (avoiding the sciatic nerve). For other bones, the proper pathway should be chosen, giving priority to the shortest and safest route, away from the neurovascular structures.

After controlling the proper position of the cementoplasty trocar, the stylet is removed, and a fluoroscopic view is obtained and used as a reference image during cement injection to watch for leakage. When needed, a bone biopsy can be performed coaxially, before the cement delivery. Venography is only performed in hypervascular tumors with active bleeding through the bone trocar; digital subtraction angiography is necessary to analyze the venous drainage and to demonstrate a possible route for cement leakage. In such cases, it is safer to wait until the cement becomes pasty before injecting it, so as to reduce the risk of intravasation.

Cement injection is slowly performed under continuous fluoroscopic control. The use of dedicated injection sets is recommended, as they provide better control of the pressure and volume of cement delivered; moreover, they reduce the radiation dose to the operator's hands.

Results

Percutaneous cementoplasty is an effective treatment for painful osteolytic bone metastases and myeloma [7, 8]. It treats pain and consolidates weight-bearing bone. During the exothermic polymerization of PMMA, temperatures may exceed 75°C; however, the cytotoxic effect is limited to 3 mm around the cement, and thus, the antitumoral effect of the cement is insufficient. Specific tumor therapy (i.e., chemotherapy, radiotherapy, or thermoablation) should be given in conjunction with cementoplasty for the tumor management where appropriate [9].

Many authors report significant pain relief in 80–97% cases after cementoplasty in cancer patients [4, 7, 9–11]. Local pain is rapidly controlled and endures at long-term follow-up.

Patients are allowed to stand a few hours after cementoplasty [12]. Overnight hospitalization is generally sufficient after percutaneous cementoplasty, but this may vary depending on the general status of the patient and the level of postprocedural analgesia.

In a series of 21 cancer patients treated with vertebroplasty, Alvarez et al. showed significant and early improvement in the functional status of patients with spinal metastases [10]. In this study, 77% of patients could walk again, 81% were satisfied or very satisfied with the results.

In cases of bone tumor with painful extension to the surrounding soft tissues, improved results can be obtained by combining thermal ablation techniques and cementoplasty [13].

Complications due to cementoplasty are mainly due to cement leakage. The incidence of leakage is higher with malignant disease compared to osteoporotic fractures, but remains often asymptomatic [14]. Cortical destruction, extension in the paraosseous soft tissues and highly vascularized tumors are likely to increase the rate of complications [15]. In case of cement leakage in contact with a nerve root, immediate active cooling of the nerve with injection of saline should be performed to prevent radiculopathy from thermal damage during the polymerization phase of the cement [16]. Additional periradicular infiltration with steroids is sometimes needed. Venous intravasation of cement limited to the basivertebral vein is usually asymptomatic when the operator recognizes it early and immediately stops injection. However, failure to notice this can cause filling of the epidural or paravertebral veins, resulting in epidural cement leakage or pulmonary embolism [17]. Minor disc leakage is common and has no further consequence.

Infection secondary to cementoplasty occurs in less than 1% cases [18]. To avoid this complication, careful preprocedural evaluation of the patients and strict asepsis are mandatory. Bleeding from the puncture site remains exceptional. Hypotension and arrhythmias have been reported during cement delivery; they may be due to small amount of fat embolism, secondary to bone marrow displacement. Anaphylactic reaction to PMMA resulting in death is exceptional, but has been reported to the Food and Drug Administration (FDA) [15].

Tumor Ablation

Tumor ablation is defined as the direct application of chemical or thermal techniques to a specific focal tumor to achieve its destruction. During the last few decades, several percutaneous ablation techniques have emerged. Considering their success rate on renal, hepatic, and lung malignancies, many authors have proposed their use for palliative or curative treatment of bone and musculoskeletal tumors. Widely adopted image-guided ablation techniques include alcohol instillation and different thermal ablation methods such as radiofrequency, microwave, cryoablation, laser photocoagulation, and low-temperature radiofrequency ionization. These different methods will be presented, highlighting their advantages and their specific indications.

General Indications of Percutaneous Musculoskeletal Ablation

The principal role of image-guided musculoskeletal tumor ablation lies on the palliative targeted minimally invasive ablation of painful metastases secondary to advanced cancer disease. Less frequently, percutaneous ablation can be considered in a curative intent, either for benign bone tumors, such as osteoid osteomas, or single metastasis in poor surgical candidates.

Fig. 17.4 Alcoholization of
a painful paravertebral
metastasis from lung cancer.
The procedure was performed
under sedation. After
injection of contrast media in
the lesion (to exclude its
intravasation), 10 ml of
opacified absolute ethanol
were injected. Note the
inhomogeneous distribution
of contrast. To increase the
pain reduction, a thoracic
sympatholysis with ethanol
was performed during the
same session

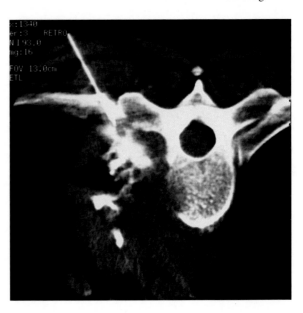

Tumors with epidural compression of the spinal cord are a significant source of morbidity in patients with systemic cancer. Surgical management should be considered first in tumors with cord compression. The surgical approach involves the early circumferential decompression of the cord with concomitant stabilization of the spine [19]. However, the treatment is mostly palliative. In such cases, the therapeutic intent has to be precisely defined on a multidisciplinary oncological basis, considering the general status of the patient and the available therapeutic options.

Alcohol Ablation

Percutaneous ethanol injection is the simplest and cheapest method of percutaneous tumor ablation. Ethanol causes tumor necrosis directly through cellular dehydration and indirectly through vascular thrombosis and tissue ischemia. A 22-gauge needle is inserted into the tumor, and a mixture of iodinated contrast (25%) and lidocaine 1% (75%) is first injected to assess the diffusion extent and achieve local anesthesia. In the absence of intravasation or diffusion in contact with vulnerable structures, a dose of 3–30 ml of 96% ethanol is injected into the tumor (Fig. 17.4). Ethanol injection in bone is very painful and requires neuroleptanalgesia. This technique has shown promising results for palliative management of painful bone tumors [20]. However, the size and shape of the induced necrosis is poorly reproducible owing to the hardly predictable distribution of ethanol. The thermal ablation techniques provide much more predictable ablation volumes and should be preferred.

Ethanol injection is still used for the treatment of aggressive vertebral hemangiomas (AVH). AVHs limited to the vertebral body are now widely treated with single vertebroplasty. More complex AVHs with paravertebral or epidural extension generally require combined therapies. Primarily the thrombosis and retraction of the AVH compartment is achieved with direct percutaneous intravertebral ethanol injection (sclerotherapy) via one or more 18-gauge spinal needles [21]. Two weeks after sclerotherapy, magnetic resonance (MR) control with dynamic injection is obtained to assess the embolization of the AVH. Subsequent vertebroplasty is performed to achieve consolidation (Fig. 17.5) [22]. In cases of major epidural extension with neurological deficit, laminectomy should be combined, and it has been reported that percutaneous treatment with sclerotherapy highly reduces the risk of perioperative hemorrhage [23].

Laser Photocoagulation

Laser photocoagulation uses the absorbed energy of infrared light to produce heat and ablate the tumor. Light energy of 2.0 W in bone produces a spherical ablation volume of 1.6 cm diameter. Higher powers result in charring and vaporization around the laser fiber tip. To ablate larger volumes, several bare fibers with a 2-cm distance apart are necessary [24]. The laser photocoagulation fibers are fully MR compatible.

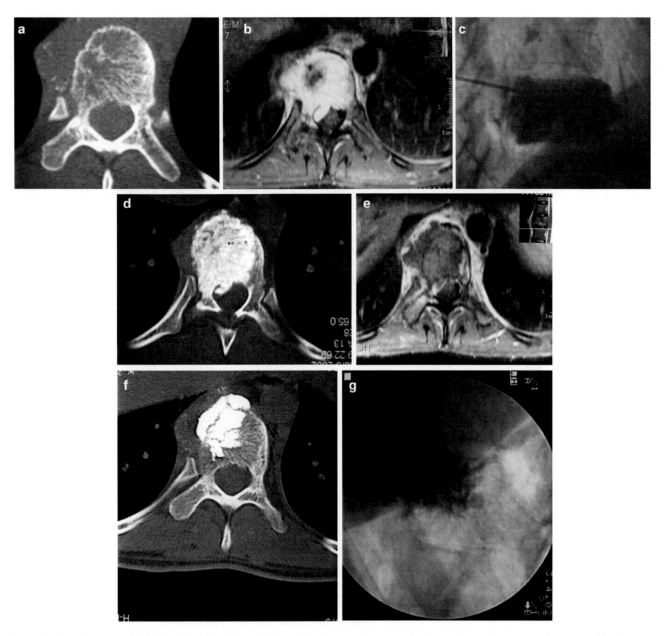

Fig. 17.5 (**a**) Axial CT and (**b**) MRI (with injection of gadolinium) image of an aggressive hemangioma with paravertebral and epidural extension. (**c**, **d**) Sclerotherapy performed with injection of ethanol and lipiodol, under CT and fluoroscopic control. Note the good filling of the hemangioma. The patient was under steroid therapy 2 days before and 3 days after the sclerotherapy. (**e**) MR-control with injection of gadolinium performed 2 weeks after the procedure showing significant reduction of the contrast enhancement and the volume of the paravertebral mass. (**f**, **g**) Vertebroplasty was performed 1 month after the sclerotherapy procedure to avoid secondary collapse of the vertebral body

Because of the small ablated volume produced by a bare tip fiber, laser is now only used for small tumors or, exceptionally, when the use of radiofrequency ablation is contraindicated, i.e., metallic implants. Osteoid osteomas which are by definition less than 1 cm in diameter are one of the best indications for bone laser ablation. The laser fiber is inserted into the nidus under CT guidance. If the osteoid osteoma is surrounded by thick cortical bone, a drill needle is used, and the fiber is inserted coaxially. For subperiosteal tumors, an 18-gauge spinal needle is used to protect the optical fiber. Once in position, the ablation is performed with continuous 2 W power for 6–10 min, depending on the nidus size. The success rate of laser ablation of osteoid osteomas is excellent and similar to radiofrequency ablation [25, 26]. Nowadays, the percutaneous minimally invasive thermal ablation of osteoid osteomas is the gold standard and has replaced the surgical approach. For tumors in close proximity to neurological structures or other vulnerable organs, thermal protection techniques are required (Fig. 17.6). Successful treatment in a single session is achieved in 95% cases. Intraarticular location of the nidus seems to be associated with a higher risk of recurrence [27]. This painful benign tumor can only be treated under deep anesthesia (general, spinal anesthesia, or regional block). Postprocedural pain is systematically controlled with nonsteroid anti-inflammatory drugs and analgesics.

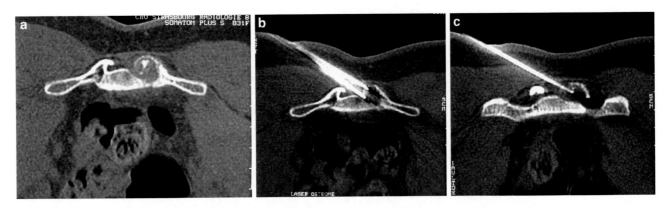

Fig. 17.6 (**a**) Axial CT-image showing an osteoblastoma of the sacrum. (**b**) Two spinal 18-gauge needles were placed inside the tumor for laser ablation of the lesion, and (**c**) a thermocouple was positioned in the foramina for thermal monitoring and cooling of the nerve root with continuous injection of saline. The temperature in the foramina during the ablation was kept below 45°C

Radiofrequency Ablation

Radiofrequency ablation (RFA) is one of the most promising thermal techniques for the treatment of localized tumors. It was first applied in the early 1990s for the treatment of hepatic tumors. RFA applicators with straight or expandable electrodes are introduced percutaneously into the target tumor. Then, a high-frequency alternating current (450–600 kHz) is delivered through the lesion, which causes agitation of the tissue ionic molecules that in turn produces frictional heat. The electrical loop is closed with grounding pads attached at the thighs. The thermal effect depends on the electrical-conducting properties of the tissue treated. Local tissue temperatures between 60 and 100°C produce protein denaturation, immediate cell death, and coagulative necrosis of the tumor. Temperatures above 100°C induce vaporization and carbonization of the tissue adjacent to the electrode, which degrade the electrical conductance and result in suboptimal treatment effect. The efficacy of RFA may be limited by adjacent high-flow vessels that act as a cooling circuitry ("heat-sink" effect). RFA produces a more controllable ablation zone than alcohol and has widely replaced its use.

The use of RFA in bone tumors is mainly palliative, but in some cases can also be curative. For palliative treatment of painful bone metastases refractory to conventional therapies, the principal aim of RFA is to ablate the bone–tumor interface, where primarily the source of pain is located. Less often, RFA can be used in a curative intent for patients with single metastasis limited in size. Of note, palliative ablation of painful sclerotic bone metastases is possible with reduced power to avoid early impedance increase [28]. Newly developed bipolar RF electrodes are of special interest in spinal and paraspinal applications; in bipolar arrays, the current flows from the tip of one electrode to the other and no grounding pad is used; thus, heat generated is mainly limited between the electrode-tips, which allows faster and better controlled ablation with improved protection of the surrounding tissues (Fig. 17.7) [13].

RFA is also an alternative efficient technique to treat osteoid osteomas; the ablation is performed with a 1-cm active tip electrode, with low power (5 W) to maintain the temperature at 90°C for 6 min inside the nidus.

For osteoid osteomas, the success rate of bone RFA is similar to laser (>85%) [25]. For painful bone metastases, significant and rapid pain relief is achieved in more than 75% cases with substantial decrease of medication. However, the RFA should be considered for patients with focal pain and limited number of metastases, and is not adapted for diffuse bone pain.

For tumors in close proximity to neurological structures or other vulnerable organs, thermal insulation and temperature monitoring techniques are required. Temperature monitoring can be achieved with thermosensors. Hydrodissection, CO_2 insufflation, or balloon interposition can displace the vulnerable organs away from the ablation zone and insulate them [29]. Large ablation volumes should be avoided near the spine to prevent nerve injury. Experimental in vivo and ex vivo studies have provided valuable insights into the distribution of RF-generated heat in the spinal canal [30, 31]. There is firm evidence that vertebral posterior cortical defects expose the nerve roots and the spinal cord to excessive heat during the RFA, with local temperature above 45°C. In the case of spinal ablation, the presence of an intact cortex to insulate the canal cannot be overstressed, and continuous thermal monitoring of the neural structures with thermosensors is highly recommended [32]. For large volumes of ablation in tumors involving weight-bearing bones, additional consolidation with cementoplasty or surgery should be considered to prevent the risk of secondary fracture. To avoid premature setting of cement, the injection is delayed until the temperature of the tumor has fallen to a normal level.

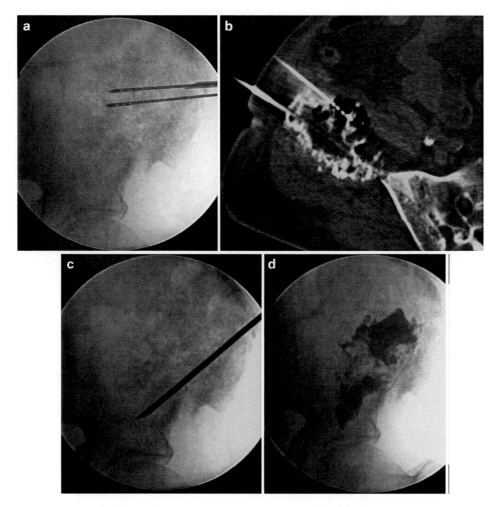

Fig. 17.7 Painful large metastasis of the iliac bone with extension to the acetabulum resisting to radiotherapy. (**a, b**) Bipolar radiofrequency (RF) ablation under general anesthesia. (**c, d**) The cementoplasty needle used as a coaxial for RF ablation was positioned in the acetabulum for cement injection

Microwave Ablation

Microwave ablation is an emerging technology that depends on the application of an electromagnetic wave (around 900 MHz) through an antenna directly inserted into the target tumor. Electromagnetic waves cause agitation of ionic molecules and produce frictional heat, which results in tissue coagulative necrosis. Microwaves are capable of propagating through many tissue types, even those with high impedance such as lung or bone, with less susceptibility to heat-sink effects near vessels [33]. Three antennas can be activated synergically to produce fast ablation of large tumors. In opposition to RFA, microwave ablation can achieve higher intratumoral temperatures and larger ablation zones in less time, and no grounding pads are necessary with microwave ablation. This technique raises interest for the percutaneous treatment of large hepatic and lung tumors. Though the use of microwave ablation has been reported to help surgical resection of osteosarcomas [34], no data are available about its percutaneous use in musculoskeletal tumors.

Cryoablation

Cryoablation is the application of extreme cold to destroy tumors. This technique has gained new interest since the development of miniaturized 17-gauge gas-driven cryoprobes that can be used percutaneously under CT or MR monitoring. Rapid expansion of high-pressure argon gas delivered through the cryoprobe produces sudden drop of temperature below −183°C

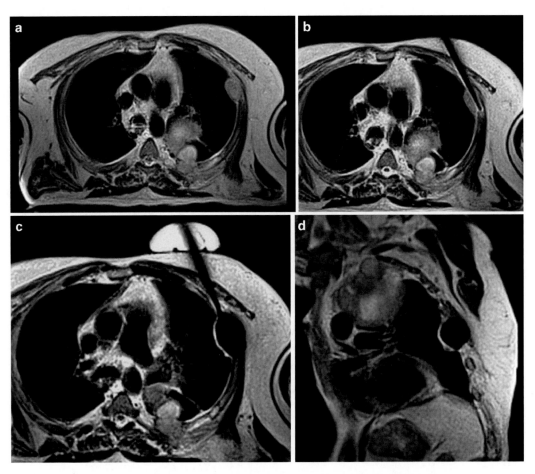

Fig. 17.8 (**a**) Patient with multiple metastases from lung cancer. (**b**) MR-guided cryoablation of the painful left intercostal metastasis. Two cryoprobes were positioned in the tumor for pain palliation. (**c**) Axial and (**d**) sagittal MR images showing the ice ball (signal-void area) covering the lesion. Note the sterile glove filled with warm saline placed on the skin surface around the cryoprobes for thermal protection of the skin

(application of the Joule–Thompson phenomenon); in opposition, fast decompression of helium gas raises the temperature to +33°C, which allows active thawing. Cellular necrosis is systematically achieved with temperatures below −40°C. To avoid uncertain cell death with temperatures between 0 and −20°C, repeated freeze–thaw cycles are needed. During the first freezing phase, the ice crystals are mainly extracellular; during the thawing phase the water diffuses into the intracellular compartment due to osmotic gradients; subsequently the second freezing phase produces intracellular ice crystals, leading to membrane rupture and cell death. The longer the duration of the thawing phase, the greater the cell damage it causes. Repetition of the freeze–thaw cycle is associated with more extensive and more certain tissue destruction [35]. In addition to this direct cell injury, intravascular ice crystals create microthrombi and cause indirect ischemia [36]. Of note, cryoablation efficacy may be compromised by tissue thawing from nearby high-flow vascular structures resulting in "cool-sink" effect.

The major advantage of cryoablation compared to RFA is the precise visual control of the aggregated ice ball with both CT and MR (Figs. 17.8–17.10) [37]. CT-reformatting and MR-multiplanar imaging are used intermittently to monitor the extension of the ice ball, to check the proper covering of the tumor and to control the safety margin with adjacent vulnerable tissues (Figs. 17.9 and 17.10). Different types of cryoprobes are available, resulting in different volumes and shapes of ice ball. Up to 25 cryoprobes can be activated simultaneously. For curative cryoablation, the margins of the ice ball should extend 3–5 mm beyond the tumor margins. In addition, cryoablation has intrinsic anesthetic properties that allow performing the procedure under mild sedation or even local anesthetic [38]. Reduction of the peri- and immediate postprocedural pain with cryoablation is a major benefit in comparison to RFA. Cryoablation is also effective in sclerotic bone lesions; however, the visual control of the ice ball is poor in these cases. In contrast to RFA, surgical metallic fixation in contact with the tumor is not a contraindication for cryoablation. As with the other thermal ablation techniques, the safety of the cryoablation can be enhanced with the use of appropriate thermosensors and insulation techniques, particularly CO_2 insufflations (Fig. 17.8) [29].

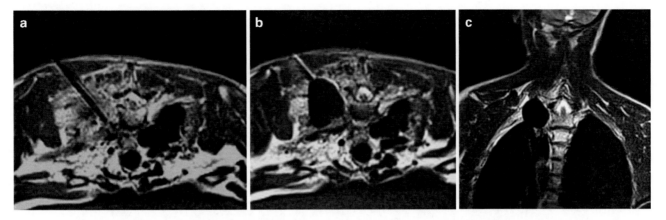

Fig. 17.9 MRI-guided palliative cryoablation of a painful Pancoast's tumor involving the lower brachial plexus. The procedure was performed under conscious sedation, and the patient was asked to move regularly his hand and fingers to avoid any damage to the brachial plexus. (**a**) Intraprocedure planning axial T2-weighted MR image shows the insertion of one of the cryoprobes into the superior edge of tumor. (**b**) Axial and (**c**) coronal T2W MR images show ice ball formation covering the tumor

Recent studies report the interest of cryoablation for the palliative treatment of bone metastases, with very promising results and low complications [39, 40]. If subsequent cementoplasty has to be performed for bone consolidation, complete thawing of the ice ball is needed. The tissue temperature should exceed +20°C before injecting the cement [41].

Radiofrequency Ionization

Radiofrequency ionization (RFI) is a low-temperature bipolar technique producing a plasma field at the tip of the electrode [42]. The high-energy ionized plasma breaks the intermolecular bonds causing cavitation inside the tissues and subsequent decompression. This process is achieved at relatively low temperatures (40–70°C), compared to the conventional thermal ablation radiofrequency devices. The ionization process consumes most of the heat and no electrical current passes directly through the target tissue. The result is volumetric removal of the tumor with minimal damage to the surrounding tissues. This technique is widely used in ear, nose, throat (ENT) surgery, cardiac surgery, arthroplasty, and spinal nucleotomy. It has been recently introduced for bone tumor decompression, especially in spinal. Unlike other intravertebral expandable systems that increase the intratumoral pressure, radiofrequency ionization creates a void without increasing the pressure or displacing the tumor.

A dedicated 16-gauge bipolar electrode is inserted into the tumor coaxially through a bone trocar. A side-arm catheter is connected to the electrode to slowly inject saline solution for activation of the plasma field. The bent tip of the electrode allows digging several channels inside the tumor by rotating the electrode around its axis. These maneuvers are monitored under fluoroscopic guidance. If there is any risk of neurological damage, combination of CT and fluoroscopic guidance is mandatory.

The best indications for this technique are nonsurgical painful spinal tumors with intracanalar bulge, or rupture of the vertebral posterior wall with risk of tumor retropulsion during vertebroplasty. RFI produces intratumoral cavitation with pressure reduction. After cavitation of spinal lesions, vertebral consolidation is achieved with subsequent cement injection. Spinal cavitation is advocated by some authors before vertebroplasty to reduce the risk of cement leakage [43, 44].

High-Intensity Focused Ultrasound Ablation

High-intensity focused ultrasound (HIFU) is a noninvasive technique that can produce coagulative necrosis at a precise focal point in the body. The ability to focus and accurately target a lesion with HIFU by using real-time US or MRI guidance allows precise ablation of lesions of any shape without damage to the surrounding structures.

The location and extent of this treatment can be monitored accurately with real-time US or MRI. There has been a general consensus that ultrasound energy cannot enter bone at an intensity level sufficient for therapeutic ablation. However, because

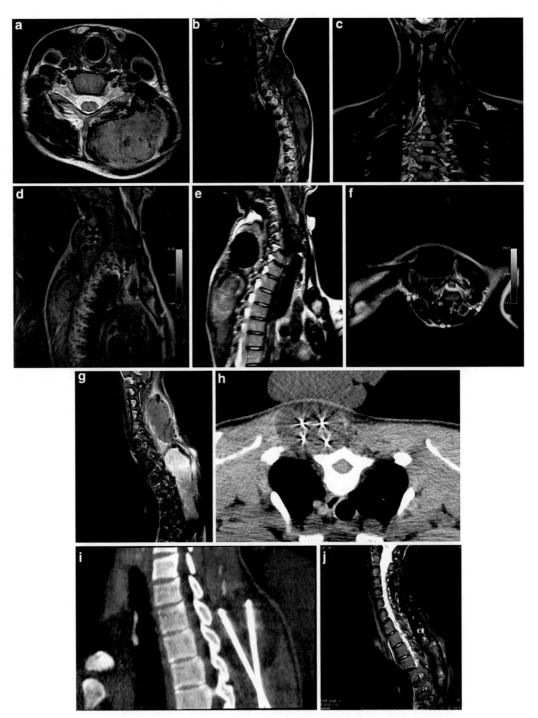

Fig. 17.10 MRI and CT-guided cryoablation of a massive cervicothoracic desmoid tumor resisting to all conventional treatment and chemotherapies in a 21-year-old female. The patient was complaining of severe cervical pain. (**a**) Axial, (**b**) sagittal, and (**c**) coronal T2W MR images show a huge cervicothoracic soft-tissue tumor, involving predominantly the paraspinal musculature. (**d**) MRI-guided sagittal T2-weighted MR image shows the positioning of five cryoprobes in the upper part of the tumor. (**e**) Sagittal and (**f**) axial T2-weighted MR images show a well-defined ice ball formation inside the tumor. (**g**) Follow-up sagittal contrast enhanced T1W MR image obtained 1 month after the cryoablation shows a large area of tumor necrosis at the site of the ablation and the residual thoracic part of the tumor. (**h**) Axial and (**i**) sagittal CT images of the cryoablation of the residual tumor with five cryoprobes positioned inside the tumor and a large well-defined ice ball. (**j**) Follow-up sagittal T2W MR image obtained 1 month after the second cryoablation shows the large necrosis of the thoracic mass and the shrinkage of the cervical tumor. Excellent clinical result with complete pain relief

of the high acoustic absorption and low thermal conductivity of bone cortex, it is possible to use a relatively low level of ultrasound energy and still achieve a localized heating effect without damaging adjacent tissue.

HIFU seems to be promising in the treatment of bone tumors. The major complications of bone HIFU ablation include skin burn (21% of cases) and nerve damage (12%). Only a few papers report the use of HIFU in bone tumors, and more studies on clinical effectiveness should precede widespread clinical use of this technique [45].

General Principles

Management of patients with musculoskeletal tumors requires consideration of many factors [46]:

- Histology of the tumor, with differentiation of benign and malignant tumors.
- Precise clinical evaluation of the patient: determination of the origin and location of pain, estimation of previous treatments applied and the type of anesthesia the patient can tolerate (general condition), understanding of the disease process and life expectancy.
- Clear definition of the therapeutic goal: curative or palliative.
- Knowledge of available treatment options.
- Appreciation of the degree of bone destruction (need for consolidation).
- Whole body three-dimensional (3D) imaging to precisely analyze the lesions and their relationship to surrounding structures.

A multidisciplinary approach is always required in order to choose the more efficient and less-disabling technique.

Treatment Strategy

1. For a painful tumor involving a flat weight-bearing bone without invasion of the surrounding tissues, associated with a risk of compression fracture, single cementoplasty is the most appropriate technique.
2. For a painful bone tumor with extension into surrounding soft tissues, thermal ablation is required to control the pain caused by the soft-tissue invasion. However, if there is a risk of pathological fracture, an additional consolidation technique is required (cementoplasty for flat bones or surgery for long bones) (Fig. 17.7).
3. For nonsurgical spinal tumors extending towards the canal with rupture of the posterior wall and epidural extension, percutaneous tumor decompression utilizing radiofrequency ionization is the best technique. After tumor decompression, the cavity created can be filled with cement (Fig. 17.11).

Curative treatment is considered for benign lesions such as osteoid osteomas or osteoblastomas. In such cases, the tumor is treated in a single session with a thermal ablation technique. Considering the small volume of the ablated zone, additional consolidation is not necessary.

Malignant nonsurgical patients with single or few slow-growing metastases (less common scenario) can be treated with percutaneous image-guided ablation techniques, generally RFA or cryoablation. Thermal ablation is able to destroy the tumor but weakens the involved bone; if weight-bearing bone is involved and there is a risk of pathological fracture, consolidation with cementoplasty or surgery is needed. However, cementoplasty should be limited to flat bones subject to compression forces.

For palliative treatment of painful bone tumors, the therapeutic goal is no longer the complete ablation but one or more of the following: tumor reduction, pain management, bone consolidation, or in some cases tumor decompression. Although small metastases may be completely eradicated, the primary goal of symptomatic pain relief is to ablate the interface between the tumor and the pain-sensitive periosteum. Though radiofrequency ablation is the most commonly used percutaneous ablation technique, cryoablation which has similar indications, offers two major advantages in musculoskeletal pathology: less peri- and postprocedural pain and precise visual monitoring of the ice ball with CT or MR. The latter results further in less risk of thermal damage to the surrounding vulnerable tissues, particularly neural structures. Cementoplasty is a cost-effective technique that achieves fast consolidation of bone tumors involving weight-bearing flat bones, particularly vertebra and acetabulum.

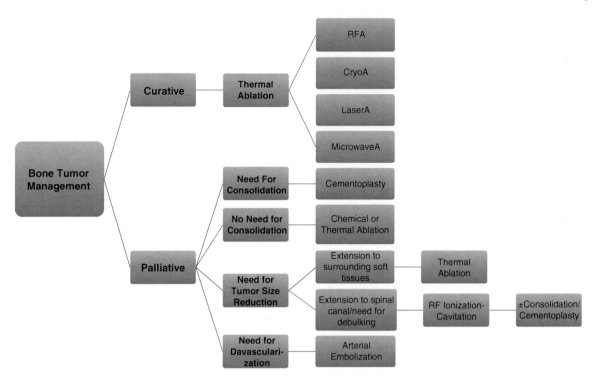

Fig. 17.11 Tumor management therapeutic option algorithm

Conclusions

A good understanding of each available technique is mandatory to obtain the best results. Combination of different techniques is required for the most complex cases, but the less-disabling technique should always be considered first. Finally, an excellent knowledge of thermal protection techniques is crucial to prevent complications, particularly when performing thermoablation procedures close to neural structures.

References

1. Coleman RE. Management of bone metastases. Oncologist. 2000;5(6):463–70.
2. Gangi A, Dietemann JL, Schultz A, et al. Interventional radiologic procedures with CT guidance in cancer pain management. Radiographics. 1996;16(6):1289–304. discussion 304–6.
3. Bickels J, Dadia S, Lidar Z. Surgical management of metastatic bone disease. J Bone Joint Surg Am. 2009;91(6):1503–16.
4. Cotten A, Dewatre F, Cortet B, et al. Percutaneous vertebroplasty for osteolytic metastases and myeloma: effects of the percentage of lesion filling and the leakage of methyl methacrylate at clinical follow-up. Radiology. 1996;200(2):525–30.
5. Gangi A, Basile A, Buy X, Alizadeh H, Sauer B, Bierry G. Radiofrequency and laser ablation of spinal lesions. Semin Ultrasound CT MR. 2005;26(2):89–97.
6. Mathis JM, Wong W. Percutaneous vertebroplasty: technical considerations. J Vasc Interv Radiol. 2003;14(8):953–60.
7. Shimony JS, Gilula LA, Zeller AJ, Brown DB. Percutaneous vertebroplasty for malignant compression fractures with epidural involvement. Radiology. 2004;232(3):846–53.
8. Aebli N, Goss BG, Thorpe P, Williams R, Krebs J. In vivo temperature profile of intervertebral discs and vertebral endplates during vertebroplasty: an experimental study in sheep. Spine. 2006;31(15):1674–8. discussion 9.
9. Weill A, Chiras J, Simon JM, et al. Spinal metastases: indications for and results of percutaneous injection of acrylic surgical cement. Radiology. 1996;199(1):241–7.
10. Alvarez L, Perez-Higueras A, Quinones D, Calvo E, Rossi RE. Vertebroplasty in the treatment of vertebral tumors: postprocedural outcome and quality of life. Eur Spine J. 2003;12(4):356–60.
11. Yamada K, Matsumoto Y, Kita M, Yamamoto K, Kobayashi T, Takanaka T. Long-term pain relief effects in four patients undergoing percutaneous vertebroplasty for metastatic vertebral tumor. J Anesth. 2004;18:292–5.
12. Klazen CA, Lohle PN, de Vries J, et al. Vertebroplasty versus conservative treatment in acute osteoporotic vertebral compression fractures (Vertos II): an open-label randomised trial. Lancet. 2010;376(9746):1085–92.
13. Buy X, Basile A, Bierry G, Cupelli J, Gangi A. Saline-infused bipolar radiofrequency ablation of high-risk spinal and paraspinal neoplasms. AJR Am J Roentgenol. 2006;186(5 Suppl):S322–6.

14. Laredo JD, Hamze B. Complications of percutaneous vertebroplasty and their prevention. Skeletal Radiol. 2004;33:493–505.
15. Nussbaum DA, Gailloud P, Murphy K. A review of complications associated with vertebroplasty and kyphoplasty as reported to the food and drug administration medical device related web site. J Vasc Interv Radiol. 2004;15(11):1185–92.
16. Kelekis AD, Martin JB, Somon T, et al. Radicular pain after vertebroplasty: compression or irritation of the nerve root? Initial experience with the "cooling system". Spine. 2003;28(14):E265–9.
17. Baumann C, Fuchs H, Kiwit J, Westphalen K, Hierholzer J. Complications in percutaneous vertebroplasty associated with puncture or cement leakage. Cardiovasc Intervent Radiol. 2007;30(2):161–8.
18. Vats HS, McKiernan FE. Infected vertebroplasty: case report and review of literature. Spine. 2006;31(22):E859–62.
19. Quraishi NA, Gokaslan ZL, Boriani S. The surgical management of metastatic epidural compression of the spinal cord. J Bone Joint Surg Br. 2010;92:1054–60.
20. Gangi A, Kastler B, Klinkert A, Dietemann JL. Injection of alcohol into bone metastases under CT guidance. J Comput Assist Tomogr. 1994;18(6):932–5.
21. Gabal AM. Percutaneous technique for sclerotherapy of vertebral hemangioma compressing spinal cord. Cardiovasc Intervent Radiol. 2002;25(6):494–500.
22. Doppman JL, Oldfield EH, Heiss JD. Symptomatic vertebral hemangiomas: treatment by means of direct intralesional injection of ethanol. Radiology. 2000;214(2):341–8.
23. Ide C, Gangi A, Rimmelin A, et al. Vertebral haemangiomas with spinal cord compression: the place of preoperative percutaneous vertebroplasty with methyl methacrylate. Neuroradiology. 1996;38(6):585–9.
24. Gangi A, Gasser B, De Unamuno S, et al. New trends in interstitial laser photocoagulation of bones. Semin Musculoskelet Radiol. 1997;1(2):331–8.
25. Rosenthal DI, Hornicek FJ, Torriani M, Gebhardt MC, Mankin HJ. Osteoid osteoma: percutaneous treatment with radiofrequency energy. Radiology. 2003;229(1):171–5.
26. Witt JD, Hall-Craggs MA, Ripley P, Cobb JP, Bown SG. Interstitial laser photocoagulation for the treatment of osteoid osteoma. J Bone Joint Surg Br. 2000;82(8):1125–8.
27. Gangi A, Alizadeh H, Wong L, et al. Osteoid osteoma: percutaneous laser ablation and follow-up in 114 patients. Radiology. 2007;242(1):293–301.
28. Moser T, Cohen-Solal J, Breville P, Buy X, Gangi A. Pain assessment and interventional spine radiology. J Radiol. 2008;89(12):1901–6.
29. Buy X, Tok CH, Szwarc D, Bierry G, Gangi A. Thermal protection during percutaneous thermal ablation procedures: interest of carbon dioxide dissection and temperature monitoring. Cardiovasc Intervent Radiol. 2009;32(3):529–34.
30. Dupuy DE, Hong R, Oliver B, Goldberg SN. Radiofrequency ablation of spinal tumors: temperature distribution in the spinal canal. AJR Am J Roentgenol. 2000;175(5):1263–6.
31. Adachi A, Kaminou T, Ogawa T, et al. Heat distribution in the spinal canal during radiofrequency ablation for vertebral lesions: study in swine. Radiology. 2008;247(2):374–80.
32. Callstrom MR, Charboneau JW, Goetz MP, et al. Image-guided ablation of painful metastatic bone tumors: a new and effective approach to a difficult problem. Skeletal Radiol. 2006;35(1):1–15.
33. Lubner MG, Brace CL, Hinshaw JL, Lee Jr FT. Microwave tumor ablation: mechanism of action, clinical results, and devices. J Vasc Interv Radiol. 2010;21:192–203.
34. Fan QY, Ma BA, Zhou Y, Zhang MH, Hao XB. Bone tumors of the extremities or pelvis treated by microwave-induced hyperthermia. Clin Orthop Relat Res. 2003;406:165–75.
35. Gage AA, Baust JG. Cryosurgery for tumors. J Am Coll Surg. 2007;205(2):342–56.
36. Theodorescu D. Cancer cryotherapy: evolution and biology. Rev Urol. 2004;6 Suppl 4:S9–19.
37. Beland MD, Dupuy DE, Mayo-Smith WW. Percutaneous cryoablation of symptomatic extraabdominal metastatic disease: preliminary results. AJR Am J Roentgenol. 2005;184(3):926–30.
38. Allaf ME, Varkarakis IM, Bhayani SB, et al. Pain control requirements for percutaneous ablation of renal tumors: cryoablation versus radiofrequency ablation–initial observations. Radiology. 2005;237(1):366–70.
39. Callstrom MR, Atwell TD, Charboneau JW, et al. Painful metastases involving bone: percutaneous image-guided cryoablation – prospective trial interim analysis. Radiology. 2006;241(2):572–80.
40. Ullrick SR, Hebert JJ, Davis KW. Cryoablation in the musculoskeletal system. Curr Probl Diagn Radiol. 2008;37(1):39–48.
41. Pritsch T, Bickels J, Wu CC, Squires HM, Malawer MM. The risk for fractures after curettage and cryosurgery around the knee. Clin Orthop Relat Res. 2007;458:159–67.
42. Belov SV. The technology of high-frequency cold-hot plasma ablation for small invasive electrosurgery. Med Tekh. 2004;2:25–30.
43. Georgy BA, Wong W. Plasma-mediated radiofrequency ablation assisted percutaneous cement injection for treating advanced malignant vertebral compression fractures. AJNR Am J Neuroradiol. 2007;28(4):700–5.
44. Jakanani GC, Jaiveer S, Ashford R, Rennie W. Computed tomography-guided coblation and cementoplasty of a painful acetabular metastasis: an effective palliative treatment. J Palliat Med. 2010;13:83–5.
45. Chen W, Zhu H, Zhang L, et al. Primary bone malignancy: effective treatment with high-intensity focused ultrasound ablation. Radiology. 2010;255:967–78.
46. Gangi A, Tsoumakidou G, Buy X, Quoix E. Quality improvement guidelines for bone tumour management. Cardiovasc Intervent Radiol. 2010;33(4):706–13.

Index

Printed by Books on Demand, Germany